AF823364

Temporomandibular Disorders

Henry A. Gremillion • Gary D. Klasser
Editors

Temporomandibular Disorders

A Translational Approach From Basic Science to Clinical Applicability

Springer

Editors
Henry A. Gremillion
School of Dentistry
Louisiana State University Health Science Center
New Orleans
Louisiana
USA

Gary D. Klasser
School of Dentistry
Louisiana State University Health Center
New Orleans
Louisiana
USA

ISBN 978-3-319-57245-1 ISBN 978-3-319-57247-5 (eBook)
https://doi.org/10.1007/978-3-319-57247-5

Library of Congress Control Number: 2017951906

© Springer International Publishing AG 2018
This work is subject to copyright. All rights are reserved by the Publisher, whether the whole or part of the material is concerned, specifically the rights of translation, reprinting, reuse of illustrations, recitation, broadcasting, reproduction on microfilms or in any other physical way, and transmission or information storage and retrieval, electronic adaptation, computer software, or by similar or dissimilar methodology now known or hereafter developed.
The use of general descriptive names, registered names, trademarks, service marks, etc. in this publication does not imply, even in the absence of a specific statement, that such names are exempt from the relevant protective laws and regulations and therefore free for general use.
The publisher, the authors and the editors are safe to assume that the advice and information in this book are believed to be true and accurate at the date of publication. Neither the publisher nor the authors or the editors give a warranty, express or implied, with respect to the material contained herein or for any errors or omissions that may have been made. The publisher remains neutral with regard to jurisdictional claims in published maps and institutional affiliations.

Printed on acid-free paper

This Springer imprint is published by Springer Nature
The registered company is Springer International Publishing AG
The registered company address is: Gewerbestrasse 11, 6330 Cham, Switzerland

We dedicate this book to our families who provided us with their unconditional support in our efforts. We would also like to dedicate this book to the various authors who unselfishly contributed the vast amount of materials that allowed us in bringing this book to print. Additionally, we dedicate the book to the many practitioners who, on a daily basis, try their utmost in improving and enhancing the quality of life of their patients who are suffering from the pain and dysfunction of temporomandibular disorders.

Foreword

The diagnosis and treatment of temporomandibular disorders is one of the most challenging problems confronting clinicians. The problems exist because there is a diverse collection of disorders affecting the masticatory system with similar symptoms and signs of pain and/or dysfunction. There are several diagnostic classification systems, which are often nonspecific and confusing. There is controversy about the appropriate treatment protocols with treatments often based on one's philosophy of etiology of the condition. Often the approach to diagnosis and treatment of the patient is more complicated than is necessary. This publication *Temporomandibular Disorders: A Translational Approach From Basic Science to Clinical Applicability* covers the topic from fundamentals and principles to management principles. The topics are beneficial to all levels of care providers, be they students, residents, academic, or clinical providers in a variety of disciplines.

This book is organized into four parts. The first part discusses the anatomy and physiology of the masticatory system in a clinically applicable manner. The second part focuses on the normal function of the masticatory muscles and temporomandibular joint. This second part establishes the foundation for discussing dysfunction of the masticatory system, which is done in Part III. In Part III, myogenous and arthrogenous disorders are discussed in a scientific, but at the same time, clinically relevant manner. Finally, in Part IV, the management of muscle-based conditions and temporomandibular joint as well as psychosocial considerations in TMD is presented.

This publication provides clinical care providers with information on several disciplines including dentistry, medicine, physical therapy, pharmacology, and psychology as a comprehensive book on Temporomandibular Disorders. It is evidence based and at the same time clinically relevant. This publication should be in the library of every person providing care to patients with TMD.

Gainesville, FL, USA M. Franklin Dolwick

Preface

When we discussed editing a book devoted to temporomandibular disorders (TMD), a key question arose. This question revolved around the notion as to whether or not the community of clinician-scientists needed an additional resource regarding this condition. There are certainly many well-written books both currently and historically that have broached this very subject. Many of the leaders in the field of TMD, much to their credit, have provided clinician-scientists with excellent resources to enhance their understanding of the complexities of this disorder. Understanding this and knowing that we have been lifelong students in this discipline, we decided to provide an evidence-based approach to the understanding, diagnosis, and management of TMD from a different paradigm. We envisioned the book as though one were taking a journey and therefore constructed the book to have a beginning, middle, and end guided by following a translational approach from basic sciences to clinical applications. We start the book with an exploration of the fundamental principles guiding the masticatory system to highlight the importance and influence of embryology on the masticatory system during function and dysfunction. We then transition into an in-depth overview of the anatomy and physiology of this system. This is followed by a comprehensive discussion as to the normal function of the masticatory system incorporating both muscles and temporomandibular joints. Now that the reader has gained an appreciation and understanding for normal we feel confident in presenting details as to the possible dysfunctions which may arise in the masticatory system. Management principles ensue, following an evidence-based or best practices approach, thereby enlightening the clinician-scientist as to the various alternatives to be considered when managing this multifactorial condition. The book concludes with a chapter devoted exclusively to the psychosocial considerations needed to better understand the complexities of the patients' total mind and body when confronted with the experience of pain.

Our goal for this book is to aid the novel practitioner in gaining recognition and an understanding of TMD to better provide assistance and direction for their patients. We believe the book will also help the experienced practitioner in enhancing their knowledge regarding the intricate mechanisms involved in the etiopathogenesis of TMD and providing useful insights as to various scientific-based interventions.

We hope that all who invest the time to read this book appreciate the importance and relevance of its contents and can envision, as weaved through our story, how basic science integrates and interplays with clinical applications. Overall, we are all health care providers who have the privilege and duty to serve our patients who put so much trust in our abilities.

Enjoy!

New Orleans, LA, USA — Henry A. Gremillion
New Orleans, LA, USA — Gary D. Klasser

Contents

Part I

Fundaments and Principles

Embryology of the Masticatory System

1

Ronald C. Auvenshine

Abstract

The temporomandibular joint (TMJ) is the most unique and complex joint in the body. The anatomy of the TMJ varies among mammals depending upon masticatory requirements. Masticatory system function demands that the mandible be capable not only of opening and closing but also of forward, backward, and lateral movements and combinations thereof. In humans, the TMJ is described as a ginglymoarthrodial type of diarthrotic joint. This means that it is not only capable of rotation (movement around a single axis) but also translation (movement around more than one axis at a time). This chapter will provide a review of the growth and development of structures of the masticatory system with special emphasis upon the osseous components.

1.1 Embryology of the Masticatory System

The temporomandibular articulation is a synovial joint. The anatomy of the temporomandibular joint (TMJ) varies considerably among mammals depending on the masticatory requirement so that a single all-embracing descriptive classification is not possible (Nanci 2008). In humans, a different situation exists. The masticatory process demands that the mandible be capable not only of opening and closing movements but also protrusive/retrusive and lateral movements and combinations thereof. To achieve these complex movements, the mandible undertakes translatory and rotational movements. Therefore, the human TMJ is described as a ginglymoarthrodial type of diarthrotic joint (Moffett 1966).

R.C. Auvenshine, DDS, PhD
MedCenter TMJ,
7505 S. Main, Ste. 210, Houston, TX, 77030, USA

Orofacial Pain Clinic, Michael E. DeBakey VA Hospital, Houston, TX, USA

Department of General Practice and Dental Public Health, University of Texas School of Dentistry, Houston, TX, USA

Visiting Faculty, Department of Diagnostic Sciences, Louisiana State University School of Dentistry, New Orleans, LA, USA
e-mail: office@medcentertmj.com

© Springer International Publishing AG 2018
H.A. Gremillion, G.D. Klasser (eds.), *Temporomandibular Disorders*,
https://doi.org/10.1007/978-3-319-57247-5_1

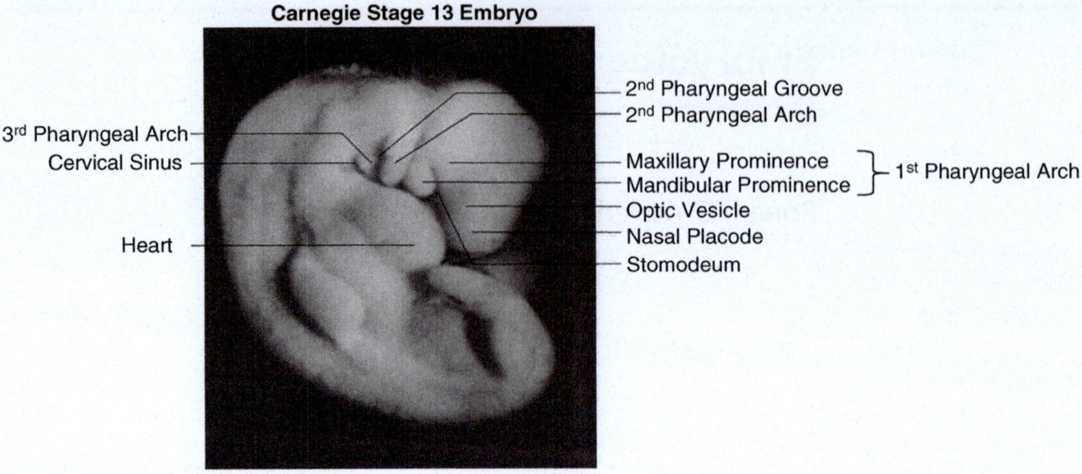

Fig. 1.1 Stage 13, 4.5-week human embryo courtesy of The Virtual Human Embryo Project. Production of the Computer Imaging Lab (CIL) in the Department of Cell Biology and Anatomy of LSU Health Sciences Center, New Orleans, LA. http://virtualhumanembryo.lsuhsc.edu (The Stages of Human Embryonic Development 2012)

The head and neck are formed by pharyngeal (branchial) arches. The pharyngeal arches begin to develop early in the fourth week as neural crest cells migrate into the future head and neck regions. They first appear as surface elevations lateral to the developing pharynx. Soon after, other arches appear as obliquely disposed, rounded ridges on each side of the future head and neck. By the end of the fourth week, four pairs of pharyngeal arches are visible externally. The fifth and sixth arches are rudimentary at this time and are not visible on the surface of the embryo. The pharyngeal arches are separated from each other by the pharyngeal grooves. Similar to the pharyngeal arches, the grooves are numbered in a rostrocaudal sequence (Fig. 1.1) (The Stages of Human Embryonic Development 2012; Auvenshine 2010).

The first pharyngeal arch (mandibular) separates into two prominences:

1. The maxillary prominence gives rise to the maxilla, zygomatic bone, and a portion of the vomer.
2. The mandibular prominence forms the mandible. The proximal mandibular prominence also forms the squamous temporal bone.

The second pharyngeal arch (hyoid) contributes, along with parts of the third and fourth arches, to form the hyoid bone.

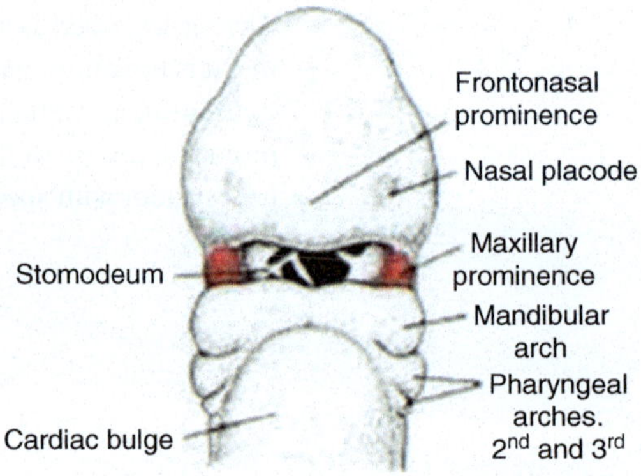

Fig. 1.2 Frontal view of a 4.5-week embryo showing the mandibular and maxillary prominences and dissolution of the oropharyngeal membrane (Sadler 2000)

The pharyngeal arches support the lateral walls of the primordial pharynx, which is derived from the cranial part of the foregut. The stomodeum (primordial mouth) initially appears as a slight depression on the surface ectoderm. It is separated from the cavity of the primordial pharynx by a bilaminar membrane, the oropharyngeal membrane, which is composed of ectoderm externally and endoderm internally. The oropharyngeal membrane ruptures at approximately 26 days bringing the pharynx and foregut into communication with the amniotic cavity (Fig. 1.2) (Sadler 2000; Moore and Persaud 2008).

1.2 Pharyngeal Arch Components

Each pharyngeal arch consists of a core of mesenchyme (embryonic connective tissue) and is covered externally by ectoderm and internally by endoderm. Originally, this mesenchyme is derived from mesoderm, but by the fourth week post-conception (PC), most of the mesenchyme is derived from neural crest cells that migrate into the pharyngeal arches. It is the migration of the neural crest cells into the arches and their differentiation into mesenchyme that produce the maxillary and mandibular prominences. Coincident with the migration of neural crest cells, myogenic mesoderm from paraxial regions moves into each pharyngeal arch forming a central core of muscle primordium. Endothelial cells in the arches are derived from lateral mesoderm. Invasive angioblasts also move into the arches.

A typical pharyngeal arch contains:

1. A pharyngeal arch artery that arises from the truncus arteriosus of the primordial heart
2. A cartilaginous rod that forms the skeletal support of the arch
3. A muscular component that differentiates into muscles in the head and neck
4. Sensory and motor nerves that supply the mucosa and muscles derived from the arch

(Table 1.1) (Fig. 1.3) (Sadler 2000; Moore and Persaud 2008).

The mandible is derived from intramembranous ossification of an osteogenic membrane which begins condensation at 36–38 days of development. Bone formation takes place lateral to Meckel's cartilage (Fig. 1.4) (Nanci 2008). A single ossification center at each half of the mandible arises in the 6-week embryo (PC) in the region of the bifurcation of the inferior alveolar nerve and artery. Ossification spreads below and around the growing inferior alveolar nerve to

Table 1.1 Structures of the Pharyngeal Arches

Arch	Nerve	Muscles	Skeletal structures	Ligaments
First (mandibular)	Trigeminal (CN V)	Muscles of mastication	Malleus	Anterior ligament of malleus
		Mylohyoid and anterior belly of digastric	Incus	
		Tensor tympani		Sphenomandibular ligament
		Tensor veli palatini		
Second (hyoid)	Facial (CN VII)	Muscles of facial expression	Stapes	Stylohyoid ligament
		Stapedius	Styloid process	
		Stylohyoid	Lesser cornu of hyoid bone	
		Posterior belly of digastric	Upper part of body of hyoid bone	
Third	Glossopharyngeal (CN IX)	Stylopharyngeus	Greater cornu of hyoid bone	
			Lower part of body of hyoid bone	
Fourth and sixth	Superior laryngeal branch of vagus (CN X)	Cricothyroid	Thyroid cartilage	
		Levator veli palatini	Cricoid cartilage	
	Recurrent laryngeal branch of vagus (CN X)	Constrictors of pharynx	Arytenoid cartilage	
		Intrinsic muscles of larynx	Corniculate cartilage	
		Striated muscles of esophagus	Cuneiform cartilage	

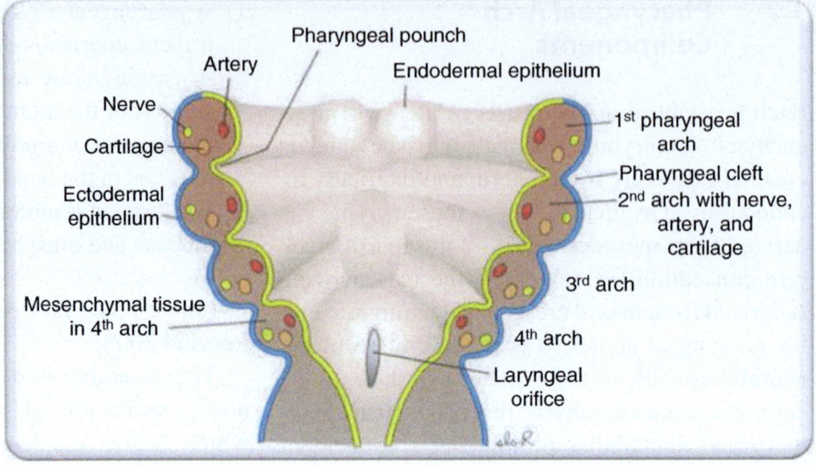

Fig. 1.3 Pharyngeal arches (Sadler 2000)

form a trough for the developing teeth. Spread of the intramembranous ossification dorsally and ventrally forms the body and ramus of the mandible. Ossification stops dorsally at the site that will become the mandibular lingula. From here, Meckel's cartilage continues into the middle ear (Fig. 1.5) (Mendez 2017a).

The prior presence of a neurovascular bundle ensures formation of the mandibular foramen and canal as well as the mental foramen. Meckel's cartilage extends forward to almost meet its fellow of the opposite side in the midline. It diverges dorsally to end in the tympanic cavity of each middle ear and ossifies to form two of the auditory ossicles, the malleus and incus (Fig. 1.6) (Merida-Velasco et al. 1999). The third ossicle, the stapes, is derived primarily from cartilage of the second pharyngeal arch (Reichert's Cartilage (Merida-Velasco et al. 1999).

Meckel's cartilage is not found in the adult mandible. Its adult remnants are present in the form of the sphenomandibular ligament and anterior malleolar ligament. Meckel's cartilage dorsal to the mental foramen undergoes resorption on its lateral surface at the same time as intramembranous bony trabecula are forming immediately lateral to the cartilage. Thus, the cartilage from the mental foramen to the lingula is not incorporated into ossification of the mandible. The interwoven bone formed along Meckel's cartilage is soon replaced by the laminar bone, and typical Haversian systems are already present at the fifth month (PC).

1.3 Formation of the Temporomandibular Joint

A great deal of research has been published on the development of the TMJ over the past several decades. However, there is disagreement about its morphological timing. The most controversial aspects concern the moment of initial organization of the condyle and squamosal part of the temporal bone, the articular disc and capsule, and also the formation of the joint spaces and onset of condylar chondrogenesis (Moffett 1966).

Merida-Velasco has identified three phases of TMJ development:

1. Blastemic stage, weeks 7–8 of development
2. Cavitation stage, weeks 9–11 of development
3. Maturation stage, after week 12 through term

His study identified the critical period of TMJ morphogenesis occurring between weeks 7–11 of development (Merida-Velasco et al. 1999).

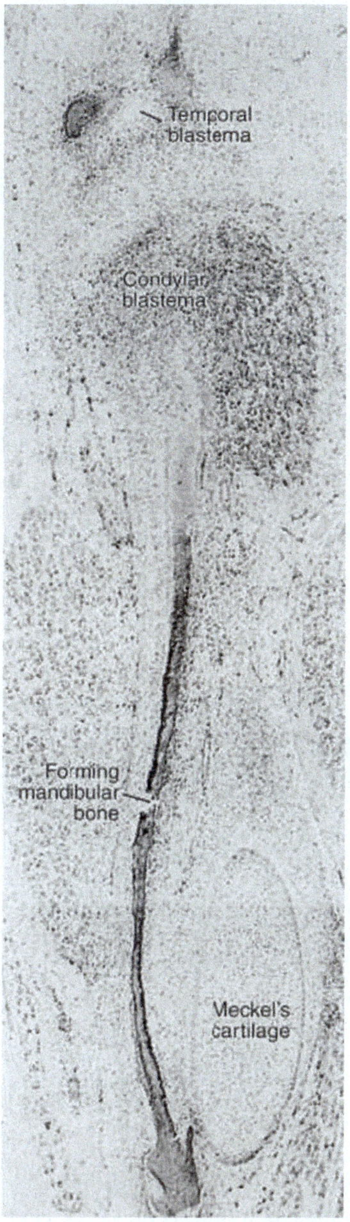

Fig. 1.4 Developing temporomandibular articulation, coronal section through a 12-week fetus. Bone formation has begun in the temporal blastema. The condylar blastema is still undifferentiated. The membranous bone forming the body of the mandibular on the lateral aspect of Meckel's cartilage is apparent (Nanci 2008). (This figure was published in Ten Cate's Oral Histology: Development, Structure, and Function, 7th ed, Nanci, A., p. 363, Copyright Elsevier, 2008)

Meckel's cartilage provides the skeletal support for the development of the mandible. In addition to skeletal support, Meckel's cartilage also provides the necessary stimulus for the initiation of cell differentiation through its relationship with the developing trigeminal nerve (Fig. 1.7) (Merida-Velasco et al. 1999).

The first structure to develop in the region of the mandible is the mandibular division of the trigeminal nerve which precedes the ectomesenchymal condensation forming the first pharyngeal arch. The prior presence of the nerve has been postulated as a requisite for inducing cellular differentiation by the production of neurotropic factors. In other words, it is the mandibular division of the trigeminal nerve which activates Meckel's cartilage, bringing about the expression of messenger RNA, which in turn initiates differentiation of undifferentiated mesenchymal cells into skeletoblasts (Fig. 1.8) (Auvenshine 1976). The skeletoblasts further differentiate into connective tissue precursors such as chondroblasts, osteoblasts, myoblasts, and fibroblasts.

The first evidence of TMJ development is the appearance of two distinct regions of mesenchymal condensation, the temporal and condylar blastema. The temporal blastema appears before the condylar blastema, and initially both are positioned some distance from each other (Nanci 2008).

The condylar blastema appears during the tenth week (PC) as a cone-shaped structure in the ramal region. This condylar cartilage is the primordium of the future condyle. Cartilage cells differentiate from its center, and the cartilaginous superior aspect of the condyle increases by interstitial and appositional growth. By the 14th week, the first evidence of the chondral bone appears in the condyle region through the process of endochondral bone formation. The condylar cartilage serves as an important center of growth for the ramus and body of the mandible. Much of the cone-shaped cartilage is replaced with bone by the middle of fetal life. The condylar process persists into adulthood acting as a growth center for the mandible for

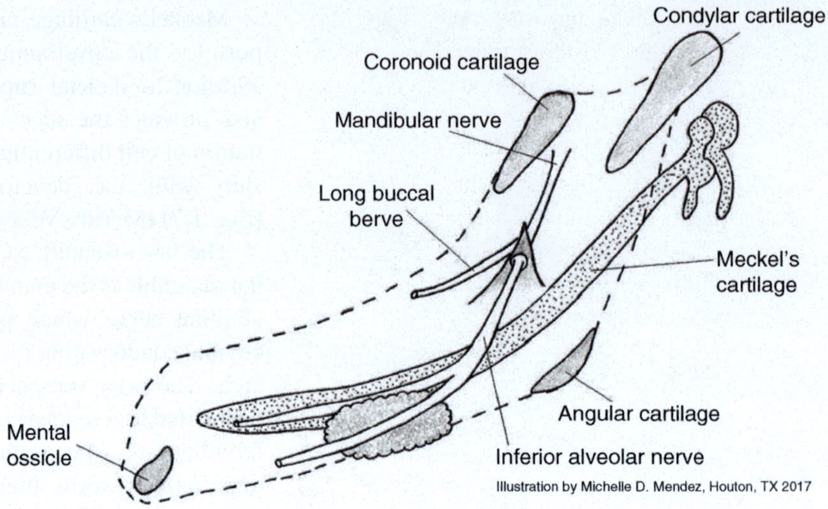

Fig. 1.5 Ossification of the mandible (Mendez 2017a)

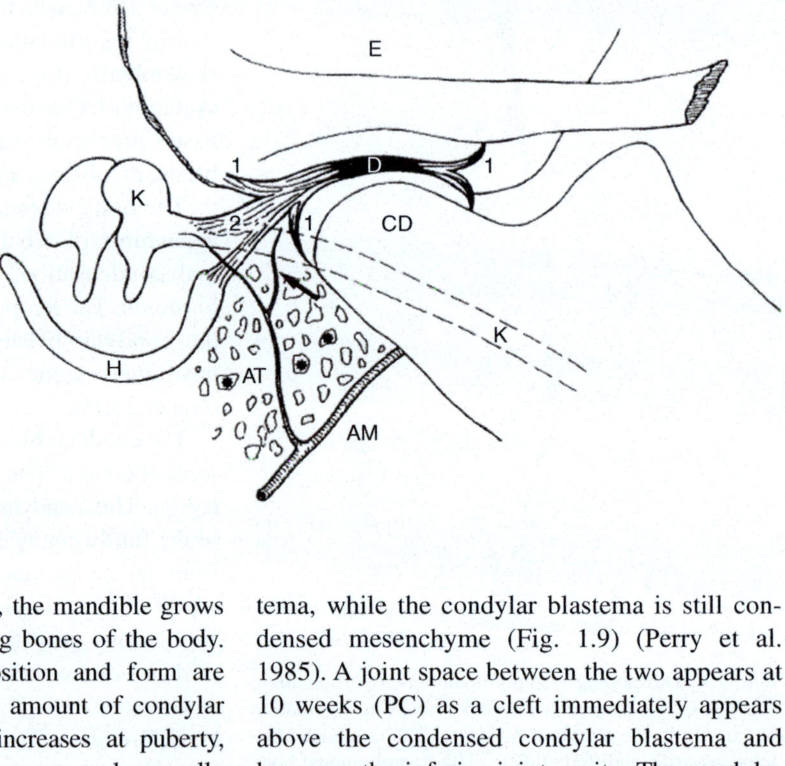

Fig. 1.6 Schematic drawing of the arrangement in the posterior joint region of the articular capsule (1) and (2) discomalleolar ligament. *CD* mandibular condyle, *K* Meckel's cartilage, *E* squamous part of the temporal bone, *D* articular disc, *AT* anterior tympanic artery, *H* tympanic bone. *Asterisk*, retrodiscal venous plexus (Merida-Velasco et al. 1999)

growth in length. Therefore, the mandible grows in length much like the long bones of the body. Changes in mandibular position and form are related to the direction and amount of condylar growth. Condylar growth increases at puberty, peaks between 12.5 and 14 years, and normally ceases at about 20 years. However, the continued presence of cartilage provides for continued growth which is realized in conditions of abnormal growth, such as acromegaly.

The condylar blastema grows rapidly in a dorsolateral direction to close the gap. Ossification begins first in the temporal blastema, while the condylar blastema is still condensed mesenchyme (Fig. 1.9) (Perry et al. 1985). A joint space between the two appears at 10 weeks (PC) as a cleft immediately appears above the condensed condylar blastema and becomes the inferior joint cavity. The condylar blastema differentiates into cartilage (condylar cartilage), and then a secondary cleft appears in relation to the temporal ossification and becomes the upper joint cavity (Edwards et al. 1994). With the appearance of the superior secondary cleft, the primitive articular disc is formed (Fig. 1.10) (Merida-Velasco et al. 1999).

Between the 10th and 14th week of gestation, another secondary blastema appears in the region of the coronoid process. Secondary cartilage of the coronoid process develops within the temporalis muscle as its predecessor. The coronoid accessory cartilage becomes incorporated into the expanding intramembranous bone of the ramus and disappears before birth. In the mental region on either side of the symphysis, one of two small cartilages appear and ossify in the seventh month (PC) to form a variable number of mental ossicles at the symphysis.

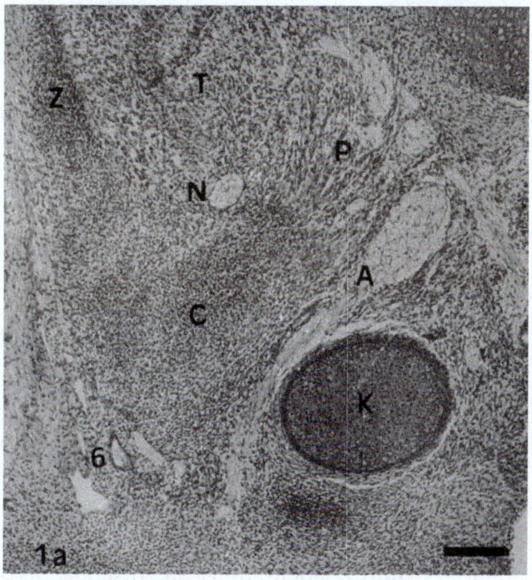

Fig. 1.7 Human embryo GIV-4, week 7 (PC) of development, frontal section. The condylar blastema (C) was associated with the lateral pterygoid muscle (P). *A* auriculotemporal nerve, *K* Meckel's cartilage, *Z* zygomatic process of the squamous part of the temporal bone, *N* masseteric nerve, *T* temporalis muscle, (6) superficial temporal artery (Merida-Velasco et al. 1999)

Shape and size of the fetal mandible undergo considerable transformation during its growth and development. The ascending ramus of the neonatal mandible is low and wide. The coronoid process is relatively large and projects well above the developing condyle. The body is merely an open shelf containing buds and partial crowns of the deciduous teeth. The mandibular canal runs low in the mandibular body. The initial separation of the right and left bodies of the mandible at the midline symphysis is gradually eliminated between the 4th and 12th months (Merida-Velasco et al. 1999).

1.4 The Role of Spontaneous and Evoked Activity on Joint Formation

Functional contractile muscle activity in the transduction of dynamic physical loads is extremely important in the formation of bones and joints. Developing limbs experience a relatively large range of movement with respect to other skeletal elements. As such, they are particularly subject to altered mechano-stimulatory cues and make for a striking example of the importance of movement for proper embryonic patterning. In other words, one of the missing factors necessary for the formation of a joint cavity is movement around two blastemas. In order to form a joint cavity, the process responsible for synovial development can be divided into two

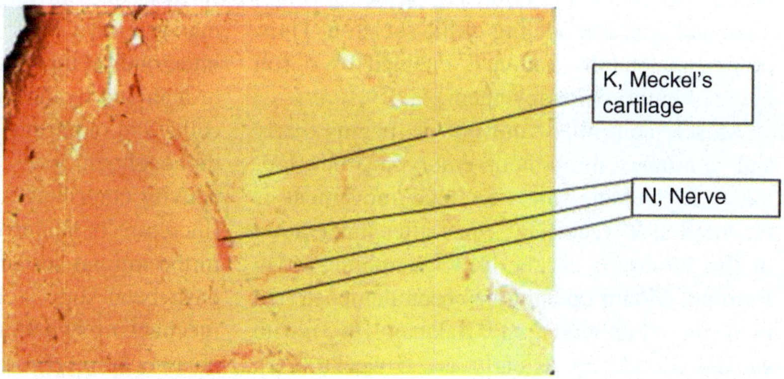

Fig. 1.8 Rat fetus, 15 days (Auvenshine 1976)

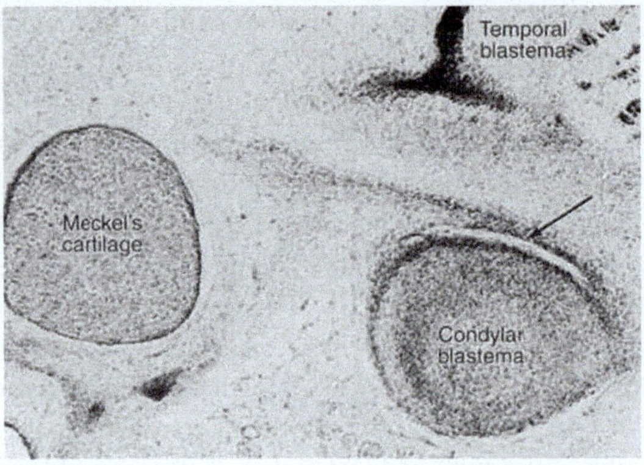

Fig. 1.9 Sagittal section of the temporomandibular joint in a fetus showing the developing inferior joint cavity (*arrow*). Bone formation has begun in the temporal blastema, but the condylar blastema still consists of undifferentiated cells. Meckel's cartilage is to the left of the developing joint (Perry et al. 1985)

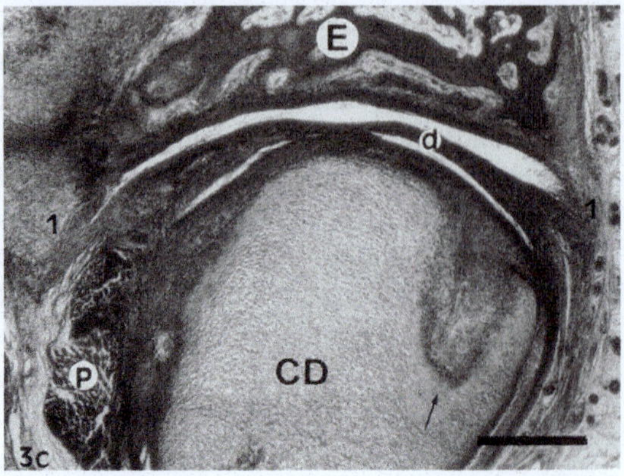

Fig. 1.10 Human fetus B-207, week 13 of development, frontal section. In the mandibular condyle, invagination of the vascular mesenchyme (*arrow*) is visible. *E* squamous part of the temporal bone, *D* articular disc, *1* articular capsule, *P* lateral pterygoid muscle, *CD* mandibular condyle. Scale bar = 500 μm (Merida-Velasco et al. 1999)

phases. The first phase involves the formation of cartilaginous anlagen and intervening interzones in which the joints will develop at a particular location—that is limb patterning.

The second phase involves the formation of the articular cartilage synovium and other related structures within the joint. This depends on elaboration of the joint cavity containing synovial fluid, a process referred to as "cavitation" (Pitsillides 2006).

A wealth of new information currently exists to support mechanical stimulation as a vital feature of healthy embryonic development particularly in the formation of joints. In the appendicular skeleton, failure of synchronization between the development of diarthroses and long bones results in an embryo with limited movement. The embryo's capacity to perform muscular movements will effectively influence further development and later remodeling of the skeleton. Thus, proper skeletal formation is enabled by a full range of embryonic movement.

Muscle-controlled movement begins early and continues throughout embryonic development. In humans, the first fetal movement is recorded at 9 weeks (PC), just after innervation of the forelimbs, as the skeletal rudiments are forming. Mouth opening has been demonstrated to occur (Hamburger and Balaban 1963) with evoked stimulation as early as 7.5 weeks (PC). The temporal relationship between movement and skeletal development hints at a close functional relationship between muscle activity and joint formation.

Synovial joint cavity formation must successfully generate new non-adherent surfaces by a process involving the assembly of a cell-free fluid-filled separation which will facilitate painless and almost frictionless articulation of the joint. As limb condensations are discrete, it is apparent that cavitation occurs between the ends of predetermined cartilaginous elements to create surfaces that are continuous with the synovial lining and associated structures, including the menisci (Pitsillides 1999).

Skeletal joint cavity development, or cavitation, occurs along planes of the future articular surfaces of synovial joints. A number of different markers have been shown to be present in the interzones at the time of cavitation, such as hyaluronan and hyaluronan synthase. Fibroblast-like cells and adjacent chondrocytes with uridine diphosphoglucose dehydrogenase (UDPGD) activity contribute to glucosamine-glycan levels (increases in hyaluronan). These cells are located in the intimal surface of the synovial lining and have been suggested as the possible cavitation mechanism switching from cellular cohesion to disassociation (Edwards et al. 1994).

A review of joint formation requires a brief overview of "limb patterning." Limb patterning involves dynamic relationships between the thickened region of ectoderm, the apical ectodermal ridge (AER), and the underlying distal limb mesenchyme or progress zone. The progress zone model predicts that the timing and location of the departure of each cell from the influence of the AER dictate its commitment to a specific fate. Therefore, limb patterning infers that different limb segments are specified as distinct domains. Therefore, when one considers the developing TMJ, the two limb segments refer to the condylar blastema and the squamosal or glenoid fossa. It is unclear why AERs develop at specific sites; however, a major supposition is that the cavitation process itself is achieved by a conserved mechanism in all joints.

The first evidence that the location for joint formation has been specified involves elaboration of an interzone of mesenchymal cells defining the boundary between the opposed skeletal elements (Shea et al. 2015). The fundamental role of intervening mesenchyme is evident when one considers that their specification interrupts what might otherwise develop into a single cartilaginous anlagen. In other words, movement is required around the two developing blastemas in order to create interzones leading to joint cavities.

The first sign of skeletal development, in limb buds, is the condensation of mesenchymal cells at the core of the bud and the location of the future skeletal elements. In the proximal forelimb bud, for example, a Y-shaped condensation represents the future humerus, radius, and ulna. Distal condensations are progressively added, and future joint sites become apparent as increased cell density, called interzones. Mesenchymal condensations prefigure immediately subsequent pattern of cartilage differentiation (chondrogenesis) indicated first by the expressions of a transcription factor (Bi et al. 1999). The merging cartilage cells (chondrocytes) build up an extracellular matrix (ECM) of collagens, primarily types I and II, and structural proteoglycans in an avascular environment. At the joint interzones, cells are organized in three territories which later form the permanent articular cartilage at the ends (epiphysis) of adjacent rudiments and the intervening joint cavity, encapsulated by a synovial membrane. Thus, formation of the limb skeleton involves coordinated endochondral ossification, differentiation of permanent cartilage at joint interfaces, and construction of functional cavitated joints in addition to the development of associated structures such as tendons, ligaments, and menisci. As with the limb skeleton, the secondary blastema of the future condyle grows through endochondral bone formation through differentiation of permanent cartilage at the joint interface. Joint cavitation is completed by movement through muscle activity creating mouth opening.

Research has now identified several important factors necessary for interzones to remain isolated from neighboring chondrogenesis. These factors include stanniocalcin, parathyroid hormone-related protein, as well as alpha 5 β-1 integrin and other factors. Current research strongly supports the notion that interzones must act to restrict local cartilage differentiation. It appears that the cellular origin of skeletal elements is initially homologous, only losing their capacity to change once they have responded to exclusive differential stimulus, such as muscle activity resulting in movement at the location of the future joint. The joint cavitation process within the interzone requires extremely precise spatial control over the position at which separation between elements will occur. This is referred to as the "plane of cleavage."

Synovial joint formation can be divided into three distinct stages (Pacifici et al. 2006): (1) definition of the joint site (specification) is followed by (2) differentiation of joint cell territories (patterning) and finally (3) formation of a joint cavity (cavitation) (Fig. 1.11) (Mendez 2017b).

The influence of movement on the process of joint formation has been demonstrated by several researchers (Murray and Drachman 1969; Narayanan et al. 1971). These studies, though done in the chick embryo, clearly show that the continuous movements of the developing embryo are not random but are specific for joint formation. Subsequently, immobilization of the developing joint has shown to produce an

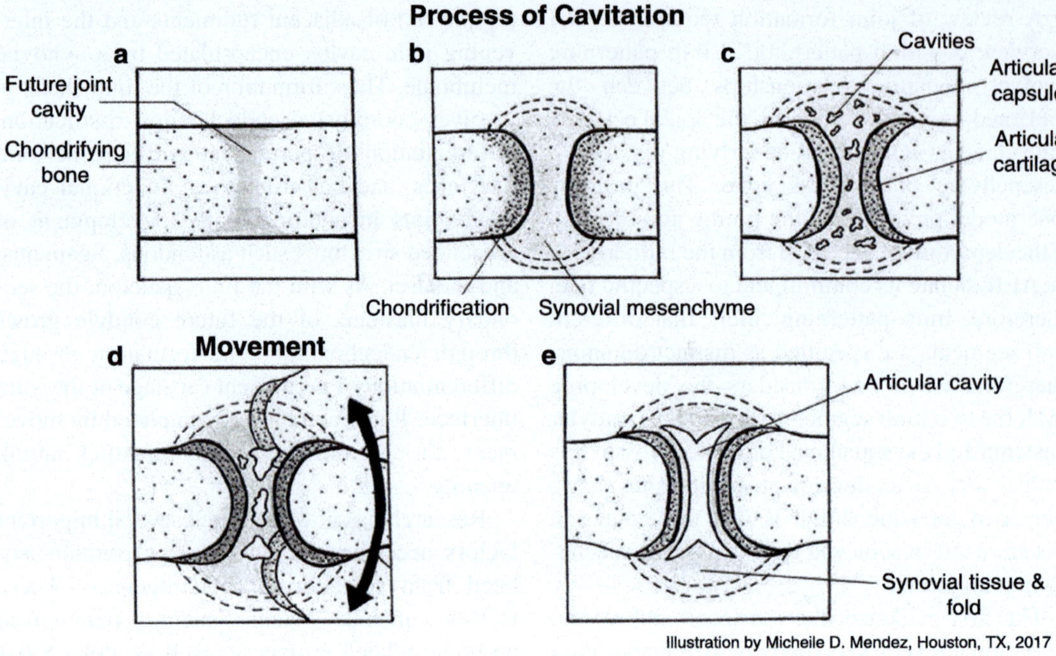

Fig. 1.11 Process of cavitation (Mendez 2017b)

absence of joint cavities and further skeletal abnormalities. Few studies have demonstrated lack of cavitation and joint formation by pure external immobilization. Most of the studies which have been performed have utilized certain drugs to bring about immobilization of the embryo. Auvenshine (1976) developed an intrauterine technique for immobilizing the TMJ by physically preventing mouth opening in the rat fetus. A suture was placed through the snout of the 16-day-old rat fetus, preventing mouth opening. Mouth opening spontaneously occurs in the developing rat at 16.5 days. The animals were reintroduced into the uterine horn and allowed to proceed in development for 24, 36, and up to 72 h of gestation. Upon sectioning of the surgerized fetuses, it was clearly shown that joint cavitation was not achieved and that ankylosis was present. In these surgerized fetuses, the animal was unable to open its mouth even with evoked stimulation. This study suggests that movement does indeed contribute to the alteration in ECM synthesis, which normally accompanies tissue separation at the cleavage site. Immobilization inhibits cavitation without affecting earlier joint specification, outgrowth, or patterning of the limb. Joint patterning is intrinsically regulated and independent of muscular activity. However, cavitation appears to be dependent on muscle activity.

Animal models of embryonic immobilization confirm that endochondral ossification in joint formation is profoundly affected by altered movement. In both chick and mouse models, immobilization causes abnormal ossification (Nowlan et al. 2008) and mechanically substandard bone. In addition, failure of cavitation to occur will result in ankylosis of the joint and failure of the joint to move (Auvenshine 1976).

The influence of movement on the process of joint formation has been demonstrated (Murray and Drachman 1969; Drachman and Sokoloff 1966), and immobilization has shown to produce an absence of joint cavities and skeletal abnormalities (Fig. 1.12) (Sperber 1989; Auvenshine 1976). Similarly, joint movement stimulates condylar chondrification (Perry et al. 1985; Sperber 1989), and the influence of the lateral pterygoid muscle on the process has been demonstrated (Petrovic 1972).

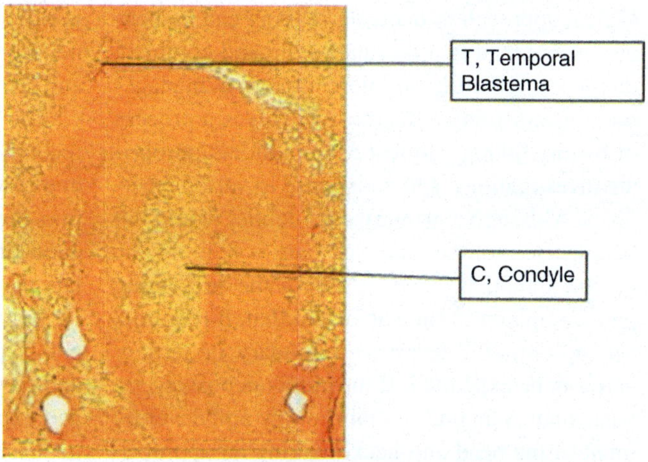

Fig. 1.12 Rat fetus, 19 days (PC), immobilized TMJ leading to the absence of joint space (Auvenshine 1976)

Buccal movements are extremely important for the organization of the structures within the TMJ. In humans, buccal movements begin during the seventh and eighth week of development (Humphrey 1968). This movement first occurs at the level of the incudomalleolar joint (Merida-Velasco et al. 1999; Merida-Velasco et al. 1990). During the maturation stage, fascicles of the lateral pterygoid muscle insert into the condyle and anteromedial two-thirds of the articular disc. During the 13th week of development, invagination of vascular mesenchyme in the external portion of the condylar cartilage occurs.

The first joint space to form is the inferior joint space. The process of joint cavitation is not synchronic since organization of the inferior joint cavity precedes that of the superior one. The inferior joint cavity begins to form at the end of the ninth week (PC) with the appearance of small spaces or clefts between the articular discs and the condyle. The superior joint cavity begins to form during week 11 of development and continues through week 12 (Merida-Velasco et al. 1999; Merida-Velasco et al. 1990).

The trigeminal nerve is one of the first nerves to begin its development in embryogenesis. Both the motor and sensory limb of the trigeminal nerve and nuclear complex are markedly mature at the time of birth. Movement of the TMJ begins during the blastemic phase of development and continues to mature through the cavitation and maturation phases. Mouth opening and tongue thrusting are important functions necessary for joint formation and feeding. The purpose for the early development of these functions is that the newborn must immediately be able to feed. This also means that tactile stimulation around the perioral area must be in place so the newborn must be able to identify the mother's mammary gland and begin sucking and swallowing. These movements and reflexes cannot wait to develop late in gestation but develop early so that they are mature and functioning at the moment of birth. The muscle activity required for suckling is complex, and coordination of 5 of the 12 cranial nerves necessitates the working in harmony with one another.

By the 26th week (PC), all of the components of the TMJ are present except for the articular eminence. Meckel's cartilage still extends through the Glaserian fissure, but by the 31st week, it has been transformed into the sphenomandibular ligament. At first, the ligament appears attached to the medial end of the temporal bone directly adjacent to the sphenoid bone, but by the 39th week, ossification of the bones in the region has proceeded to the point where the ligament gains its apparent attachment to the spine of the sphenoid bone just lateral and posterior to the foramen spinosum.

1.5 Clinical Implications

A correct diagnosis is the key to managing orofacial pain. Differentiating the many causes of orofacial pain can be difficult for practitioners, but a logical approach to decision-making can be beneficial and lead to a more accurate and complete diagnosis resulting in more effective management. Confirming a diagnosis involves a process of history taking, clinical examination, appropriate investigations, and a response to various therapies. Although a primary care dentist would not be expected to diagnose rare pain conditions, he or she should be able to assess the presenting pain complaint to such an extent that, if required, an appropriate referral to secondary or tertiary care can be expedited. If the clinician possesses a basic understanding of embryology and development of the head and neck, making an appropriate and correct diagnosis becomes much more simplified and orderly.

Not all pain in the facial and oral regions is temporomandibular related. Knowledge of embryology will help the clinician understand the segmentation of the face and the distribution of the sensory innervation of the head and neck. Even though the head develops from neuroectoderm and maintains a close relationship to the somatosensory and association cortex, there is a segmentation of the face and head which is established through embryological development.

The site of the pain is not necessarily the source of the pain. This is a principle that is prevalent in its clinical expression for orofacial pain. Again, a knowledge of embryology will facilitate being able to accurately pinpoint the origin of the pain through various techniques such as diagnostic nerve blocks.

1.6 Neuralgia

Neuralgia is defined as an irritation or inflammation of a sensory nerve ganglion. Therefore, the involved nerve must have a ganglion in order to meet the criteria for neuralgia. Of the 12 cranial nerves, the trigeminal nerve (V cranial nerve) has the largest ganglion. Therefore, the majority of cranial neuralgias are of trigeminal nerve origin. Other cranial nerves which have a ganglion are the VII, IX, and X. Neuralgia of the VII cranial nerve is called a geniculate neuralgia. Neuralgia of the IX and X cranial nerve is called glossopharyngeal or superior laryngeal neuralgia, respectively (Okeson 2014; QuBayer and Stenger 1979).

The neuralgia will be experienced in the receptive field of the affected nerve. Therefore, due to the segmentation of the trigeminal nerve into three divisions, a neuralgia can be experienced in the ophthalmic division (V1), the maxillary division (V2), and/or the mandibular division (V3). The receptive field for a geniculate neuralgia is principally a small area of the external auditory meatus and ear canal. The receptive field and expression of neuralgia of the glossopharyngeal and superior laryngeal nerves are the ear, base of the tonsillar fossa, and below the angle of the mandible. It can be precipitated by swallowing, talking, or coughing.

1.7 Burning Mouth Syndrome

Burning mouth syndrome is characterized by continuous burning pain of the oral mucosa. Symptoms include a burning sensation of the tongue, palate, gingiva, lips, and pharynx. The tongue, embryologically, is derived from the endodermal contributions of the four pharyngeal pouches. The innervation of tongue consists of contributions from cranial nerves V, VII, IX, X, and XII. Knowledge of the formation and development of the tongue enables the clinician to better diagnose the origin of the pain through application of various techniques such as diagnostic nerve blocks (Fortuna et al. 2013; Klasser et al. 2011).

1.8 Temporomandibular Disorders

Temporomandibular disorders encompass pain affecting the masticatory muscles and/or the temporomandibular joints. They consist of muscular pain, TMJ disc-interference disorders, and TMJ degenerative joint disease to name a few. Underlying causes of TMD are wide ranging and complex. The greater one's understanding of the biomechanics and proprioception of jaw function through development, the more enabled the clinician will be to better establish a more accurate diagnosis and, therefore, allow for a more relevant management with predictable outcomes.

1.9 Ear Symptoms

Many patients appear in the office of an otolaryngologist complaining of pain, pressure, stuffiness, hearing loss, dizziness, and ringing in the ears. It is not uncommon for the specialist upon examination to determine that there is an external factor causing the symptoms for which the patient complains (Costen 1997). A referral is then made to the dentist with the diagnosis of TMD. Embryologically, the mandible develops from Meckel's cartilage which contributes two of the three middle ear ossicles: the malleus and the incus. The adult remnant of Meckel's cartilage is the condylar-malleolar ligament or Pinto's ligament. This ligament passes through the petrotympanic fissure to the malleus. Thus, an adult relationship is established between the ear and the TMJ. One's knowledge of this relationship will not only help to better render appropriate care but will enable the dentist to better explain to the patient why their symptoms are not within the ear itself but are associated closely with a dysfunctional relationship of the TMJ.

1.10 Hyoid Syndrome

The hyoid bone has been identified with a specific but not well-recognized pain syndrome for over 40 years (Lim 1982). The painful symptoms are generally caused by trauma at the greater cornu of the hyoid bone with pain radiating to other sites. The pain usually radiates to the throat, mandible, mandibular molar teeth, zygomatic arch, condyle, face, ear, and temporal region. Anteriorly, it can radiate to the neck, clavicle, shoulder, arm, and scapula. The condition is not well known in medicine and dentistry for at least two reasons: (1) the diffuse and seemingly unrelated radiation of symptoms and (2) the absence of histopathological evidence of injury (Robinson et al. 2013).

Even though the hyoid bone has no direct contact with any other bone in the human body, it is held in place by twenty muscles, ten on each side. Therefore, the hyoid bone has connections with muscles of the mandible, tongue, skull, thyroid cartilage, sternum, and to the medial border of the scapula as well as the pharyngeal median raphe.

The hyoid bone, embryologically, is derived from the second pharyngeal arch with contributions from the third and fourth pharyngeal arches. Due to the innervation in the area (both sensory and motor), pain can be referred to locations distant from the site of a possible injury or dysfunction (Stern et al. 2013).

1.11 Summary

Knowledge of the embryology of the head and neck as well as that of the temporomandibular joint forms the foundation or basic building blocks for a complete understanding of the adult structure. This will allow the clinician to accurately determine the root cause of the patient's complaints and enable the clinician to apply appropriate treatment modalities to resolve the problem. The fact that the TMJ is similar to other synovial joints allows it to be included in the broad category of orthopedic disorders. These disorders have no treatment that results in a complete cure. Therefore, orthopedic problems must be managed correctly in order for the patient to enjoy as pain-free and functionally complete life as possible. The clinician's understanding of how the head and neck develops is critical for treatment success and education of the patient.

References

Auvenshine RC. Relationship between structure and function in the development of the squamosal mandibular joint in rats. Unpublished dissertation, on file at LSU, Medical School, School of Graduate Studies. 1976.

Auvenshine RC. Anatomy of the airway: an overview. Sleep Med Clin. 2010;5:45–7.

Bi W, Deng J, Zhang Z, Behringer R, de Crombrugghe B. Sox9 is required for cartilage formation. Nat Genet. 1999;22:85–9.

Costen J. A syndrome of ear and sinus symptoms dependent upon disturbed function of the temporomandibular joint. Ann Otol Rhinol Laryngol. 1997;106:805–19.

Drachman D, Sokoloff L. The role of movement in embryonic joint development. Dev Biol. 1966;14:401–20.

Edwards J, Jones H, Jones H. The formation of human synovial joint cavities: a possible role for hyaluronan and CD44 in altered interzone cohesion. J Anat. 1994;185(Pt2):355–67.

Fortuna G, Di Lorenzo M, Pollio A. Complex oral sensitivity disorder: a reappraisal of current classification of burning mouth syndrome. Oral Dis. 2013;19(7):730–2.

Hamburger V, Balaban M. Observations and experiments on spontaneous rhythmical behavior in the chick embryo. Dev Biol. 1963;7:533–45.

Humphrey T. The development of mouth opening and related reflexes involving the oral area of human fetuses. Ala J Med Sci. 1968;5:126–57.

Klasser G, Epstein J, Villines D. Diagnostic dilemma: the enigma of an oral burning sensation. J Can Dent Assoc. 2011;B146:77.

Lim RY. The hyoid bone syndrome. Otolaryngol Head Neck Surg. 1982;90(2):198–200.

Mendez MD. Ossification of mandible. Houston, TX. 2017a.

Mendez MD. Process of cavitation. Houston, TX. 2017b.

Merida-Velasco J, Rodriguez-Vazquez J, Jimenez-Collado J. Meckelian articular complex. Eur Arch Biol. 1990;101:447–53.

Merida-Velasco J, Rodriguez-Vazquez J, Merida-Velasco J, Sanchez-Montesinos I, Espin-Ferra J, Jimenez-Collado J. Development of the Human Temporomandibular Joint. Anat Rec. 1999;255:20–33.

Moffett B. The morphogenesis of the temporomandibular joint. Am J Orthod. 1966;52:401–15.

Moore KL, Persaud T. The developing human: clinically oriented embryology. Philadelphia: Saunders Elsevier; 2008.

Murray P, Drachman D. The role of movement in the development of joints and related structures: the head and neck in the chick embryo. J Embryol Exp Morpholog. 1969;22:349–71.

Nanci A. Ten cate's oral histology: development, structure, and function. 7th ed. St. Louis: Mosby Elsevier; 2008.

Narayanan C, Fox M, Hamburger V. Prenatal development of spontaneous and evoked activity in the rat. Behaviour. 1971;40(1):100–33.

Nowlan N, Murphy P, Prendergast P. A dynamic pattern of mechanical stimulation promotes ossification in avian embryonic long bones. J Biomech. 2008;41:249–58.

Okeson J. Bell's oral and facial pain. 7th ed. Chicago: Quintessence; 2014.

Pacifici M, Koyama E, Shibukawa Y. Cellular and molecular mechanisms of synovial joint and articular cartilage formation. Ann N Y Acad Sci. 2006;1068:74–86.

Perry HT, Xu Y, Forbes DP. The embryology of the temporomandibular joint. Cranio. 1985;3(2):125–32.

Petrovic A. Mechanisms and regulation of mandibular condylar growth. Acta Morphol Neerl-Scand. 1972;10:25–34.

Pitsillides A. The role of hyaluronan in joint cavitation. In: Archer C, Caterson B, Benjamin M, Ralphs J, editors. Biology of the synovial joint. Singapore: Harwood Academic Publishers; 1999. p. 41–62.

Pitsillides AA. Early effects of embryonic movement: 'a shot out of the dark'. J Anat. 2006;208:417–31.

QuBayer D, Stenger T. Trigeminal neuralgia: an overview. Oral Surg Oral Med Oral Pathol. 1979;48(5):393–9.

Robinson P, Davis J, Fraser J. The hyoid syndrome: a pain in the neck. Ann Otol Rhinol Laryngol. 2013:159–62.

Sadler T. Langman's medical embryology. Baltimore: Lippincott Williams & Wilkins; 2000.

Shea C, Rolfe R, Murphy P. The importance of foetal movement for co-ordinated cartilage and bone development in utero. Bone Joint Res. 2015;4(7):105–16.

Sperber G. Craniofacial embryology. 4th ed. Cambridge: Wright; 1989.

Stern N, Jackson-Menaldi C, Rubin A. Hyoid bone syndrome: a retrospective review of 84 patients treated with triamcinolone acetonide injections. 2013

The Stages of Human Embryonic Development. Retrieved 2017, from The Virtual Human Embryo: http://virtual-humanembryo.lsuhsc.edu (2012)

Anatomy of the Masticatory System

2

Homer Asadi and Alan Budenz

Abstract

In order to appreciate the normal function and dysfunction of any system, and more specifically the stomatognathic system, the starting point should involve a complete and thorough understanding of the anatomy of this system. The masticatory system is composed of an array of rather complex anatomical structures that often operate in unison to provide unique and selective daily functions. The orchestration and coordination of the muscles, bones, nerves, and vessels allow human beings to perform functions only capable by our species. However, when this finely tuned arrangement is upset, the outcome, in some individuals, may involve pathosis involving dysfunction, dysregulation, and/or pain. This chapter provides a descriptive anatomical review of the masticatory system. Ultimately, this knowledge will assist the clinician in recognizing specific disorders, their signs and symptoms, diagnosis and treatments, and the relationship to the anatomic structures of this intricate system.

2.1 Osteology of the Mandible

The mandible is a "u" shaped, one-piece bone, bilaterally symmetrical in its normal state. It consists of the vertically oriented ramus posteriorly and the horizontally oriented body anteriorly on each side of the mandible. The ramus has two projections arising from its superior aspect, the condylar and the coronoid processes. The condylar process arises from the ramus of the mandible

H. Asadi, DDS (✉)
Department of Biomedical Sciences, University of the Pacific, Arthur A. Dugoni School of Dentistry, 155 Fifth Street, San Francisco, CA 94103, USA

Interim-Chair of Department of Preventive and Restorative Dentistry, University of the Pacific, Arthur A. Dugoni School of Dentistry, 155 Fifth Street, San Francisco, CA 94103, USA
e-mail: hasadi@pacific.edu

A. Budenz
Department of Biomedical Sciences and Vice Chair of Diagnostic Sciences and Services, San Francisco, CA 94103-2919, USA

Department of Dental Practice and Community Service, San Francisco, CA 94103-2919, USA
e-mail: abudenz@pacific.edu

© Springer International Publishing AG 2018
H.A. Gremillion, G.D. Klasser (eds.), *Temporomandibular Disorders*,
https://doi.org/10.1007/978-3-319-57247-5_2

posteriorly and consists of a head and a neck. There is a shallow depression on the anterior aspect of the condylar neck, the pterygoid fovea, which serves as the attachment for the inferior head (belly) of the lateral pterygoid muscle and the majority of the superior head (belly). The anteriorly located coronoid process is the site of attachment of the temporalis muscle of mastication. The curved depression between the two processes on each side is the mandibular (sigmoid) notch (Fig. 2.1). The posterior-inferior corner of the mandible is the angle (gonion) of the mandible. Anterior to the gonial angle along the inferior border of the mandible, there is an upward depression of the inferior border, the antegonial notch. The masseter muscle attaches to the entire lateral surface of the ramus and may produce roughness at the sites of insertion or a tuberosity at the insertion at the angle of the mandible. The internal surface of the ramus shows a similar roughness in the region of the gonial angle due to the attachment of the medial pterygoid muscle of mastication.

The anterior border of the coronoid process descends vertically and becomes the anterior border of the ramus. This edge has a distinct curved indentation just below the coronoid process, the coronoid notch. As the anterior border continues inferiorly, it thickens into an oblique ridge that gently curves anteriorly and inferiorly as it blends into the body of the mandible. The anterior border of the ramus and oblique ridge on the external surface of the body are referred to as the external oblique line or ridge.

The upper portion of the mandibular body contains the bony support for the teeth, the alveolar process, in which individual bony sockets house the mandibular teeth. Other features on the external body of the mandible are the mental foramen and the mental ridges and prominences of the chin (mental region). Although there are variations, the mental foramen is usually found in close proximity to the apex of the second premolar tooth (Fig. 2.2).

The inner surface of the mandibular ramus has a second ridge that descends vertically just inside from the anterior border/external oblique ridge. This second ridge is the internal oblique ridge. The depression that lies between the internal and external oblique ridges is the retromolar fossa. Like the external oblique ridge, the internal oblique ridge gently curves anteriorly and inferiorly as it blends into the body of the mandible. This portion of the internal oblique ridge is also known as the mylohyoid line or ridge because it is the origin of the mylohyoid muscle, which forms the floor of the mouth (Fig. 2.3). Inferior to the mylohyoid ridge and posteriorly is a depression in the bone referred to as the submandibular fossa, which houses the superficial portion of the

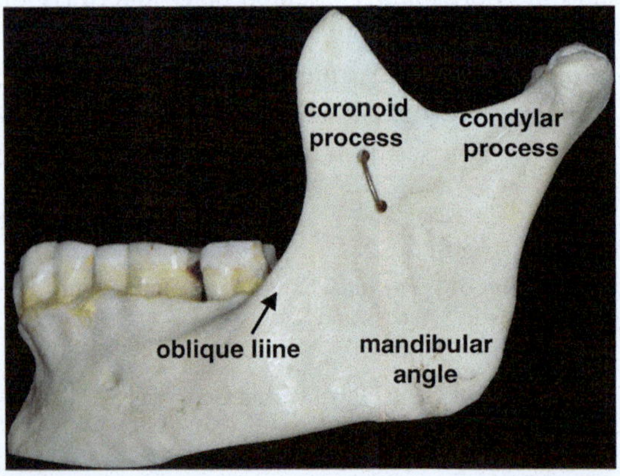

Fig. 2.1 Lateral view of the mandible

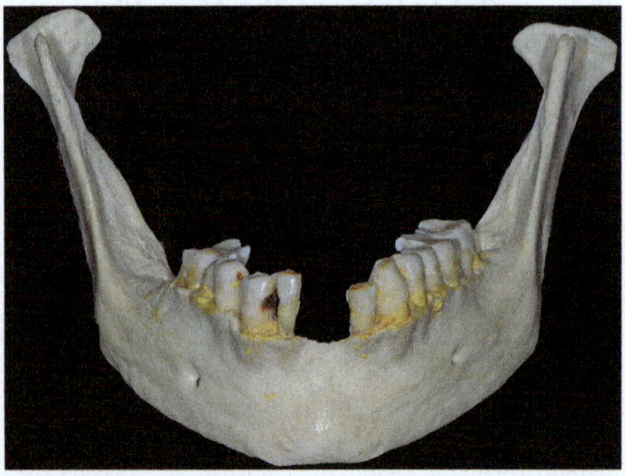

Fig. 2.2 Anterior view of the mandible

submandibular gland. Anteriorly, on the medial aspect of the mandible in the mental region is a small depression located inferior to the mylohyoid ridge which is termed the digastric fossa. This is the location where the anterior belly of the digastric muscle attaches to the mandible. Superior to the mylohyoid ridge on either side of the midline on the medial aspect of the mandible are two projections, a superior and an inferior mental spine (genial tubercle). The superior spine is the site of attachment of the genioglossus muscle, and the inferior spine is the site of attachment of the geniohyoid muscle.

The blood supply and innervation of the mandibular teeth are from the inferior alveolar neurovascular bundle. This bundle enters the bone of the mandible through the mandibular foramen, an opening on the medial surface of the ramus. The lingula is a bony projection just medial to the mandibular foramen which serves as the attachment of the sphenomandibular ligament. Inferior to the mandibular foramen, a bony groove, the mylohyoid groove, runs inferiorly and anteriorly, housing the mylohyoid neurovascular bundle as it courses anteriorly to supply the mylohyoid and anterior belly of the digastric muscles.

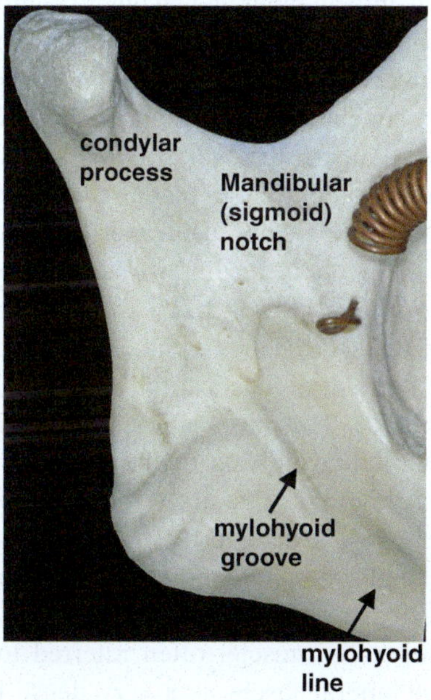

Fig. 2.3 Medial (inner) view of the mandible

2.2 Osteology of the Temporal Bone

The bilateral temporal bones form the lower lateral surfaces of the cranium and the cranial base. Each temporal bone articulates with the zygomatic bone anteriorly, the frontal bone anterosuperiorly, the parietal bone posterosuperiorly, and the occipital bone posteriorly. The temporal bones also articulate with the condyle bilaterally (Fig. 2.4).

Based upon its embryological origins from three separate centers of ossification, the temporal bone is comprised of the squamous, the petrous, and the tympanic portions. The squamous portion forms the flat lateral wall of the lower cranial vault and projects anteriorly as a thin process to form the zygomatic arch in combination with the zygomatic bone. The petrous portion forms the dense base of the cranial vault which houses the auditory and vestibulocochlear structures and separates the posterior cranial fossa from the middle cranial fossa. The mastoid process, with its air cells communicating with the middle ear cavity, projects inferiorly from the petrous portion of the temporal bone. The anteriorly located tympanic portion of the temporal

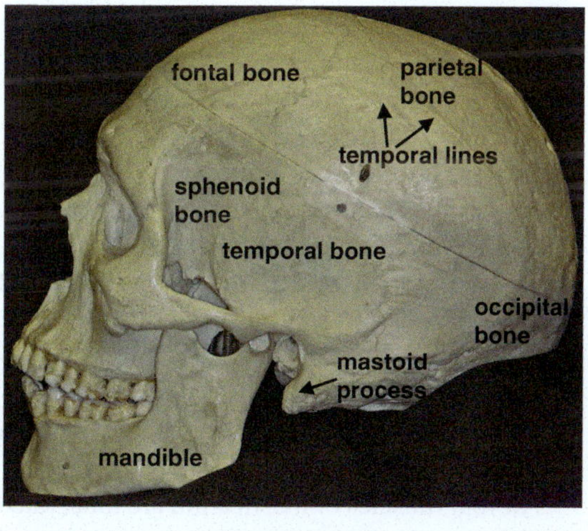

Fig. 2.4 Lateral view of the cranium and mandible

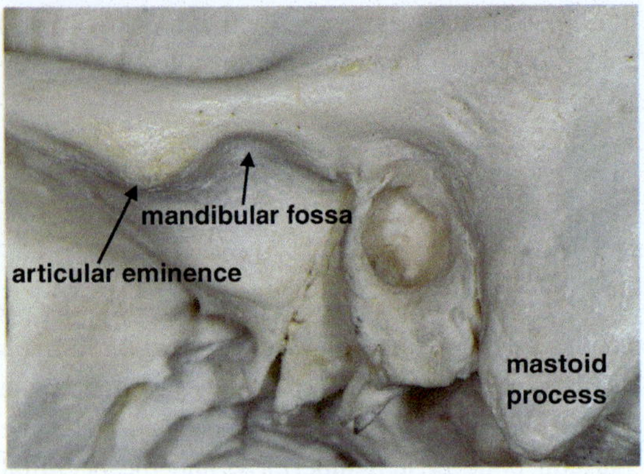

Fig. 2.5 Lateral view of the bones within the TMJ structure

bone contains the external auditory meatus and the depression of the mandibular (glenoid) fossa just anterior to that. Lying between the external auditory meatus and the mandibular fossa is the tympanic plate, and anterior to the mandibular fossa is the thickened bony prominence of the articular eminence. The roof of the mandibular fossa is a thin bone which is clearly not structurally suitable as a load bearing surface with the condyle; rather, load bearing occurs against the posterior slope of the much thicker articular eminence (Fig. 2.5).

2.3 Muscles of Mastication

The muscles of mastication are responsible for chewing movements of the mandible. Because these muscles are attached directly to the mandible, they are sometimes referred to as the mandibular muscles.

Bilaterally, there are four pairs of muscles directly involved in mastication. The four muscles on each side are the masseter, the temporalis, the medial pterygoid, and the lateral pterygoid muscles. Upper cervical muscles, or suprahyoid muscles, are also inferiorly attached to the mandible and are considered to be accessory masticatory muscles because of their secondary role in mandibular movement and stabilization.

All four muscles of mastication are innervated by the mandibular division of the trigeminal nerve (cranial nerve V), which is described in greater detail later in this chapter. The mandibular division of the trigeminal nerve also provides the sensory innervation for the mandibular mucosa and teeth. The blood supply to the muscles of mastication is via the maxillary artery, one of the two terminal branches from the external carotid artery. As the external carotid artery rises above the gonial angle of the mandible posteriorly, it enters into the parotid gland, which cups the posterior border of the mandibular ramus and lies over its lateral surface. The external carotid artery splits into its two terminal branches within the parotid gland at a level slightly below the neck of the condyle. The maxillary artery branch passes anteriorly, deep to the ramus, while the superficial temporal branch continues superiorly in close approximation to the anterior aspect of the tragus. The superficial temporal branch provides cutaneous blood supply to the lateral scalp region and to the retrodiscal tissues.

2.3.1 The Masticator Space

All of the muscles of mastication are contained within an envelope of investing fascia arising from the deep cervical fascia. This investing fascia splits into an inner and an outer layer of fascia at the lower border of the mandible. The outer layer covers the superficial aspect of the masseter muscle, attaches to the zygomatic arch, and then continues superiorly over the lateral surface of the temporalis muscle to blend into the gala aponeurosis of the scalp. The inner layer of fascia covers the deep, or medial, surface of the medial pterygoid muscle as it rises up to attach to the base of the skull. This fascial envelope, containing the muscles of mastication, is named the masticator space. The masticator space also contains the mandibular division of the trigeminal nerve and the maxillary artery. The deep cervical investing fascia also forms the capsules of the parotid and submandibular salivary glands.

Deep to the layer of investing fascia overlying the temporalis muscle, often referred to as the parietotemporal fascia, is a very dense layer of fascia, the temporalis fascia proper. The temporalis muscle arises in part from this very dense fascial layer, which originates from the superior temporal line of the skull. At the lower end, as the temporalis fascia approaches the zygomatic arch, it splits into a superficial and a deep layer. The superficial layer passes superficially over the arch, while the deep layer follows the temporalis muscle inferiorly to its attachment to the coronoid process of the mandible. The temporal fat pad is positioned between these two layers of the temporalis fascia.

2.3.2 The Masseter Muscle

The masseter muscle arises from the inferior border of the zygomatic arch from two heads. The larger, more superficial head arises from the anterior two-thirds of the inferior border of the zygomatic arch, and the smaller, deeper head arises from the more posterior one-third. The fibers of the superficial head extend inferiorly and posteriorly from the arch to the ramus, while the more posterior deep head fibers run in a strictly vertical direction. The two heads of the masseter muscle attach to the entire lateral aspect of the ramus, extending inferiorly to the gonial angle and the inferior border of the mandible (Fig. 2.6a, b).

The masseter muscle is substantially covered by the parotid gland, which is cupped around the posterior border of the mandibular ramus and projecting anteriorly over the masseter muscle. The parotid duct arises from the anterior border of the parotid gland, crosses to the anterior border of the masseter muscle one to two fingerbreadths below the zygomatic arch, and then dives deep to pass through the buccinator muscle to open into the buccal vestibule through the parotid papilla adjacent to the first to second maxillary molar tooth. The transverse facial artery, arising from the superficial temporal artery, is within a fingerbreadth inferior to the zygomatic arch and also crosses the masseter muscle. Additionally, branches of the facial nerve (cranial nerve VII), motor branches to the muscles of facial expression, emerge from the anterior border of the parotid gland to pass anteriorly to enter the deep surfaces of the more centrally located muscles of facial expression. The facial artery, the chief blood supply to the superficial face, crosses the inferior border of the mandible within the antegonial notch to traverse onto the face just anterior to the superficial masseter muscle.

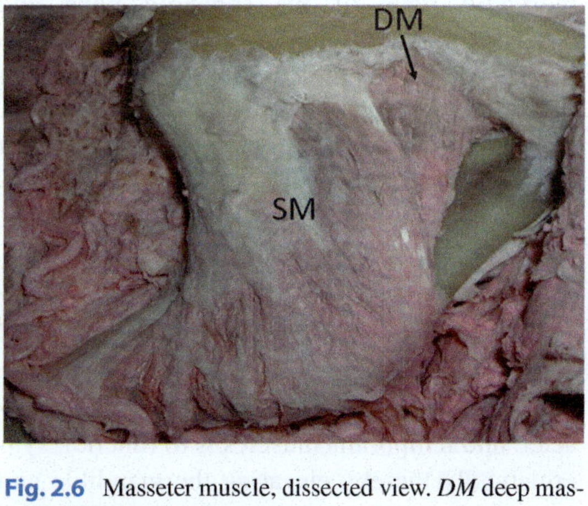

Fig. 2.6 Masseter muscle, dissected view. *DM* deep masseter, *SM* superficial masseter

The neurovascular bundle supplying the masseter muscle enters the deep surface of the muscle by passing through the mandibular notch of the ramus. The masseteric nerve originates from the mandibular division of the trigeminal nerve. The masseteric artery is a branch of the maxillary artery within the infratemporal fossa, and the masseteric vein drains into the pterygoid venous plexus, which coalesces into the maxillary vein.

The masseter muscle is a primary elevator of the mandible. Because the fibers of the superficial head are also angled posteriorly, they aid in protrusion of the mandible. The deep head of the masseter, being more vertically oriented, also has a minor role in retrusion of the mandible. It is always important to remember that although the muscles of mastication are bilaterally paired, they all insert onto a single bone, the mandible, and therefore all movements of the mandible require coordination of both sets of masticatory muscles.

2.3.3 The Temporalis Muscle

The temporalis muscle is often described as a large, fan-shaped muscle which originates from the broad temporal fossa of the lateral skull. The muscle arises in part from the inferior temporal line and in part from the overlying dense temporalis fascia, as previously described. The temporalis muscle can be functionally divided into three different fiber groups: anterior, middle, and posterior. The anterior groups of fibers are oriented almost straight vertically, the middle group of fibers is angled posterior-superiorly, and the posterior group of fibers is almost completely horizontal in their orientation. The temporalis muscle becomes tendinous before passing deep to the zygomatic arch and inserting onto the coronoid process of the mandibular ramus. The attachment of the temporalis muscle is limited to the coronoid process except on the medial aspect, where the insertion may extend down the retromolar fossa between the external and internal ridges all the way to the occlusal plane of the mandibular posterior teeth (Fig. 2.7).

The primary action of the temporalis muscle, like the masseter, is elevation of the mandible. This is readily evident in the near-vertical orientation of its anterior fibers. The middle and posterior fibers not only assist in elevation but also provide retrusive force due to the diagonal and horizontal orientation of these fibers.

The innervation of the temporalis muscle is provided by the deep temporal nerves and branches from the mandibular division of the trigeminal nerve within the infratemporal fossa. There are usually two deep temporal nerves, an anterior and a posterior, although there may be only one or there may be three. These nerves traverse through the infratemporal fossa travelling between the skull and the superior head of the lateral pterygoid muscle to enter onto the deep side of the temporalis muscle. These nerves are accompanied by deep temporal arteries which arise from the maxillary artery within the infratemporal fossa.

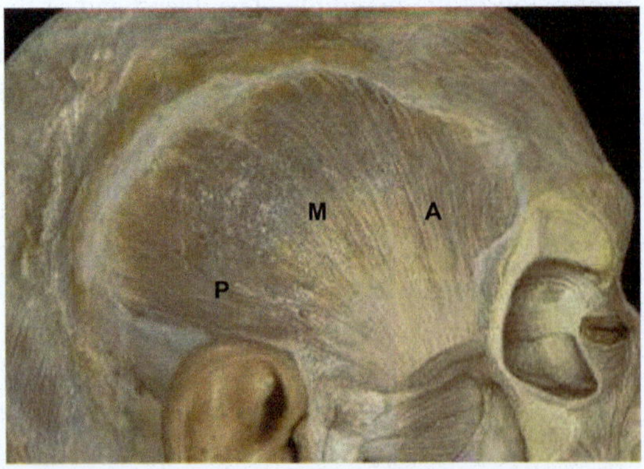

Fig. 2.7 Temporalis muscle, lateral dissected view. *A* Anterior temporalis, *M* middle temporalis, *P* posterior temporalis

2.3.4 The Pterygoid Muscles

There is a pair of pterygoid muscles on each side of the mandible, named the medial and lateral pterygoid muscles based upon their origins from the medial side and the lateral side of the lateral pterygoid plate of the sphenoid bone, respectively. They reside within the infratemporal fossa, inferior to the ramus of the mandible.

2.3.4.1 The Medial Pterygoid Muscle

The medial pterygoid muscle is often described as a mirror image of the masseter muscle, a convenient but rather inaccurate description. The similarity is that, like the masseter muscle, the medial pterygoid muscle fibers are also oriented diagonally, inferiorly, and posteriorly and attach to the ramus of the mandible. However, the attachment of the medial pterygoid muscle is to the medial surface of the ramus of the mandible rather than the lateral surface as occurs with the masseter muscle. The medial pterygoid muscle originates from the medial surface of the lateral pterygoid plate of the sphenoid bone and descends posteriorly, inferiorly, and laterally to insert onto the medial surface of the ramus of the mandible from just inferior to the mandibular foramen down to the inferior border and gonial angle of the mandible. The fibers of the masseter and medial pterygoid muscles intertwine around the inferior border of the mandible to form a muscular sling (pterygomasseteric sling) that structurally allows for an enhanced elevation of the mandible. So it is clear that the primary function of the medial pterygoid, masseter, and temporalis muscles is to function synergistically thereby elevating the mandible and provide the massive forces required to affect

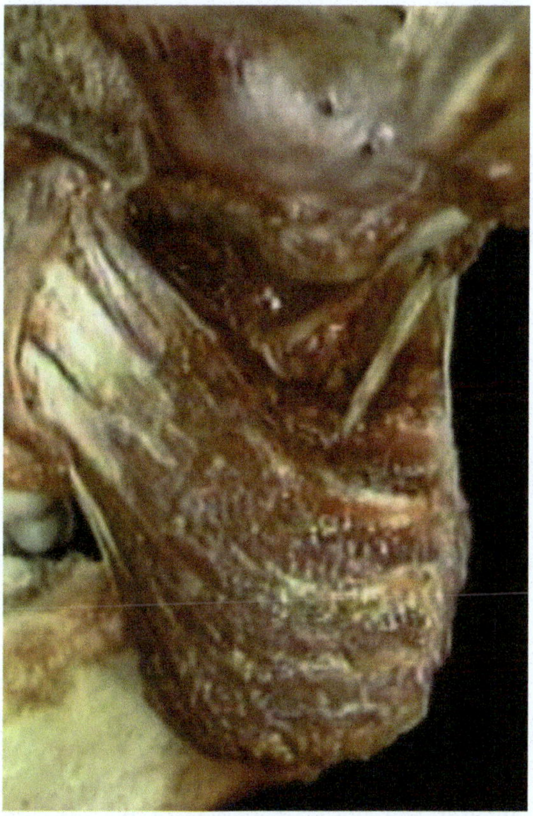

Fig. 2.8 Medial pterygoid muscle, lateral dissected view

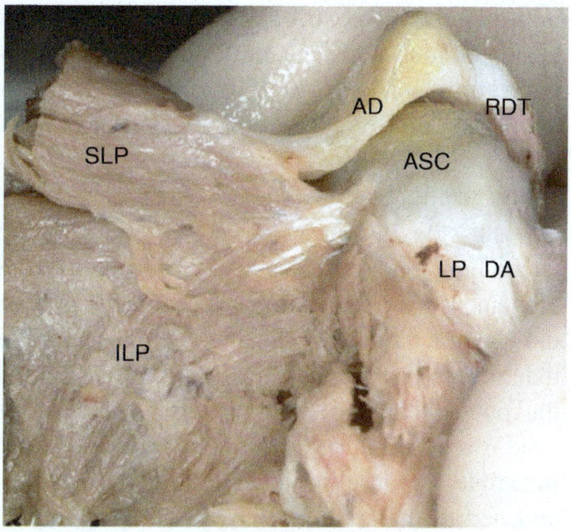

Fig. 2.9 Lateral pterygoid muscle, dissected view. *SLP* superior lateral pterygoid, *ILP* inferior lateral pterygoid, *AD* articular disc, *RDT* retrodiscal tissue, *ASC* articular surface of condyle, *LP DA* lateral pole discal attachment

closure of the mandible when biting into and chewing food. These three muscles also maintain the normal mandibular resting position with the maxilla and mandible slightly apart and the condyle held against the posterior slope of the articular eminence of the temporal bone. The medial pterygoid muscle also contributes to bilateral protrusion and contralateral excursive movements of the mandible (Fig. 2.8).

Innervation of the medial pterygoid muscle is via the medial pterygoid nerve, which arises from the mandibular division of the trigeminal nerve as it enters the infratemporal fossa through foramen ovale. The medial pterygoid artery, a branch of the maxillary artery, accompanies the nerve into the muscle.

2.3.4.2 The Lateral Pterygoid Muscle

The fibers of the lateral pterygoid muscle lie in a horizontal orientation, and the muscle has two distinct heads, a superior and an inferior head. The superior head is smaller in cross-sectional dimensions. It arises from the roof of the infratemporal fossa (the base of the greater wing of the sphenoid bone of the lateral skull). It extends in a relatively inferior and posterior direction with variable degrees of insertion into the condylar neck (pterygoid fovea), anteromedial aspect of the articular disc, and/or the medial capsule of the temporomandibular joint. The inferior head is larger in cross-sectional dimensions and originates from the lateral surface of the lateral pterygoid plate of the sphenoid bone. The fibers run laterally and posteriorly and insert into the pterygoid fovea on the anterior aspect of the neck of the mandibular condyle. There may be some merging of the fibers of the two heads as they approach their insertions (Fig. 2.9a, b).

The function of the lateral pterygoid muscle is differentiated between the two heads, which facilitate contrasting movements. The larger inferior head is the primary protractor of the mandible during opening movement of the mandible. This action is readily understood due to the largely horizontal orientation of the fibers and the insertion of the inferior heads unto the bony neck of the condyle bilaterally. Perhaps not as easily understood is the contribution of the inferior head to depression of the mandible as the condyle is pulled forward over the height of the articular eminence of the temporal bone. The inferior head of the lateral pterygoid muscle when active unilaterally facilitates mandibular excursion to the opposite side. In contrast, the superior head of the lateral pterygoid muscle is relaxed during opening movements of the mandible. The superior head is only contracting during closing movements of the mandible, when the teeth encounter food (termed the power stroke of mastication). The inferior head is relaxing during closing movements of the mandible. Because the superior head is generally attached to the articular disc, disc-capsule complex, and condylar neck of the temporomandibular joint, it plays an important role in stabilizing the temporomandibular joints during mastication. The complex actions of the two heads of the lateral pterygoid muscles will be described in greater detail elsewhere in this text.

The nerve to the lateral pterygoid muscle itself passes from the mandibular division of the trigeminal nerve into the deep surface of the muscle and divides into two separate branches serving each of the heads of the muscle. Each of these nerves is accompanied by an arterial branch from the maxillary artery. The maxillary artery runs on the superficial aspect of the two heads of the lateral pterygoid muscle in approximately 70% of patients or may pass deep to the inferior head and emerge between the two heads in the remaining 30% of patients.

All four pairs of muscles of mastication are innervated by the mandibular division of the trigeminal nerve (CN V_3). The mandibular division of the trigeminal nerve also carries sensory innervation from all of the mandibular mucosa and teeth as well as the motor innervation for the muscles of mastication.

The myriad of possible movements of the mandible requires that the masseter, temporalis, and medial and lateral pterygoid muscles work synergistically in bilateral coordination. The fundamental masticatory movements of elevation, depression, protrusion, retrusion, and medial and lateral excursions must be blended into smooth chewing, speaking, and breathing actions. Additionally, the suprahyoid and infrahyoid muscles of the neck function as accessory muscles of mastication, contributing primarily to depression and/or stabilization of the mandible, while the tongue muscles and the buccinator muscle of the cheek assist to position and maintain a bolus of food centered over the teeth during chewing.

2.4 Upper Cervical Muscles

In addition to the four pairs of muscles of mastication, there are other muscles in the upper cervical region that are involved in masticatory movements of the mandible. These cervical muscles primarily assist in depression of the mandible when opening and in stabilization of the tongue and mandible during chewing and swallowing. These cervical muscles are grouped into suprahyoid and infrahyoid muscle groups.

The suprahyoid groups of muscles are attached to the hyoid bone and pass between the hyoid and the mandible. There are five pairs of muscles bilaterally in the suprahyoid group: the anterior and posterior bellies of the digastric muscles, the stylohyoid muscles, the mylohyoid muscles, and, most superior, the geniohyoid muscles (Fig. 2.10a, b).

The mylohyoid muscles form the floor of the oral cavity. They originate from the mylohyoid ridge or line on the medial aspect of the body of the mandible on either side, with the fibers passing inferiorly toward the midline to insert into a midline raphe with the fibers from the opposite side of the mandible. The most posterior fibers also insert onto the body of the hyoid

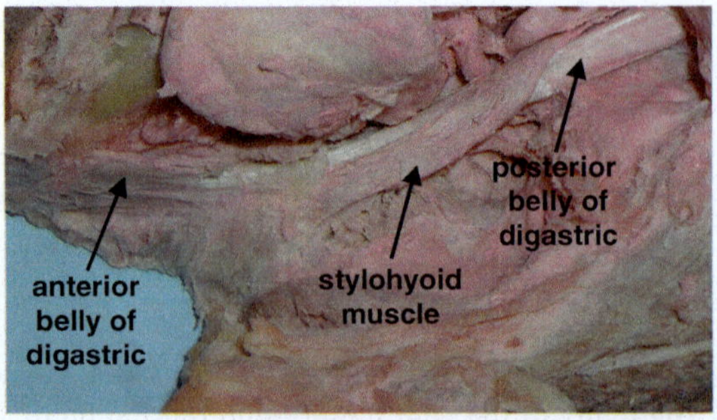

Fig. 2.10 Suprahyoid group of muscles, dissected view

bone. The function of the mylohyoid muscle is elevation of the hyoid bone and in turn elevation of the base of the tongue and the floor of the mouth. It is innervated by the mylohyoid nerve, a branch of the inferior alveolar nerve that arises before that nerve dives into the mandibular foramen. The mylohyoid nerve closely approximates the lingual surface of the mandible, creating a trough in the bone (the mylohyoid groove), as it descends to innervate the mylohyoid muscle from its superficial side. The mylohyoid nerve also innervates the anterior belly of the digastric muscle. The mylohyoid nerve is accompanied by a small artery and vein of the same name passing to the mylohyoid muscle. The mylohyoid muscle also receives a significant blood supply from the lingual artery within the floor of the mouth.

The geniohyoid muscles are located superior to the mylohyoid muscles within the floor of the mouth. The geniohyoid muscles originate from the inferior genial tubercle (inferior mental spine) of the anterior medial surface of the mandible and insert onto the body of the hyoid bone posteriorly. The geniohyoid muscles share some of the functionality of the mylohyoid muscle in that they too elevate the hyoid bone, but they may also protract the hyoid bone. Innervation of the geniohyoid muscles is by the first cervical spinal nerve, C_1.

The posterior belly of the digastric muscle originates from the digastric groove on the medial aspect of the mastoid process of the temporal bone, and runs inferiorly and anteriorly, eventually melding into a tendinous junction with the anterior belly of the digastric muscle. The intermediate tendon is loosely attached to the greater horn of the hyoid bone by a fascial sling. The anterior belly of the digastric muscle, originating from the intermediate tendon, inserts into the digastric fossa on the lower anteromedial aspect of the mandible.

The stylohyoid muscle arises from the styloid process on the base of the temporal bone and passes inferiorly-anteriorly to split around the intermediate tendon of the digastric muscles and blend its insertion into the fascial sling attaching to the greater horn of the hyoid bone.

The function of both digastric muscles and the stylohyoid muscle is elevation of the hyoid bone. Because the two bellies of the digastric muscle are derived from two distinctly different embryological origins, the innervation of the bellies is from two different cranial nerves. The first brachial arch gives rise to the anterior belly of digastric, and so the innervation arises from the mandibular division of the trigeminal nerve (cranial nerve V). The posterior belly of the digastric, and the stylohyoid muscle, arises from the second brachial arch and is therefore innervated by the facial nerve (cranial nerve VII).

The infrahyoid muscles as a group attach to the hyoid bone and therefore provide minor assistance in depression of the mandible when opening and in stabilization of the tongue and mandible during chewing and swallowing movements.

2.5 Nerves and Vessels of the Mandible and the Maxilla

All sensory innervation of the maxilla and mandible arises from cranial nerve V (the trigeminal nerve). Within the middle cranial fossa of the cranial vault, the trigeminal ganglion gives rise to three branches, or divisions, to the face. Uppermost is the ophthalmic division (V_1) which provides sensory innervation to the skin of the upper eyelid, the forehead, and the anterior scalp. The middle division is the maxillary (V_2), which provides sensory innervation to the middle face region: the lower eyelid, the lateral surfaces of the nose and adjacent cheek, the upper lip, and the maxillary teeth and gingiva, including the hard and soft palates. The mandibular division (V_3) provides sensory innervation to all structures of the mandible, including all of the mandibular teeth and gingiva along with the tongue and floor of the mouth, and also provides the motor innervation to the muscles of mastication.

The maxillary division of the trigeminal nerve leaves the middle cranial fossa through the foramen rotundum, passing anteriorly to enter into the roof of the pterygopalatine fossa (Fig. 2.11).

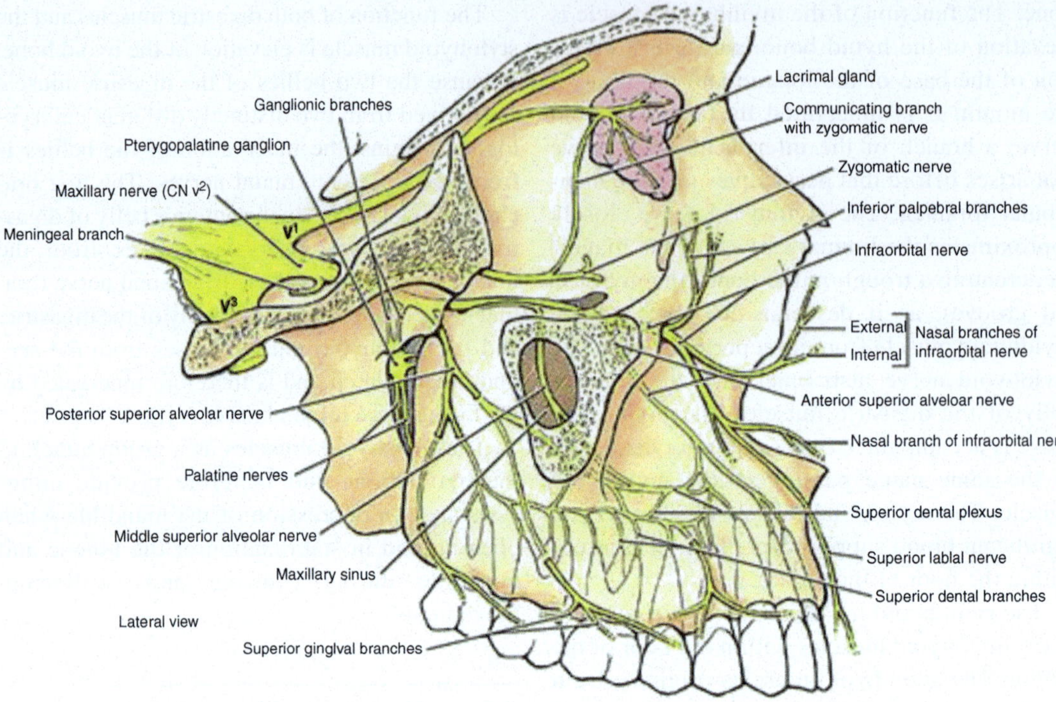

Fig. 2.11 Maxillary division of the trigeminal nerve

A few branches are given off in this region before the majority of the nerve bundle continues anteriorly through the inferior orbital fissure as the infraorbital nerve. As the infraorbital nerve traverses the floor of the orbit, it usually gives off a middle superior alveolar nerve branch (approximately 70% of patients have this branch), which descends in the lateral wall of the maxillary sinus to innervate the premolar teeth, the mesiobuccal root of the first molar, and the adjacent buccal gingiva. As the infraorbital nerve continues forward on the floor of the orbit, it enters a groove in the bone, the infraorbital groove, which gradually closes over to become the infraorbital canal. Just before the infraorbital nerve emerges out of the canal onto the midface, it gives off the anterior superior alveolar nerve, which descends in the anterior wall of the maxillary sinus to innervate the central and lateral incisor and cuspid teeth and their buccal gingiva. Upon emerging from the infraorbital canal onto the midface through the infraorbital foramen, approximately 1 cm below the inferior orbital rim, the infraorbital nerve splits into three cutaneous branches: the inferior palpebral branch to the lower eyelid, the lateral nasal branch to the lateral nose and the adjacent anterior cheek, and the superior labial branch to the upper lip.

There are several branches of the maxillary division of the trigeminal nerve within the pterygopalatine fossa. The first branches given off are ganglionic branches which connect to the pterygopalatine parasympathetic ganglion, the "relay" station for secretomotor innervation to the mucous glands of the palate and the nasal cavity, the lacrimal gland of the orbit, and the sweat glands of the midface. Descending from the ganglion within the pterygopalatine fossa are the greater and lesser palatine nerve branches to the hard and soft palates, respectively, and the palatal gingiva. Superiorly, the maxillary nerve gives off a zygomatic nerve branch. This branch gives rise to the zygomaticotemporal and zygomaticofacial nerves, small cutaneous branches to the skin just posterior to the orbit, and over the zygomatic (malar) eminence of the cheek. The zygomatic branch also carries the secretomotor nerve branches from the pterygopalatine ganglion to the lacrimal gland via a communicating branch to the lacrimal nerve within the superior lateral orbit. Branching off the medial aspect of the maxillary division of the trigeminal nerve within the pterygopalatine fossa are the nasopalatine nerve (long sphenopalatine nerve), the posterolateral nasal branches (short sphenopalatine nerves), and pharyngeal branches. These branches all exit the pterygopalatine fossa through the sphenopalatine foramen to enter into the posterior aspect of the nasal cavity. The nasopalatine nerve travels across the posterior roof of the nasal cavity and then turns down and forward across the nasal septum to reach the incisive canal. The nerve will emerge onto the anterior palate through the incisive foramen just palatal to the two maxillary central incisive teeth. This nerve provides sensory innervation to the nasal septum and to the anterior hard palate from cuspid to cuspid tooth. The last branch of the maxillary division of the trigeminal nerve to arise within the pterygopalatine fossa is the posterior superior alveolar nerve, which enters into the posterior aspect of the maxillary tuberosity, usually as three or four small branches, to innervate the maxillary molar teeth and buccal gingiva.

The mandibular division of the trigeminal nerve descends from the middle cranial fossa through the foramen ovale into the roof of the infraorbital fossa to lie deep to the medial and lateral pterygoid muscles. Immediately after exiting from the foramen ovale lies the otic ganglion, a parasympathetic autonomic relay station that is attached to the medial surface of the mandibular division of the trigeminal nerve at this point. The preganglionic parasympathetic secretomotor fibers from the lesser petrosal nerve synapse here and then transmit the postganglionic fibers which travel with the auriculotemporal nerve to the parotid gland.

Just inferior to the otic ganglion, V_3 quickly splits into an anterior and a posterior division. The anterior division gives off all of the motor branches to the muscles of mastication and carries with it the long buccal nerve sensory branch. The long buccal nerve branch and the anterior deep temporal motor nerve branch often pass between the two heads of the lateral pterygoid muscle. The long buccal nerve runs anterior and inferior from the lateral pterygoid muscle to innervate the skin and mucosa of the cheek. This nerve also extends to the buccal gingiva of the mandibular molar teeth and frequently supplies accessory sensory innervation to these molars. The masseteric nerve branch and the posterior deep temporal nerve branch(es) of the anterior division traverse the superior head and the bony roof of the infratemporal fossa. The masseteric nerve passes laterally through the mandibular notch to reach the deep surface of the masseter muscle.

The posterior division of V_3 gives rise to three primary branches: the auriculotemporal, the inferior alveolar, and the lingual nerves. The inferior alveolar and the lingual nerves are the two largest of these branches, and they appear together from under the inferior border of the lateral pterygoid muscle, passing inferiorly over the medial pterygoid muscle. The lingual nerve travels more anterior and medial relative to the position of the inferior alveolar nerve. The auriculotemporal nerve is a posterior branch of V_3 which passes deep to the lateral pterygoid muscle. It characteristically comes off of V_3 in two roots going around the middle meningeal artery, a branch of the maxillary artery, then coalesces to pass deep to the neck of the condyle and the temporomandibular joint, and then finally turns superiorly in front of the ear to provide cutaneous innervation to the lateral scalp.

The major sensory nerve supply to the mandible and the mandibular teeth is the inferior alveolar nerve of V_3. This nerve descends from the foramen ovale deep to the lateral pterygoid muscle and passes between the lower head of the lateral pterygoid and the medial pterygoid muscle as it angles laterally toward the mandibular ramus. Near the ramus, the inferior alveolar nerve passes posteriorly and laterally behind the sphenomandibular ligament and its attachment to the lingula to enter into the mandibular foramen of the medial ramus. Once through the mandibular foramen and into the inferior alveolar bony canal, the inferior alveolar nerve provides sensory branches to each tooth until it reaches the region of the second premolar tooth and the mental foramen. Although the exact location of the mental foramen varies, it is almost always located near the apex of the second mandibular premolar tooth. At the mental foramen, the inferior alveolar nerve splits into two terminal branches. The incisive branch continues anteriorly in the bony canal to innervate the remaining lower anterior teeth (the first premolar, cuspid, lateral, and central incisor) and the facial gingiva of these teeth. The other terminal branch, the mental nerve, carries the sensory innervation to the skin and mucosa of the lower lip and chin area. Just before the inferior alveolar nerve enters the mandibular foramen, it gives rise to the mylohyoid nerve branch. This nerve lies in the bony mylohyoid groove on the medial aspect of the mandible to descend below the mylohyoid muscle. It then travels anteriorly between the mylohyoid and the anterior belly of the digastric muscles. The mylohyoid nerve provides motor innervation to these two muscles and may also provide accessory sensory innervation to any of the mandibular teeth.

The lingual nerve provides the sensory innervation to the body of the tongue, the floor of the mouth, and the lingual gingiva. This nerve descends in a position close to the region of the mandibular third molar teeth. Because of its close relation to the mandibular third molars, the lingual nerve is at risk during surgery. The nerve then passes inferior to the submandibular duct as it turns medially away from the mandible to rise up into the body of the tongue. Higher up within the infratemporal fossa, the lingual nerve is joined by the chorda tympani nerve, a branch of cranial nerve VII, the facial nerve. The chorda tympani nerve conveys parasympathetic secretomotor fibers to the submandibular and sublingual salivary glands and special sensory taste fibers from the anterior two-thirds of the tongue. The parasympathetic fibers are relayed through the submandibular ganglion, which is juxtaposed with the lingual nerve as it descends into the floor of the mouth.

As previously stated, the blood supply to the muscles of mastication is via the maxillary artery, one of the two terminal branches from the external carotid artery of the neck. As the external carotid artery rises above the gonial angle of the mandible posteriorly, it enters into the parotid gland, which cups the posterior border of the mandibular ramus and lies over the lateral surface of the ramus and the masseter muscle. The external carotid artery bifurcates into its two terminal branches within the parotid gland at a level slightly inferior to the neck of the condyle. The maxillary artery branch passes anteriorly and deep to the ramus, while the superficial temporal branch continues superiorly in front of the ear to provide cutaneous blood supply to the lateral scalp region.

The blood supply for the entire infratemporal fossa region is from the maxillary artery. The maxillary artery passes anteriorly deep to the ramus of the mandible, traversing the infratemporal fossa until it reaches the pterygomaxillary fissure just posterior to the maxillary tuberosity. The pathway of the maxillary artery within the infratemporal fossa is divided into three portions based upon the artery's relationship to the lateral pterygoid muscle (Fig. 2.12). The first portion, from its origin to the inferior border of the lateral pterygoid muscle, is the mandibular portion. The second portion usually lies deep to the inferior head of the lateral pterygoid muscle and is appropriately named the pterygoid portion. The third and final portion enters into the pterygopalatine fossa and is named the pterygopalatine portion.

Shortly after the maxillary artery arises, the first, or mandibular, portion of the artery gives rise to two small arteries, the deep auricular artery and the anterior tympanic artery. These arteries ascend superior and posterior to supply the temporomandibular joint, the middle ear cavity, and external auditory meatus. The next branch is the middle meningeal artery which passes superiorly through the foramen spinosum to provide the major blood supply to the dura mater covering the lateral aspect of the brain. Characteristically, the auriculotemporal nerve leaves V_3 as two roots encircling the middle meningeal artery and then coalesces to form the auriculotemporal nerve trunk as it continues posteriorly toward the temporomandibular joint. There may also be a smaller accessory middle meningeal artery branch which passes superiorly through the foramen ovale to the dura mater. The final branch from this portion of the maxillary artery is the inferior alveolar artery which descends to approximate the inferior alveolar nerve shortly before it enters into the mandibular foramen.

The second portion of the maxillary artery, the pterygoid portion, is primarily involved in

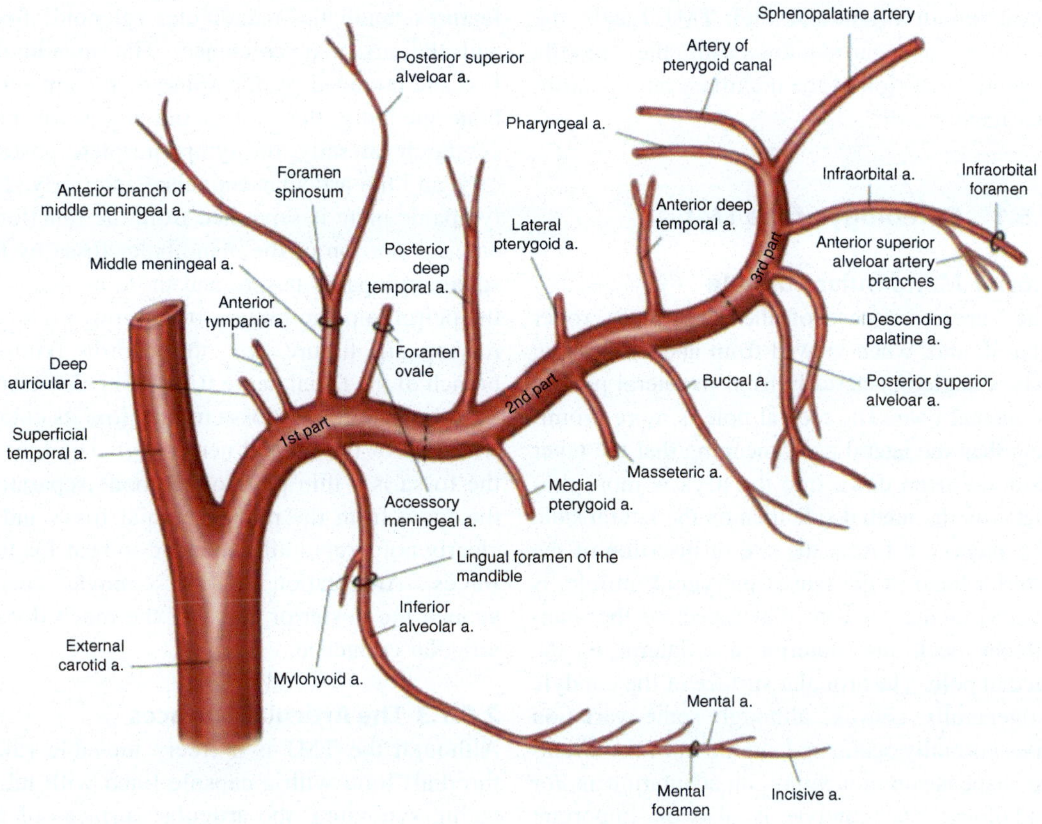

Fig. 2.12 Pathway of the maxillary artery

supplying blood to the four muscles of mastication. An anterior and a posterior deep temporal artery are the first branches from this portion, and they ascend superiorly into the deep surface of the temporalis muscle. Multiple small branches pass into the adjacent lateral and medial pterygoid muscles, and a small masseteric branch passes laterally through the mandibular notch between the neck of the condyle and the coronoid process to enter the deep surface of the masseter muscle. One additional small branch, the buccal branch, passes inferiorly and anteriorly to approximate the long buccal nerve to the cheek region.

As the maxillary artery exits the infratemporal fossa and passes through the pterygomaxillary fissure to enter the pterygopalatine fossa, it gives rise to branches which accompany the terminal branches of the maxillary division of the trigeminal nerve (V_2).

The pterygoid plexus of veins is a meshwork of small venules that closely approximate the muscles of mastication within the infratemporal fossa. This mesh of venules gradually coalesces posteriorly to form the maxillary vein, which passes deep to the mandibular ramus. The maxillary vein, in turn, joins the superficial temporal vein to form the retromandibular vein within the parotid gland.

2.6 The Temporomandibular Joint

The temporomandibular joint (TMJ) is one of the most complex joints in the human body. First, it is not just a simple articulation between two bones, the mandibular condyle and the temporal bone; rather, there is an articular disc interposed between these two bones that divide the joint into two separate joint spaces allowing for complex movement. Second, the single bone of the mandible articulates bilaterally with the base of the skull, the two temporal bones, through both a right and a left TMJ. Lastly, the mandible also articulates with the maxilla through occlusion of the maxillary and mandibular teeth.

2.6.1 Osteology of the TMJ

2.6.1.1 Mandibular Condyle

The superior aspect of the condyle is roller shaped, and, when viewed from above, the long axis is angled posteriorly from its lateral pole to its medial pole. The medial pole is more prominent than the lateral pole, meaning that the taper from the head down into the neck is more dramatic on the medial side than on the lateral side. The pterygoid fovea, the site of insertion of the inferior head of the lateral pterygoid muscle, is located at the anteromedial aspect of the mandibular neck just anterior and lateral to the medial pole. The articular surface of the condyle is generally convex, although some variation does normally occur, and alteration of the articular shape is common with joint adaptation and/or pathology. The condyle is also an important growth center for the mandible up until the mid- to late teen years (Fig. 2.13a, b).

2.6.1.2 The Temporal Bone

The temporal bone contributions to the TMJ are from the tympanic portion, with the two primary features being the mandibular (glenoid) fossa and the articular eminence. The mandibular fossa is bounded by the spine of the sphenoid bone medially, the root of the zygomatic process/arch laterally, the tympanic plate posteriorly, and the articular eminence anteriorly. The tympanic plate is separated from the functional anterior portion of the mandibular fossa by the squamotympanic fissure and more medially by the petrotympanic fissure. It is through the petrotympanic fissure that the chorda tympani branch of the facial nerve (CN VII) gains access to the infratemporal fossa to then join its course with that of the lingual nerve (V_3). The roof of the fossa is a thin plate of the bone separating the fossa from the middle cranial fossa and is clearly not structurally intended to bear loading forces. Articulation of the condyle occurs against the posterior slope of the much denser articular eminence.

2.6.1.3 The Articular Surfaces

Although the TMJ is a freely movable (diarthrodial) joint with a capsule lined with lubricating synovium, the articular surfaces of the condyle and the articular eminence are not covered with hyaline cartilage, as is the characteristic of this type of joint elsewhere in the human body. Rather, the articular surfaces of the TMJ are covered with a double layer of dense, fibrous connective tissue and/or fibrocartilage.

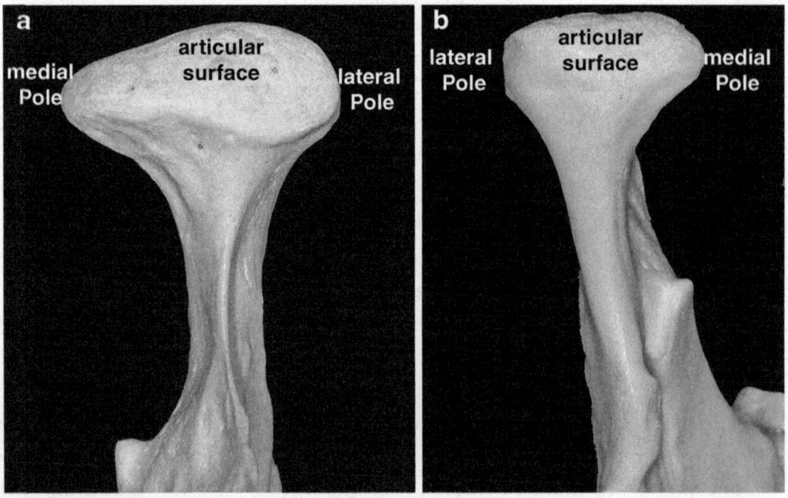

Fig. 2.13 (**a**) The condyle, anterior view. (**b**) The condyle, posterior view

The fibers of the outer layer run parallel to the surface of the underlying bone, while the inner layer consists of more obliquely oriented fibers that help to bind the outer layer to the bone. This unique articular surface provides some distinct advantages to the TMJ, which is undoubtedly the most used, and sometimes overused, joint of the body. Dense, fibrous connective tissue and/or fibrocartilage allows a greater degree of resilience to deformation under loading pressures without damage or permanent loss of shape or surface integrity. Dense, fibrous connective tissue and/or fibrocartilage also has a more rapid regenerative capacity if damage to the surface does occur. However, just as with all other articular joint coverings, the articular surfaces are devoid of blood vessels and nerves so all nourishment must come from the epiphyseal vessels of the underlying bone or from the synovial fluid of the joint space, so integrity of the supporting joint structures is paramount to joint health.

2.6.2 The Joint Capsule, Articular Disc, and Ligaments of the TMJ

2.6.2.1 The Joint Capsule

Like all synovial joints, the TMJ is completely encapsulated. This encapsulation is complex and is composed of the capsule, the retrodiscal tissue, and the insertion of the superior belly of the lateral pterygoid muscle. Superiorly, the capsule attaches to the boundaries of the mandibular fossa. Specifically, the capsule extends from the anterior edge of the squamotympanic fissure posteriorly all the way anteriorly to the anterior slope of the articular eminence. The medial and lateral attachments are to the rim of the mandibular fossa. Inferiorly, the capsule attaches to the neck of the mandible just below the articular surfaces and just inferior to the medial and lateral poles of the condyle. The capsule is lined by synovial cells which produce synovial fluid that is secreted into the joint cavity. Synovial fluid provides lubrication as well as nutrition and waste removal functions to the articular surfaces.

2.6.2.2 The Articular Disc

Interposed between the two bones of the TMJ is an articular disc composed of dense, fibrous connective tissue. The attachment of the disc to the medial and lateral poles of the TMJ results in division of the joint space into two separate joint cavities, a superior joint cavity between the temporal bone and the articular disc, and an inferior joint cavity between the disc and the condyle. These joint cavities serve very different functions during movement of the TMJ. Translational (sliding) movements occur in the superior cavity, while hinge-like (rotational) movements occur in the inferior (Fig. 2.14).

The articular disc is biconcave in shape, thin in the center and thicker around its periphery. The posterior edge or band of the disc is the thickest portion and, at rest, sits on top of the condyle and fills the space between the condyle and the roof of the fossa. The anterior edge, thinner than the posterior, lies in front of the condyle and just behind the height of the articular eminence at rest. The medial edge of the disc is thicker than the lateral edge. During typical movements of the mandible, the condyle is nestled into the center (intermediate zone) of the disc, positioned against the posterior slope of the articular eminence, an arrangement that provides stability to the joint (Fig. 2.15).

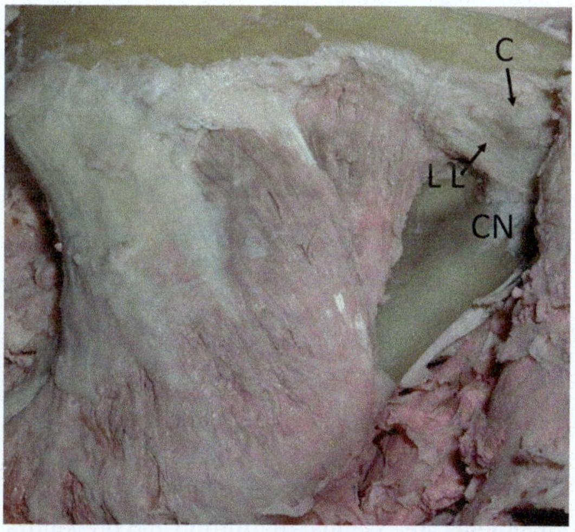

Fig. 2.14 The joint capsule, lateral dissected view. *C* temporomandibular joint capsule, *LL* lateral tempromandibular ligament, *CN* condylar neck

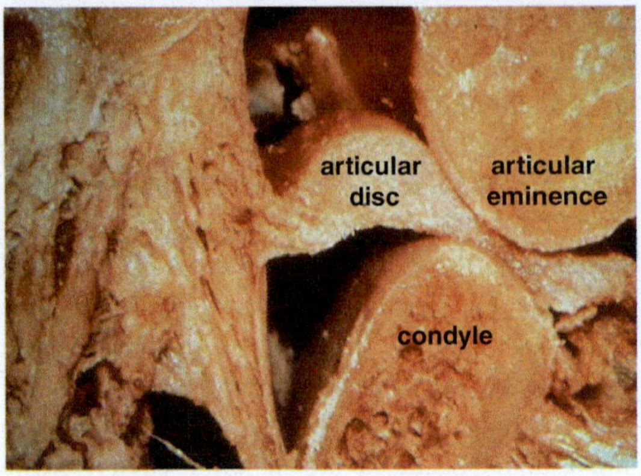

Fig. 2.15 The articular disc, lateral view

Since there are no attachments of the disc to the temporal bone, the disc is allowed to freely translate anteriorly and posteriorly over the articular eminence on opening and closing movements. In contrast, the attachments of the disc to the condyle just inferior to the medial and lateral poles are very tight. The disc therefore moves in coordination with the condyle. The retrodiscal tissues (posterior attachment) are composed of the superior and inferior retrodiscal lamina. These lamina are all composed of collagen fibers with the exception of the superior retrodiscal lamina, which has elastic fibers attaching it to the anterior edge of the squamotympanic fissure. This means that the superior retrodiscal lamina can stretch, while the other attachments of the disc to the capsule have limited ability to do so. Posterior to the disc within the capsule, the superior and inferior retrodiscal lamina are divergent, sandwiching loose connective tissue in this retrodiscal space. This space is also referred to as the bilaminar zone, and this loose connective tissue contains the primary nerve and blood supply to the TMJ. The innervation is via articular branches from the auriculotemporal nerve of V_3; articular branches from the superficial temporal artery provide the blood supply, with accompanying venules draining to the superficial temporal vein.

2.6.2.3 Ligaments of the TMJ

Ligaments are essential in limiting and preventing excessive movement and potential displacement or dislocation of any joint. Ligaments are passive in function and primarily protective in action. There are five ligaments that support the functions of the temporomandibular joint: the temporomandibular, the medial and lateral discal, the sphenomandibular, and the stylomandibular ligaments.

1. The temporomandibular ligament is a lateral thickening of the joint capsule itself. The fibers arise from the lateral surface of the articular eminence and pass diagonally posteriorly and inferiorly to insert onto the posterior aspect of the neck of the condyle. The temporomandibular ligament prevents posterior and inferior displacement of the condyle away from the articular eminence.
2. The medial and lateral discal (collateral) ligaments are derived from the joint capsule as well and attach the medial and lateral aspects of the disc to the condylar neck just below the medial and lateral poles, respectively. These two ligaments prevent any significant medial or lateral movement of the disc over the condyle, but they allow free rotation of the disc anterior-posteriorly over the condyle, an action often analogized with a bucket handle swinging over the top of a bucket.
3. The sphenomandibular ligament runs from the sphenoid spine, just posterior to the foramen ovale on the base of the sphenoid bone, inferiorly and anteriorly to insert unto the lingula which lies immediately anterior to the mandibular foramen on the medial surface of the mandibular ramus. This attachment serves as a passive center of rotation for the mandible during protraction.
4. The stylomandibular ligament extends inferiorly and anteriorly from the styloid process of the temporal bone to the gonial angle of the mandible. The stylomandibular ligament minimally resists excessive protrusion of the mandible.

2.6.3 Innervation of the TMJ

The primary innervation of the TMJ is supplied by the articular sensory branches of the auriculotemporal branch of V_3 as this nerve passes medial to the TMJ capsule. The masseteric and the posterior deep temporal nerves of V_3 also provide small sensory nerve branches to the TMJ which are primarily proprioceptive in nature.

The primary sensory outputs from the TMJ are proprioception and pain sensation. The proprioceptive fibers provide feedback on joint movement and position; the pain fibers provide feedback that limits excessive movements in any direction.

2.6.4 Blood Supply of the TMJ

Small articular branches from the superficial temporal artery to the retrodiscal tissue of the TMJ provide the major blood supply. Small arterial branches from the branches of the maxillary artery to the muscles of mastication also provide a minor source of blood supply. Venules accompanying the arterial branches provide the venous drainage into the pterygoid venous plexus and then into the maxillary vein.

2.7 Summary

Understanding the anatomy of the masticatory system is an essential starting point in the study of stomatognathic function and critical in the recognition of pathosis. The intricate and complex composition of the muscles, nerves, and vessels which form the region must be fully and deeply understood before specific disorders, their symptoms, diagnosis, and treatment are considered. As in any other scientific area related to the human body and study of medicine, the practitioner must be able to visualize and see the interaction among all anatomical systems and subparts in a healthy state of functionality prior to assessment of dysfunction and/or pain.

Bibliography

Antonopoulou M, Latrou L, Paraschos A, Anagnostopoulou S. Variations of the attachment of the superior head of human lateral pterygoid muscle. J Craniomaxillofac Surg. 2013;41:e91–7.

Aziz MA, Cowie RJ, Skinner CE, Abdi TS, Orzame G. Are the two heads of the human lateral pterygoid separate muscles? A perspective based on their nerve supply. J Orofac Pain. 1998;12(3):226–39.

Chang Y, Cantelmi D, Wisco J, Fattah A, Hannam A, Agur A. Evidence for the functional compartmentalization of the temporalis muscle: A 3-dimensional study of innervation. J Oral Maxillofac Surg. 2013;71:1170–7.

Davies JC, Charles M, Cantelmi D, Liebgott B, Ravichandrian M, Ravichandrian K, Agur AM. Lateral pterygoid muscle: a three- dimensional analysis of neuromuscular partitioning. Clin Anat. 2012;25: 576–83.

Hollinshead HW. Textbook of anatomy. 4th ed. NewYork: Harper & Row; 1985.

Kim JK, Cho JH, Lee YJ, Kim CH, Bae JH, Lee JG, Yoon JH. Anatomical variability of the maxillary artery, findings from 100 Asian cadaveric dissections. Arch Otolaryngol Head Neck Surg. 2010;136(8):813–8.

Liebgott B. The anatomical basis of dentistry. St. Louis: Mosby Elsevier; 2001.

Muraleedharan A, Veeramani R, Chand P. Variations in the branching pattern of posterior division of mandibular nerve: a case report. Surg Radiol Anat. 2014;36:947–50.

Naidoo LC, Juniper RP. Morphometric analysis of the insertion of the upper head of the lateral pterygoid muscle. Oral Surg Oral Med Oral Pathol Oral Radiol Endod. 1997;83:441–6.

Pearson W. G. Jr., Langmore S. E. Ann C. Zumwalt A. C. (2011). Evaluating the structural properties of suprahyoid muscles and their potential for moving the hyoid, Dysphagia 26:345-351.

Verma S, Fasil M, Muruga M, Sakkarai J. Unique variation in the course of maxillary artery in infratemporal fossa: a case report. Surg Radiol Anat. 2014;36:507–9.

Physiology of the Masticatory System

3

Greg M. Murray and Christopher C. Peck

Abstract

This chapter is a review of the physiology of the masticatory system from both a peripheral and central perspective. From the peripheral perspective, important components include the muscles that drive movements and the associated somatosensory and motor nerves. The basic functional unit of muscle is the motor unit. Most mandibular muscles have a complex internal architecture, and selective activation of regions within the muscles is thought to contribute to the complex array of finely controlled forces and movements that are characteristic of orofacial function. From the central perspective, the extensive array of orofacial somatosensory receptors encodes peripheral information (about, e.g., tooth contacts, food bolus consistency, mandibular position and movement) that is transmitted to higher centers of the brain to allow us to sense our environment and also to provide continual feedback to refine orofacial movements. The face primary motor cortex plays a key role in the generation of voluntary orofacial movements, and the masticatory central pattern generator is important in the generation of masticatory (i.e., chewing) movements. The orofacial sensorimotor regions of the brain are in receipt of extensive orofacial somatosensory inputs and are capable of considerable adaptability (through neuroplastic changes) in response to changes to the peripheral motor apparatus (e.g., dentures, implants). The peripheral and central nociceptive pathways can become sensitized and responsive even to non-noxious (non-painful) stimuli. These effects can contribute to the allodynia and hyperalgesia seen in acute and chronic pain states. Older models of the effects of pain on motor activity are being superseded by more complex models that emphasize a complex reorganization of muscle activity in the presence of pain as well as emphasizing a role for psychological aspects.

G.M. Murray (✉) • C.C. Peck
Faculty of Dentistry, University of Sydney, Sydney, NSW, Australia
e-mail: greg.murray@sydney.edu.au; dentistry.dean@sydney.edu.au

© Springer International Publishing AG 2018
H.A. Gremillion, G.D. Klasser (eds.), *Temporomandibular Disorders*,
https://doi.org/10.1007/978-3-319-57247-5_3

3.1 Physiology of the Masticatory System: Peripheral Aspects

3.1.1 The Muscles

The muscles involved in mastication are the masticatory, facial, and tongue muscles. Swallowing involves these muscles and also other muscles such as those controlling the palate, pharynx, and esophagus. The masticatory, facial, and tongue muscles are driven by α-motoneurons located within, respectively, the trigeminal, facial, and hypoglossal motor nuclei within the brainstem; many motoneurons involved in swallowing are located in the nucleus ambiguus, also within the brainstem. The functional anatomy of the masticatory muscles as well as the morphology and physiology of masticatory muscles and motor units have been described in detail in previous reviews (Hannam and McMillan 1994; Korfage et al. 2005a, b; Miller 1991; van Eijden and Turkawski 2001). The following summarizes some of the main features and will concentrate on the masticatory muscles, with reference to the facial and tongue muscles as needed.

The masticatory muscles are capable of generating high forces necessary for breaking down tough foods in chewing but also are capable of generating low forces with precision as required, for example, in the precise positioning of the upper and lower anterior tooth incisal edges as required in clearly articulated speech sounds such as the "s" sound. How do the muscles work to achieve this remarkable flexibility? In this first section, the anatomy and physiology of the masticatory muscles will be described, and aspects of the complex central neural control will be described in the next section.

3.1.1.1 The Motor Unit

Muscles exert force by contracting or shortening. The smallest contractile element of a muscle is termed the motor unit. A motor unit consists of an α-motoneuron plus all the muscle fibers innervated by (i.e., connected to and activated by) that α-motoneuron. The trigeminal motor nucleus in the brainstem contains the cell bodies of masticatory muscle α-motoneurons (see below). Each cell body gives rise to an efferent axon that travels out in motor nerves to then branch and terminate at special synapses called neuromuscular junctions on all the muscle fibers of that motor unit (Fig. 3.1). Action potentials travelling along each α-motoneuron axon pass to all the muscle fibers of that motor unit to cause them all to contract in unison (Fig. 3.1b). As the action potentials arrive at the presynaptic terminal, calcium ions enter the neuronal terminal and cause vesicles containing acetylcholine (a neurotransmitter) to fuse with the presynaptic membrane and release acetylcholine. The acetylcholine then binds to nicotinic acetylcholine receptors on the muscle membrane (the sarcolemma) which allow ionic flow (sodium ions) into the muscle fiber. This ionic flow results in the generation of action potentials which travel the length of the muscle fiber; the action potentials enter the muscle fibers via a system of T-tubules, and this is followed by a sudden release of calcium ions from the sarcoplasmic reticulum. The calcium ions, together with ATP, result in successive cycling of actin and myosin filaments within the sarcomeres, which are the contractile elements of a muscle fiber. Each sarcomere contains overlapping myosin and actin filaments that are the basic structural elements that work to pull the z bands on either side of the sarcomere closer to each other in a muscle contraction. Many sarcomeres are in series in any one muscle fiber so that they can generate adequate force and length change during contraction, and with functional changes the sarcomere numbers can change to reestablish optimal overlap of filaments (Goldspink 1998). The masticatory muscles contain "superfast myosin," not generally seen in limb or trunk muscles, and which has very high ATPase activity which allows the masticatory muscles to contract very quickly and very forcefully.

3.1.1.2 There Are a Range of Sizes of Motor Units

The size of a motor unit is defined in terms of its innervation ratio which is the number of muscle fibers innervated by the α-motoneuron of the motor unit. Small motor units consist of only a few muscle fibers, for example, motor units in the

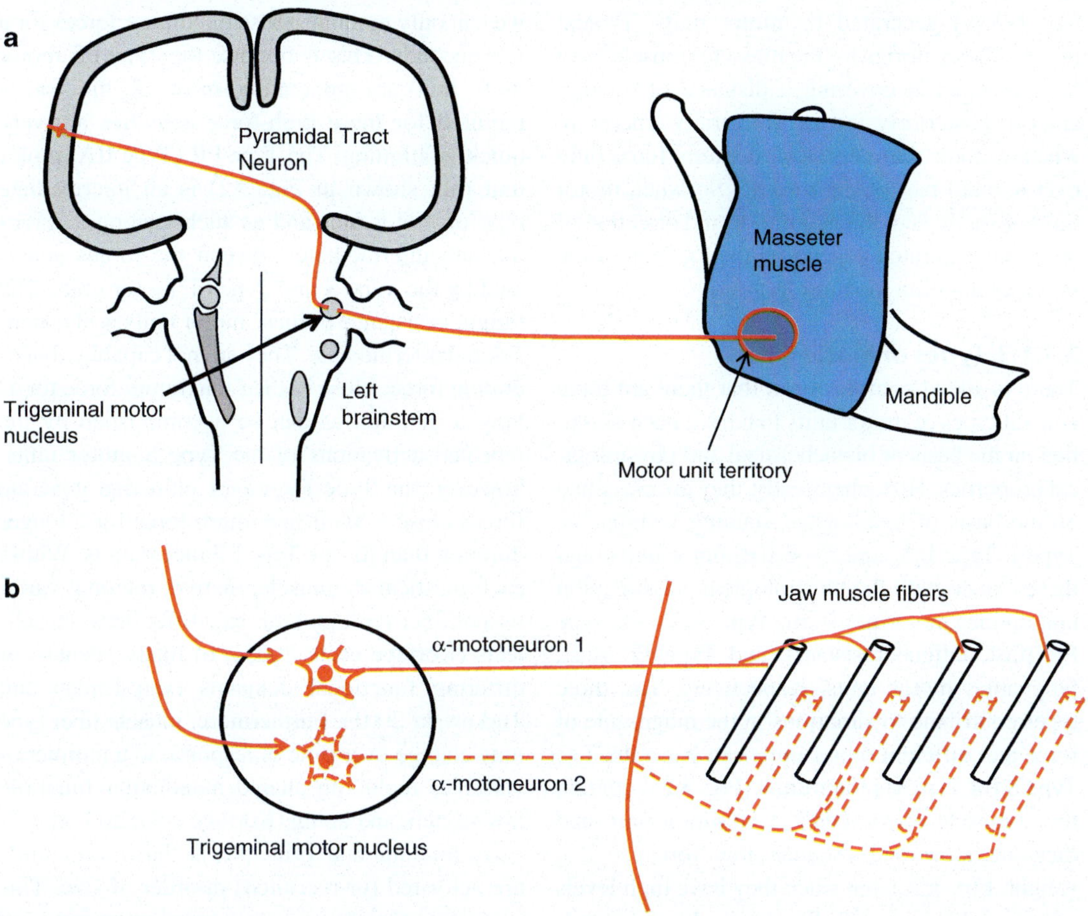

Fig. 3.1 The upper panel (**a**) shows a diagrammatic brain (hemispheres not to scale) with a pyramidal tract neuron passing to an α-motoneuron in the trigeminal motor nucleus in the brainstem. This α-motoneuron passes to innervate (i.e., drive) a motor unit in the masseter muscle. The lower panel (**b**) is a higher detail of the trigeminal motor nucleus with 2 α-motoneurons sending axons to innervate two groups of four muscle fibers within the masseter muscle. The combination of α-motoneuron one plus the four muscle fibers in black constitutes one motor unit; α-motoneuron two plus the four muscle fibers in *dotted red outlines* constitutes another motor unit. Therefore two motor units are shown. The muscle fibers of one motor unit are interleaved with muscle fibers of the other motor unit. Only four muscle fibers are shown, but for the masticatory muscles, there can be many hundreds of muscle fibers activated when one motor unit becomes activated

extraocular muscles controlling the eyeball may contain only 5–10 muscle fibers for each α-motoneuron in each motor unit. When these motor units are activated, they generate only low forces as required for fine positioning of the eyeball for small and precise eye movements. The lower limb muscles (e.g., the quadriceps femoris muscle), on the other hand, have high innervation ratios of, for example, >1000 muscle fibers for each α-motoneuron of a motor unit, and therefore when one motor unit activates, much larger forces are generated as required for the much larger forces that lower limb muscles need to generate in supporting the weight of the body. Masticatory muscles have intermediate innervation ratios of ~500–1000 muscle fibers per motor unit.

The muscle fibers of a motor unit are contained within the motor unit territory, and there are multiple territories within a muscle (Fig. 3.1a). As indicated in Fig. 3.1b, the muscle fibers of one motor unit are intermingled with the muscle fibers of other motor units. This intermingling of muscle fibers of one motor unit with fibers of other motor units may help to smooth out the twitch forces (see below) generated by motor units. Typical motor unit territories for the masseter muscle have been mapped at covering a distance of ~5 mm anterior-posteriorly and mediolaterally. Therefore when a motor unit contracts, it exerts force only over a small part of the muscle. So when motor units are activated, the magnitude and direction of the force generated depend on the location of the motor unit within the muscle.

3.1.1.3 Types of Motor Units

There is added complexity in that there are three general types of motor units that have been classified on the basis of histochemical and physiological properties. Histochemically, they are classified on the basis of histological staining features, as Type I, Type IIA, and Type IIB motor units, and these equate with the physiological classification that divides motor units into Type S (slow), Type FR (fast, fatigue resistant), and Type FF (fast, fatiguable) motor units, respectively. The three types contribute to variations in the magnitude of force that different motor units can generate. The Type S (or Type I) motor units (Fig. 3.2a) contain fewer muscle fibers within each motor unit, and they are slow and produce low forces (~2 g weight, Fig. 3.2c), but since they have high levels of myoglobin and mitochondria and a rich capillary bed (and are therefore termed red muscle fibers), they are fatigue resistant. Fatigue resistance means that these motor units will generate the same force repeatedly every time they are activated, and they can do this for sustained periods (hours). These motor units are therefore good for the generation of low forces for a long time as required for postural support as, for example, in keeping us sitting upright or keeping our mandible in the postural rest position. At the other end of the spectrum are the Type FF (Type IIB) motor units (Fig. 3.2b) which are fast contracting and produce the highest forces (~10 g weight, Fig. 3.2c). They, however, fatigue rapidly, that is, these motor units cannot generate the same force repeatedly every time they are activated, and over even a few seconds of repeated activation, the force they are able to generate rapidly decreases. When we clench as hard as we can or sprint down an athletic track, we can generate high forces, but we can only maintain these maximum forces for a few seconds. This is because the Type FF motor units that are generating most of the forces required for these high-force activities are very quickly fatiguing. The Type FR (Type IIA) motor unit (not shown in Fig. 3.2) is an intermediate type of motor unit and as such generates forces that are intermediate between the forces generated by the Type S and Type FF motor units. The fatigue resistance of these motor units is also considered intermediate. They are not capable of generating forces close to their maximum force for as long a duration as can be accomplished by the repeated activations of the Type S motor units; however, the Type FR motor units can generate forces close to their maximum force for a longer duration than for the Type FF motor units. Within each masticatory muscle, there is regional variation of fiber type, and this can differ between subjects (Korfage et al. 2005a, b) likely because of differing functional demands (van Eijden and Turkawski 2001). Furthermore, muscle fiber type may change over time in response to a number of variables including altered mandibular function, jaw stretch, and aging (Korfage et al. 2005a).

A fundamental principle is that motor units are activated (or recruited) in order of size. This size principle of motor unit recruitment was proposed by Elwood Henneman in the 1950s. It means that the smallest motor units of a muscle, the Type S motor units, are recruited first in a muscle contraction, and then with larger forces, larger motor units of the Type S class are recruited followed by the Type FR and Type FF motor units. Therefore, it is only at the higher forces in a contraction that the Type FF motor units become activated. It is important to note that in the masticatory muscles, some motor units are heterogeneous and contain different fiber types (van Eijden and Turkawski 2001).

There is good evidence now that the centers of the brain that activate muscles are able to selectively activate specific regions or subcompartments within the masticatory muscles independently of other regions. This ability of subcompartments of the masticatory muscles to be selectively activated independently of other regions is called functional heterogeneity

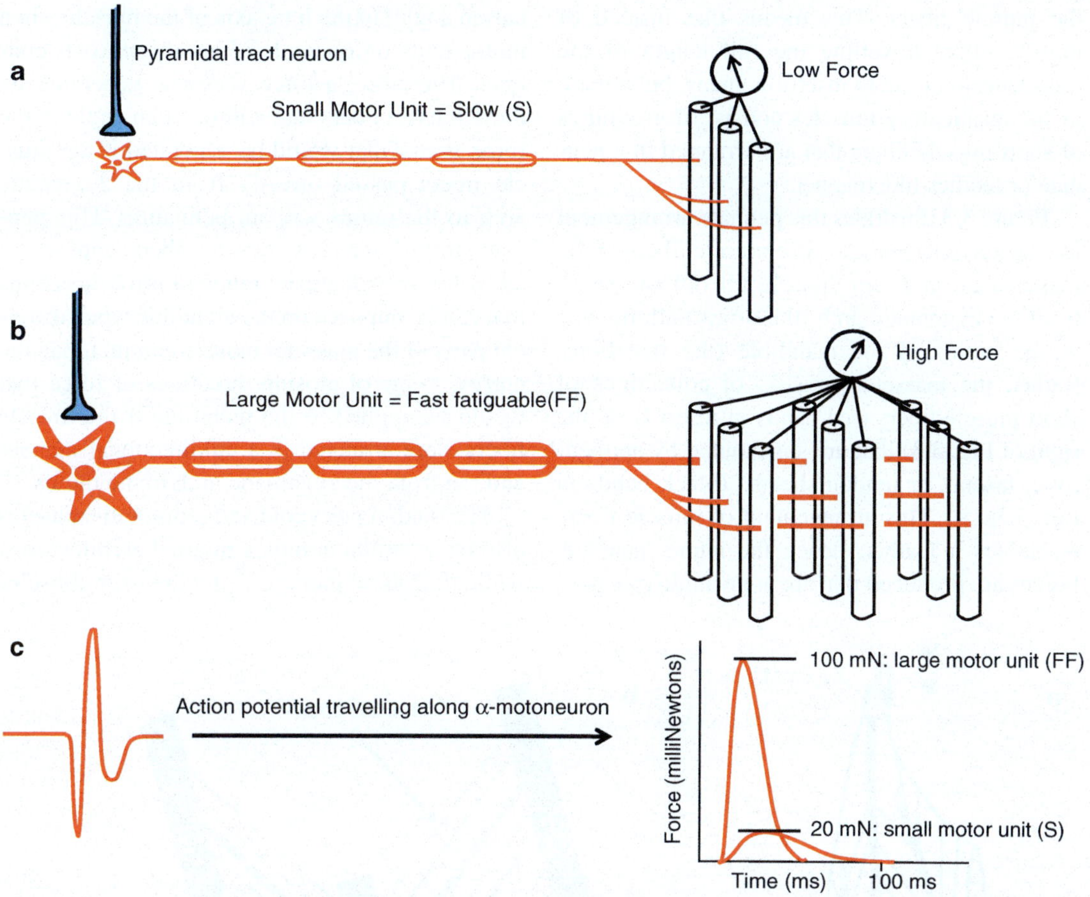

Fig. 3.2 Panel (**a**) shows a small Type S (slow) motor unit where the α-motoneuron innervates only a few muscle fibers (3 shown here). When this Type S motor unit activates, it generates low forces, but because it is fatigue resistant, the motor unit can keep generating the same forces for a long time. Panel (**c**) shows an action potential travelling along the α-motoneuron of this small, slow motor unit to cause a single brief contraction of the muscle fibers of this motor unit, the so-called twitch contraction. The force generated by a single twitch contraction of this slow motor unit is about 20 mN (~2 g of force) as shown in the graph on the right. Panel (**b**) shows a large Type FF (fast, fatiguable) motor unit where the α-motoneuron innervates many muscle fibers (can be many hundreds). When it contracts, it generates large forces, but because it rapidly fatigues, the motor unit can only keep generating the same forces for a few seconds before the force being generated from this motor unit rapidly decreases. An example of the large force generated by this Type FF motor unit is shown in panel (**c**) where a force of about 100 mN (~10 g of force) is shown in the graph on the right

(Blanksma and van Eijden 1990, 1995; Phanachet et al. 2001, 2003; Weijs and Kwa 1995). The concept contrasts with anatomical views that a muscle contraction involves increasing levels of evenly distributed activity throughout a muscle. Rather, it appears that in many muscles of the body and probably all of the masticatory muscles, the brain can selectively activate those regions of a muscle that are biomechanically best suited to contribute forces in the required direction (i.e., generate a required force vector) to allow a particular movement or force to be generated. The next section explains how many of the masticatory muscles are organized to allow this selective activation.

3.1.1.4 Muscles Have a Complex Internal Architecture

Further complexity arises by the fact that most of the masticatory muscles have a complex internal architecture, that is, a complex arrangement of the muscle fibers. This means that instead of muscle fibers travelling the full length of the muscle from origin to insertion, many, but not all, of the masticatory muscles consist of groupings of short muscle fibers that are arranged in a pennate or feather-like manner.

Figure 3.3 illustrates this pennate arrangement for the masseter muscle. The muscle fibers of the masseter are not long muscle fibers that extend from the zygomatic arch (the origin) all the way to the ramus of the mandible (the insertion). Rather, the masseter consists of collections of short muscle fibers (red bands in insert B on the right of Fig. 3.3) that are surrounded by aponeurotic, fascial, or tendon sheaths (black bands in Fig. 3.3a, b). This arrangement of muscle fibers resembles a feather, hence the name, pennate. Forces are produced that are at an angle (the pennation angle) to the long axis of the muscle when motor units on one side of an aponeurosis contract. Therefore, a force vector is generated by these muscle fibers that will be at an angle to the force vector that would be generated if the muscle fibers passed directly from the zygomatic arch to the ramus without pennation. This pennate arrangement of muscle fibers appears to allow for a much greater range of force directions that can be imposed on the mandible when different parts of the masseter muscle contract than the narrow range of closing directions of force that would be applied to the mandible if the muscle fibers were arranged in a unidirectional manner and ran from the zygomatic arch to the ramus.

The medial pterygoid and temporalis muscles also have similar complex internal architectures, while the lateral pterygoid and digastric muscles

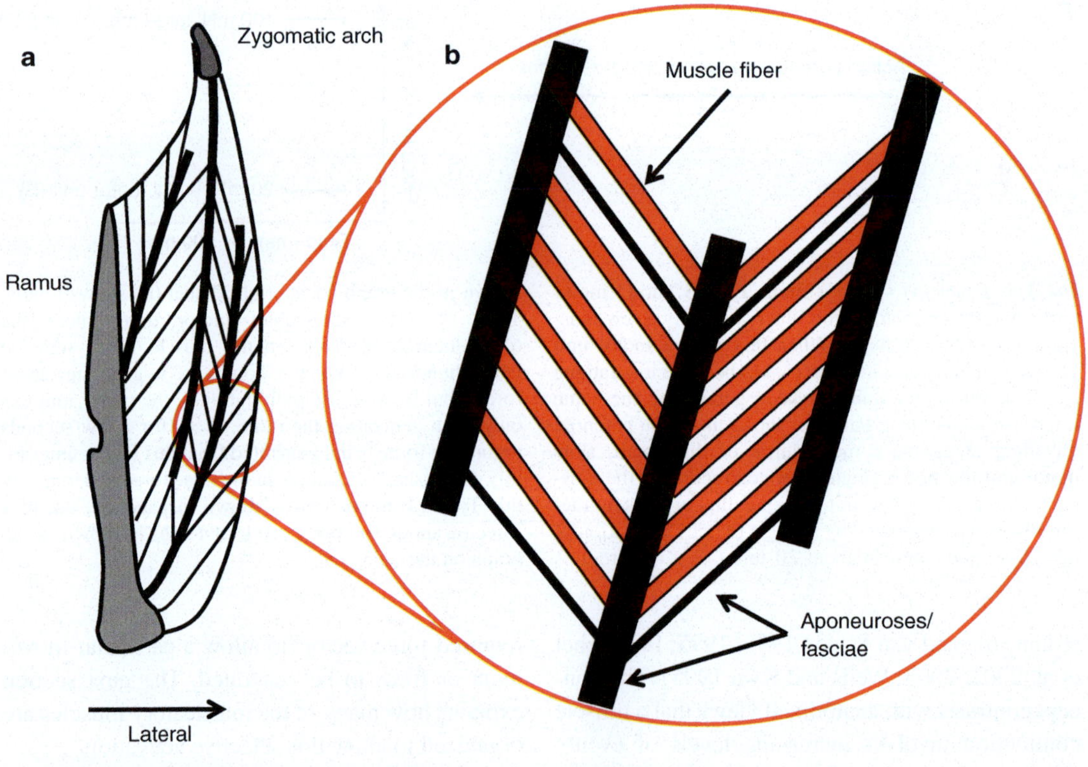

Fig. 3.3 Panel (**a**) shows a coronal section through the left masseter muscle (looking from the front). The *black bands* (3 are shown) represent aponeurotic sheaths that pass from the zygomatic arch or the ramus of the mandible into the muscle. These aponeurotic sheaths are connected by smaller sheaths or fasciae (**b**). Muscle fibers do not run from the zygomatic arch down to the ramus of the mandible but rather run from one aponeurotic sheath to another. So when muscle fibers of a motor unit on one side of an aponeurosis contract, they exert forces at a markedly different angle to those on the other side of the same aponeurosis. A wide range of force vectors (different magnitudes and directions of force) are therefore possible depending on how the brain activates the range of motor units available within the masseter muscle. A similar complexity of force directions appears to occur also in the medial and lateral pterygoid muscles and the temporalis muscles

appear to have simpler internal muscle fiber arrangements with many of the muscle fibers passing the full length of the muscle. Nonetheless, these complexities of muscle fiber architecture within most of the masticatory muscles provide the possibility for a wide range of directions with which forces can be applied to the mandible. Selective activation of these regions, or subcompartments, provides a range of forces and movements enabling a wide range of mandibular tasks.

The above description points to a considerable flexibility in the activation of motor units within muscles. Higher centers of the brain appear capable of activating those motor units in whatever muscles that are most ideally placed for the task at hand. Therefore, in the production of mandibular, facial, or tongue movement, the higher brain centers (i.e., sensorimotor cortical regions; see below) that drive voluntary movements are not organized in terms of muscles but rather the elemental components of muscles, namely, the motor units. Rather than sending command signals to activate muscles in sequence or simultaneously, the higher centers of the brain only "think" in terms of activating those motor units, wherever they may be located, that are biomechanically best suited to generate the force vector required for that particular mandibular movement. Thus, for example, a grinding movement of the mandible to the left side from intercuspal position and with the teeth together might be best achieved by activation of some motor units in the inferior head of the right lateral pterygoid, some motor units in the left posterior temporalis to prevent the left side of the mandible moving forward, and some units in the left masseter and anterior temporalis to help pull the mandible to the left side and to keep the teeth together while doing so. The activation of these motor units will produce a force on the mandible that moves the jaw to the left side. The important point to note is that the entire muscle does not have to become activated to generate the forces for the task at hand. This feature of muscle activation that different parts of a muscle become active for different tasks may be a reason why muscle tenderness can become localized within a muscle if these regions become overworked or strained for some reason.

The pennate arrangement of the muscle fibers together with fiber type composition and selective activation within the masticatory muscles means that there are a wide range of force vectors and durations that can be generated at different locations within the muscle and which enables functional heterogeneity to contribute to the generation of a wide range of mandibular tasks. Generation of contraction forces is complex, and while underpinned by the Henneman size principle where motor units are activated in order of size, other factors including selective activation of regions of a muscle and the rate of motor unit activation are important contributors.

3.1.2 Somatosensory Receptors

The orofacial tissues (e.g., facial skin, intraoral mucosa, periodontal ligaments, muscles, temporomandibular joints—TMJs) are extensively supplied with somatosensory receptors that transduce the energy from a physical stimulus (e.g., mechanical, thermal) on the orofacial tissues into action potentials that travel along the nerve fibers to which they are connected. This information enters the brain and is used for perception as well as motivational, affective, and cognitive functions. The information also plays an important role in the control of orofacial movements. Orofacial somatosensory receptors have been extensively reviewed (Capra 1995; Sessle 2006, 2016).

All movements are critically dependent on sensory feedback in order for them to be executed properly. Take, for example, the difficulties encountered with properly coordinated movements of the tongue and lips during mandibular nerve block local anesthesia targeting the sensory nerves to the teeth, bone, lips, and tongue. The *somatosensory* system refers to that part of the sensory system that processes information about touch, pressure, pain, temperature, position, and movement applied to the skin, mucosa, teeth, muscles, or TMJs. The word was coined to distinguish it from other forms of sensory information that is processed by the visual, auditory, and vestibular sensory systems. In the somatosensory system, stimuli (e.g., touch, pressure, pain, tem-

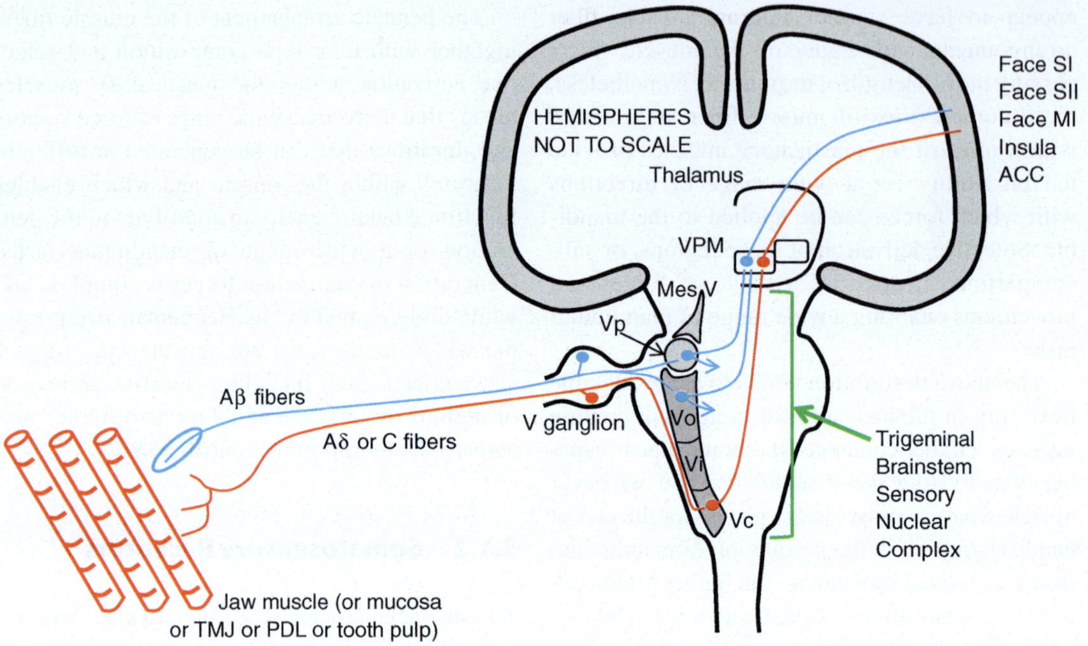

Fig. 3.4 This shows the basic somatosensory pathway for transmitting information about touch, pressure, pain, temperature, position, and movement from the orofacial area. A section of muscle is shown on the left, but any orofacial tissue can be substituted here (tooth pulp afferents may be nociceptive only). Most somatosensory information travels as action potentials along axons toward the trigeminal brainstem sensory nuclear complex (TBSNC) where the axons terminate via synapses on 2nd order neurons. *Blue* pathways are for pathways (along Aβ fibers) conveying information about non-noxious stimuli (e.g., touch, pressure) and which mainly terminate on 2nd order neurons in the more rostral (*upper*) parts of the TBSNC. *Red* is for pathways (C fibers) conveying nociceptive information and which mainly terminate on 2nd order neurons in the more caudal (*lower*) parts of the TBSNC. *TMJ* temporomandibular joint, *PDL* periodontal ligament, *V* trigeminal, *Vc* subnucleus caudalis of TBSNC, *Vi* subnucleus interpolaris, *Vo* subnucleus oralis, *Vp* principal sensory nucleus of V, *Mes V* mesencephalic nucleus of V, *VPM* ventroposteromedial subnucleus of the thalamus, *SI* primary somatosensory cortex, *SII* secondary somatosensory cortex, *MI* primary motor cortex, *ACC* anterior cingulate cortex

perature changes) are transduced by mechanoreceptors, nociceptors, and thermoreceptors into action potentials that pass mainly through the trigeminal nerve to enter the brainstem (Fig. 3.4).

3.1.2.1 Nociceptive (i.e., Pain-Related) Information

A noxious stimulus at the periphery (e.g., overstretching a masticatory muscle or the TMJ) will be transduced by the muscle and/or the TMJ nociceptors into action potentials that will pass along Aδ and C afferent nerve fibers. The axons of these nerve fibers pass through the trigeminal ganglion, and this nociceptive information descends to terminate via synapses on 2nd order neurons within the subnucleus caudalis (Vc) of the trigeminal brainstem sensory nuclear complex (TBSNC; see Fig. 3.4). The terminals of these primary afferent nociceptive nerve fibers release neurotransmitters (e.g., substance P, glutamate) which bind to receptors (e.g., neurokinin receptors; *N*-methyl-D-aspartate (NMDA) receptors) on the membranes of the 2nd order neurons; the cell body of a 2nd order neuron is represented as a small red dot within the subnucleus caudalis in Fig. 3.4. When the neurotransmitter binds to these receptors, there is an influx of positive ions into the 2nd order neuron, which if large enough causes excitation of the neuron in the form of action potentials which travel along the axon of the 2nd order neuron. The properties of these neurons as well as the pathway ascending to higher centers will be discussed in section 3.2.

It is worth mentioning here that the TBSNC also receives somatosensory input from other cranial nerves, such as the VII, IX, X, and XII nerves and upper cervical nerves. This convergence of input from these other sites may contribute to some of the referral pain patterns observed in patients with pain, e.g., angina referring to the left mandible, the pain of temporomandibular disorders (TMD) referring to the neck.

It is also important to note that only some of the Aδ and C fibers convey nociceptive information, as other Aδ and C fibers are for sensory and motor autonomic functions (see below). The Aδ nociceptive afferents are fast conducting and are responsible for the first and sharp pain experienced following an initial noxious stimulus, e.g., pinprick. The C nociceptive afferents are much slower conducting and are responsible for the slow and dull pain that is experienced several seconds after an initial noxious stimulus. Under inflammatory conditions such as with damaged muscles or a mucosal ulcer, local immune cells at the site release a range of chemicals (e.g., bradykinin, H+, nerve growth factor (NGF), cytokines) that sensitize the terminals of the nociceptive afferents. These terminals can now become activated even with non-noxious stimuli, such as touching an ulcer or an area of sunburn, or normal muscle contractions during normal mandibular movements in patients with myalgia. The result of this is a sensation of pain in response to normally non-painful stimuli. This phenomenon is called *allodynia*. These sensitized nociceptive somatosensory afferents also can generate many more action potentials in response to a noxious (i.e., painful) stimulus, and the term *hyperalgesia* refers to an increased pain response to a normally painful stimulus. These changes to the excitability of the nociceptive afferent terminals are part of what is called *peripheral sensitization*. One mechanism whereby nonsteroidal anti-inflammatory (NSAID) drugs, such as aspirin, exert their analgesic affects is through interfering with the process of peripheral sensitization. With healing, this peripheral sensitization usually resolves, and, clinically, the allodynia and hyperalgesia also resolve, although with chronic pain (e.g., persistent arthritis, neuropathic pain) these may persist. There is also some evidence for sex differences in these peripheral sensitization mechanisms (Cairns et al. 2014). The increased nociceptive barrage of action potentials associated with peripheral sensitization (particularly along C nociceptive fibers) is also thought to contribute to neuroplastic changes in the brain, and this is termed *central sensitization* (see below).

3.1.2.2 Information About Touch and Pressure

Information about touch, pressure, position, and movement is conveyed mostly by the larger diameter, faster conducting nerve fibers called Aβ fibers (blue fibers in Fig. 3.4). Many of these fibers are connected with mechanoreceptors located within the mucosa, skin, periodontal ligaments, muscle spindles, and TMJ capsule, and these mechanoreceptors are mostly exquisitely sensitive to touch, pressure, and stretch stimuli applied to the tissues. Food contacting the mucosa or the teeth or the maxillary teeth contacting the mandibular teeth as in chewing will activate mucosal and periodontal mechanoreceptors and result in action potentials travelling along these Aβ fibers in the trigeminal nerve to enter the brainstem. Movement of the mandible can also activate mechanoreceptors in the TMJs, muscle spindles, as well as mechanoreceptors in the facial skin and intraoral mucosa (see below). Mandibular movements are therefore associated with a barrage of somatosensory information that travels along many afferent nerves that enters the brainstem and into the TBSNC (Lund and Olsson 1983).

The axons of these nerves conveying non-noxious information (blue lines in Fig. 3.4) terminate on 2nd order neurons mostly in the more rostral parts of the TBSNC, such as the principal sensory nucleus (Vp) and subnucleus oralis (Vo) (see Section 3.2). These 2nd order neurons send their information via the thalamus to higher centers for the perception of touch, pressure, and stretch of orofacial tissues at the periphery and also for motivational, affective, and cognitive functions. Some of the information, particularly from muscle spindle afferents and TMJ mechanoreceptors, can be used for kinesthetic perception (i.e., mandibular position sense or proprioception). Periodontal, muscle spindle, and TMJ afferents appear to convey information that plays a particular role in interdental size discrimination and for the modulation of motor activity.

Periodontal mechanoreceptors are particularly important and have been extensively reviewed (Trulsson 2007; Trulsson et al. 2012). These mechanoreceptors are located in the periodontal ligaments around the roots of the teeth, and they generate action potentials when forces are applied to the teeth. They signal the magnitude and also the direction of the forces applied to the teeth from tooth-to-tooth contact and also food-to-tooth contact or tongue-to-tooth contact. They also assist other mechanoreceptors (e.g., muscle spindles and possibly TMJ mechanoreceptors) in providing interdental size discrimination. Most individuals are able to detect between 10 and 35 μm (i.e., less than the thickness of a hair) between the teeth (Dubner et al. 1978).

Loss of teeth means therefore a loss of periodontal mechanoreceptors and therefore a loss of the perceptual and motor functions performed by these mechanoreceptors. The somatosensory and motor systems of patients with partial and complete dentures and patients with implant-supported prostheses will therefore be more reliant (or totally reliant if all teeth have been lost) on other orofacial receptors and particularly those that may be less efficient in providing reliable information as to tooth contacts. Thus, in partial and complete denture patients and patients with implants, activity in muscle spindle and TMJ mechanoreceptors as well as mucosal and even cutaneous mechanoreceptors will likely be used by the somatosensory system to take over largely or completely the role of periodontal mechanoreceptors in the perception of tooth contacts as well as in modulating motor activity as in chewing (Klineberg and Murray 1999; Trulsson 2007; Trulsson et al. 2012).

3.1.2.3 Information About Position and Movement: The Muscle Spindle, the Golgi Tendon Organ, and TMJ Mechanoreceptors

Muscles not only have receptors within them for pressure, pain, and temperature, but they also have sophisticated receptors that provide information about their length and how fast their length is changing, as well as the force they are generating. The muscle spindle, located in series with the main fibers of the muscle, provides information about length and length change; and the Golgi tendon organ, located at the end of the muscle fibers before the fibers insert into the bone or tendon, provides information about the forces generated by muscles.

The muscle spindle is a very complicated and very sensitive sensory receptor, and it provides detailed information about length and velocity changes in a muscle over the entire working range of the muscle. It can detect micrometer changes in length. Such a sensitive receptor would easily saturate over the wide range of length changes that most muscles operate if the muscle spindle did not have a system to maintain its optimal sensitivity to avoid saturation. The muscle spindle does indeed have such a system so that it can provide high sensitivity to length and rate of length change throughout the full range of mandibular movements. This maintenance of optimal sensitivity is achieved by the γ-motoneuron innervation of muscle spindles, and the phenomenon is illustrated in Fig. 3.5.

Muscle spindle sensitivity is optimized for all lengths of a muscle which means that the muscle spindle can provide detailed information on lengths and velocities over a wide range of muscle lengths. During a muscle contraction, both α- and γ-motoneurons are activated, and this is termed α-γ-coactivation. The α-motoneurons cause contraction of the main (extrafusal) muscle fibers and are responsible for the force produced by muscles (Fig. 3.5). There is added complexity here in that all muscle spindles have their own motor supply to specialized muscle fibers located within the muscle spindle, and these fibers are called intrafusal muscle fibers. These intrafusal

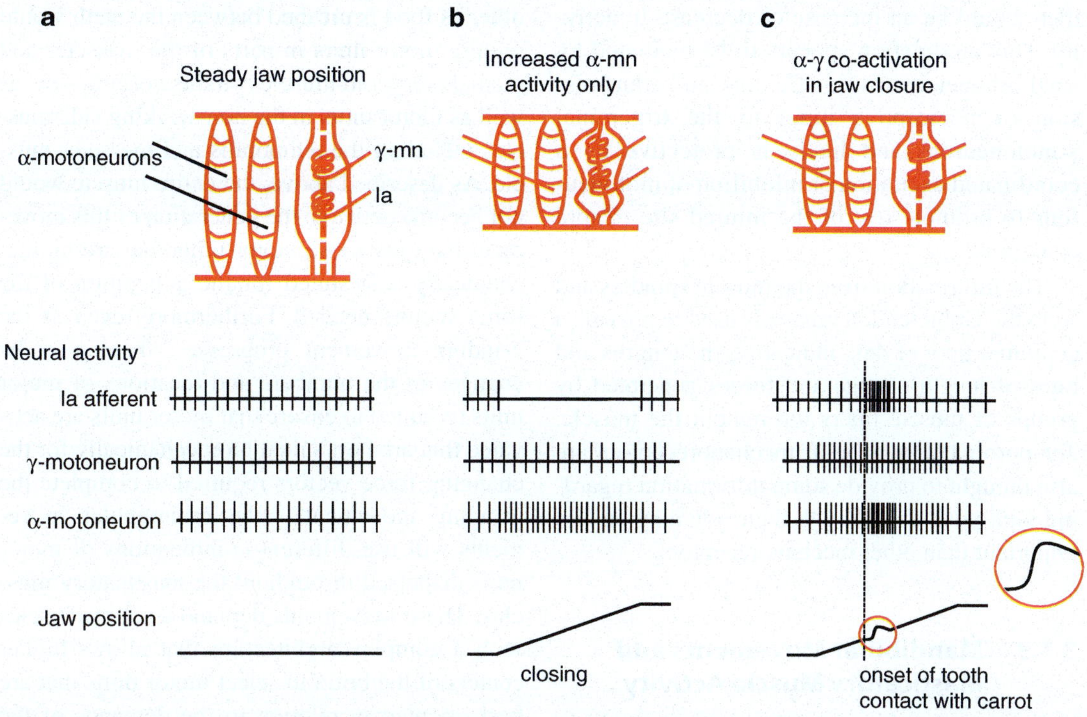

Fig. 3.5 The *top diagram* in each panel (**a**, **b**, **c**) represents the medial pterygoid muscle showing two extrafusal muscle fibers (innervated by α-motoneurons) and a muscle spindle that contains one intrafusal muscle fiber (continuous *dashed line*; innervated by a γ-motoneuron) supporting the mandible. The sensory part of the muscle spindle is the Group Ia primary afferent that responds to the length and changes in length of the muscle spindle; there are also Group II sensory endings (not shown). Panel (**a**) shows the normal α-γ-coactivation that occurs in any contraction so that α-motoneurons are activated (each short *vertical line* in the neural activity traces represents a single action potential) to induce extrafusal muscle fiber contraction. The simultaneous γ-motoneuron activation results in a slight stretch of the intrafusal muscle fibers so that there is a continuous barrage of action potentials along the Ia afferents from the muscle spindle; these Ia afferents are therefore able to encode or signal any changes in muscle length. Panel (**b**) shows an artificial situation where only α-motoneurons increase their firing to cause a muscle contraction during mandibular closing. The absence of an increased activity in the γ-motoneurons leads to a reduction in the tension within the muscle spindle, and the Group Ia afferents cease to fire action potentials for the duration of the contraction (top neural activity traces, (**b**)). During this period, the Ia afferents are unable to provide any information about unexpected changes in muscle length, and in effect the sensory function of the spindle becomes disabled. Panel (**c**) shows the normal operation of a muscle spindle during a muscle contraction with α-γ-coactivation. The intrafusal muscle fibers contract at the same rate as the extrafusal muscle fibers to maintain the tension at the terminals of the Ia afferents so that they maintain their firing and are able to respond to and signal irregularities in the movement. Contact with a hard nut in a muffin, for example, causes a brief cessation in mandibular closing which stops muscle shortening. However, the γ-motoneuron activity continues to increase and thereby leads to a stretch of the central terminal region of the intrafusal muscle fibers and then a resultant increase in activity of the Ia afferents. As these Ia afferents are connected to α-motoneurons via a monosynaptic reflex arc, the increased Ia afferent discharge causes a very fast, reflex increase in α-motoneuronal activity and an increase in muscle activity to help overcome the increased resistance encountered because of the nut in the muffin. Therefore, this mechanism of α-γ-coactivation maintains the sensitivity of the muscle spindle throughout a muscle contraction, and the spindle is therefore always able to detect small changes in muscle length irrespective of the length of the muscle

muscle fibers are driven by the γ-motoneurons. The γ-motoneurons are activated at the same time as the α-motoneurons, and they cause contraction of the intrafusal muscle fibers within the muscle spindle and therefore maintain the sensitivity of the spindles as the muscle and spindles shorten. Figure 3.5 explains how this comes about.

It should be noted that noxious input to the masticatory muscles can influence the sensitivity of spindles to muscle length changes, so that there could be an increase or decrease in activity. This modulation appears to be mediated by small-diameter muscle afferents and transmission of nociceptive input to the trigeminal γ-motoneurons and likely is protective by a coordinated excitation or inhibition of motoneurons to promote rest of the injured site (Capra et al. 2007).

The information from the muscle spindles and from the Golgi tendon organs is used to provide a continual flow of data indicating the lengths and rates of length change and forces generated by groups of muscle fibers throughout the muscle. Temporomandibular joint mechanoreceptors are also thought to provide some information regarding joint position although their role may be less important than other mechanoreceptors.

3.1.3 Mandibular Movements and Masticatory Muscle Activity

The anatomy of the TMJ is described in detail in Chap. 2. Basic mandibular movements are also described in Chap. 4. The following will briefly review some aspects of mandibular movements and masticatory muscle activity during mastication.

Mastication in the human is not a simple open–close mandibular movement. Animals with large cuspid teeth have such hinge-like mandibular movements. Because of our small cuspid teeth, however, as well as the ability of our mandible to translate forward as well as rotate, masticatory mandibular movements are characterized by varying degrees of lateral displacement particularly during the grinding movements associated with crushing food. As indicated above, these mandibular movements are controlled by motor units in many of the masticatory muscles, so that command signals from the brain do not "think" in terms of which muscles to activate but rather "think" in terms of activating those combinations of motor units, wherever they may be located, that are biomechanically best suited to generate the force vector required for that particular mandibular movement. For example, a grinding movement of the teeth against each other as food is crushed between the teeth would require motor units in parts of the masseter and medial pterygoid muscles on the working side, as well as motor units in the non-working side muscles including the temporalis and masseter muscle. As described above, the entire muscle would not become active in the generation of this movement but only those motor units that are biomechanically best suited for the generation of the force vectors needed. Furthermore, even as the grinding movement progresses, there may be changes in the numbers and locations of motor units recruited to ensure that motor units are activated that are best suited biomechanically for the changing force vectors required to complete the grinding movement. Other mandibular movements will use different combinations of motor units dispersed throughout the masticatory muscles. These movements demand a set of muscles with a complex architecture that allows higher centers of the brain to select motor units that are best oriented in relation to the demands of the movement required.

Dentists have often had an interest in mandibular movements and have described these movements with the use of devices such as pantographs and other jaw-tracking devices. These systems typically provide kinematic information of a single point, by usually recording the movement of the anterior midline of the mandible at the mandibular mid-incisor point. As the mandible is a three-dimensional object, these single point tracings may therefore provide misleading information if used for diagnostic purposes or in the evaluation of treatment outcomes. Furthermore, descriptions of the mandible's movement have not aided clinical diagnosis or management beyond simple range of movement information (i.e., opening, lateral, and protrusive directions) obtained from routine clinical assessment. Attempts have also been made to use the electrical activity of muscles, electromyography, in clinical diagnosis and/or treatment. Unfortunately the recording of electromyographic (EMG) activity from human participants provides data that is highly variable between participants irrespective of whether there is a clinical diagnosis of pain or not. As a diagnostic tool, like kinematic recordings, electromyography simply does not possess the required sensitivity and specificity to allow clinicians to provide an aid to diagnosis. It is worth quoting from the American Association for Dental Research policy statement on TMD: *the consensus of recent scientific literature about currently available technological diagnostic devices for TMD is that, except for various imaging modalities, none of them shows the sensitivity and specificity required to separate normal subjects from TMD patients or to distinguish among TMD subgroups* (Greene 2010).

3.1.3.1 Masticatory Mandibular Movements

Masticatory movements are complex and consist of mandibular, facial, and tongue movements that are driven by masticatory, facial, and tongue muscles as mentioned below. The facial and tongue muscles are involved because the lips, cheeks, and tongue help control the food bolus in the mouth and keep the food contained over the occlusal table for effective comminution (the effective reduction of the size of the food bolus).

Masticatory mandibular movements usually occur well within the classical border movement pathways except when the mandible approaches or makes tooth contact toward the end of chewing. In the frontal plane, the masticatory cycle is described as "teardrop" in shape. At the beginning of opening, the mid-incisor point moves first downward, and at the end of opening, it moves laterally and upward toward the working side (or chewing side). The mid-incisor point then moves upward and medially, and the food is crushed between the teeth.

While these mandibular movements during chewing are the classical description, the masticatory movements tend to be highly variable from cycle to cycle in a subject chewing the same or different foods and from subject to subject (Lund 1991). Part of this variability relates to the changing consistency of the food bolus from cycle to cycle as the food breaks down. The movement of the mandible toward intercuspal position is less variable. The masticatory muscles must move the mandible precisely toward the teeth at the end of the chewing cycle, so that the teeth glide smoothly along cuspal inclines and generate the required force to crush and break down the food. Mechanoreceptors (particularly periodontal, but also muscle spindle afferents; see above) provide a continual source of afferent input to the CNS to ensure that the chewing cycle is harmonious with existing tooth guidance (see above). These modulatory effects on motoneuronal activity will be mediated via local reflex circuits and also by modulatory influences on the masticatory central pattern generator (CPG), as well as providing modulatory influences on higher motor centers such as the motor cortex (see below) (Lund 1991).

There are several different phases of each masticatory cycle (Trulsson et al. 2012). The preparatory phase is the phase in which the mandible, tongue, lips, and cheeks prepare the bolus for effective food comminution. The reduction phase is the phase where food comminution is associated with salivary flow and mix of food and saliva, and the pre-swallowing phase is where the comminuted food is brought together with saliva as a bolus, in preparation for swallowing.

There are a number of intrinsic and extrinsic factors responsible for variations in the masticatory cycle (Woda et al. 2006). Intrinsic factors include age, gender, and dental status, and extrinsic factors include the hardness, rheological properties (plasticity/elasticity), and size of the food. For example, harder foods of larger size are associated with more cycles of longer duration and higher EMG activity, while older age and tooth loss are also associated with more cycles of longer duration and higher EMG activity (Van der Bilt 2011; Woda et al. 2006). A significant factor in modifying the chewing cycles would be changes in the somatosensory inputs associated with foods of different sizes, hardness, and textures (Van der Bilt 2011; Woda et al. 2006). The activity in periodontal, muscle spindle, mucosal, and possibly TMJ mechanoreceptors associated with different foods can modify, as noted above, motoneuronal activity via brainstem and higher pathways.

It is noteworthy that the tongue is largely made of muscle which during mastication positions the food bolus but does not itself get bitten, usually. The face motor cortex may play an important role here by strongly inhibiting mandibular closing muscle activity during tongue and indeed facial movements that move the food bolus over the occlusal table. The tongue is most active during the opening phase of the chewing cycle when food is required to be collected and repositioned for effective comminution on the occlusal table.

The movement of the condyle and disc during normal mandibular movements is complex. The lateral pterygoid muscle plays an important role because it is a major contributor to opening, lateral, and protrusive jaw movements and inserts near the TMJ, with the inferior head inserting exclusively into the condylar neck and the superior head inserting largely into the condylar neck. Some fibers of the superior head do insert into the disc–capsule complex of the TMJ, but the long-held view (still held by some) that the superior head inserts exclusively into the disc is not correct. Further, the view that the superior and inferior heads of the lateral pterygoid muscle exhibit reciprocal patterns of activity is not supported by current data (Murray et al. 2007; Murray 2012). The superior head and the inferior head of the lateral pterygoid muscle have very similar functions in that both are active in contralateral, protrusive, and open–close jaw movements. However, there is evidence for functional heterogeneity within each head of the lateral pterygoid muscle so that it appears that the brain is able to activate independently those motor units of each head of the muscle to provide a force vector onto the condyle that is biomechanically best suited to generate the movement required.

Changes to the occlusion may have an influence on the movement of the mandible and the TMJ and the function of the masticatory muscles, and these effects have been extensively reviewed (Van der Bilt 2011; Woda et al. 2006). Thus, restoring teeth, in such a way that necessitates a change to the normal pathways of a chewing cycle, will lead to different levels of firing of orofacial afferents (e.g., periodontal afferents, but also muscle spindle and possibly TMJ mechanoreceptors and Golgi tendon organs). This information will feed back to the CNS (see below) and can cause a variety of changes to neural activity, including reflex changes in muscle activity, changes in the activity of the CPG controlling mastication as well as changes in the activity of the primary motor cortex. These changes in neural activity brought about by an altered afferent input can result in immediate functional changes and can also contribute to longer-term structural changes. The resultant effects will be a change to the activity of particular motor units, in particular subcompartments of muscles, so that the appropriate modification to the chewing cycle can occur so as to accommodate to the change in the occlusion. The new chewing cycle will now accommodate to the changed occlusion unless the interference is too large and beyond the adaptive capacity of the CNS and muscles. Of note is that normal tooth contact occurs for only approximately 10–20 min daily with eating and swallowing (Sheppard and Markus 1962) and together with neuroplasticity (the ability of the nervous system to adapt; see below) results in an individual tending to adapt to occlusal changes rather rapidly in the majority of the population; some individuals may not adapt as well, and this lack of adaptability may be a factor contributing to impaired jaw function.

3.2 Physiology of the Masticatory System: Central Aspects

Up to now, we have been mostly describing the complex peripheral apparatus that allows us to perceive our environment and to generate mandibular movements. How does the brain process the somatosensory information from the periphery and how does the brain drive the muscles to generate the range of movements and forces possible by the orofacial motor system? To answer these questions, the following will review the central pathways for the processing of somatosensory information as well as the central pathways responsible for the generation of movements.

3.2.1 Processing of Somatosensory Information Within the Brain

Low-threshold, non-noxious stimuli applied to mechanoreceptors in the orofacial area result in action potentials travelling along nerves to terminate on 2nd order neurons mostly within the more rostral components of the TBSNC such as the Vp and the Vo. Other receptors in the orofacial area respond to innocuous temperature changes (hot and cold thermal receptors), and they terminate on 2nd order neurons in the subnucleus caudalis.

As shown in Fig. 3.4, this information is relayed through the thalamus (the ventroposteromedial subnucleus) to terminate within the face region of the primary somatosensory cortex (face SI), the face region of the secondary somatosensory cortex (face SII), as well as other centers such as the insula (Haggard and de Boer 2014). These projections to face SI and face SII are likely important for our perception of tooth contacts. The possible projections to the insula may play a role in the awareness associated with orofacial sensory stimuli, for example, the pleasurable aspects associated with the enjoyment of food textures, or an excessive awareness of occlusal contacts.

Somatosensory information can be used for the local modulation of motor activity through reflex pathways and via the masticatory CPG. When encountering harder food during chewing, the harder food will activate periodontal mechanoreceptors, and this information can be used not only for fast reflex increases in activity in parts of the masticatory muscles but also for modulation of the masticatory CPG so that the mandible is moved so as to generate the required forces between the teeth to crush the food with greater consistency. These pathways from the 2nd order neurons for fast reflex changes in muscle activity and also for modulation of the masticatory CPG are indicated by the blue arrows arising from the 2nd order neurons within Vp and Vo in Fig. 3.4.

Orofacial somatosensory information ascends to higher centers of the brain such as the face region of the primary motor cortex (face MI) for the modulation of voluntary motor activity. For example, we can voluntarily increase the force on an object between the teeth (e.g., food bolus, cotton roll), and this ability would require continual monitoring of the activity of periodontal afferents, particularly, that would be fed back to the face MI and face SI and allow us to finely adjust the amount of force exerted.

In the previous section describing peripheral aspects of nociceptive somatosensory processing, it was noted that primary afferents terminate on 2nd order neurons in the subnucleus caudalis (Vc) of the TBSNC. There are two main types of nociceptive 2nd order neurons. The nociceptive-specific (NS) neurons receive only Aδ or C fiber input conveying nociceptive information that is evoked when noxious stimuli are applied to the receptive fields of these neurons. [A receptive field of a neuron is the region of the skin, mucosa, or deep tissue over which a stimulus can be applied, and the neuron will respond by generating action potentials.] The other type of nociceptive 2nd order neuron is called a wide dynamic range (WDR) neuron, and these neurons not only receive Aδ or C fiber input conveying nociceptive information but also low-threshold non-noxious input conveyed along Aβ fibers, such as tactile input. These WDR 2nd order neurons therefore not only respond by generating action potentials when noxious stimuli are applied to their receptive fields but also can generate action potentials when tactile and other low-threshold inputs are applied to their receptive fields. Another feature of each of these 2nd order neurons is that many receive the so-called convergent somatosensory inputs from a number of different regions of the orofacial area, such as masticatory muscles, the TMJs, tooth pulp, facial skin, mucosa, etc. Under normal physiological conditions, these inputs may be inconsequential and may only become *unmasked* under pathological conditions (see below). This convergence of somatosensory inputs is thought to contribute to the poor localization and referral so characteristic of orofacial pain.

Under conditions where there is long-lasting and/or intense noxious stimulation of the periphery (Mense and Hoheisel 2008; Sessle 2008), such as a blow to the jaw or stretching of the masticatory muscles as with a prolonged dental appointment, these 2nd order NS and WDR neurons can undergo *central sensitization*. This sensitization consists of neuroplastic changes to these 2nd order neurons that result in increased levels of neuronal excitability. Recent evidence suggests that the glial cells in the vicinity play a key role in these central sensitization processes (Chiang et al. 2011; Sessle 2011b). Since these 2nd order neurons convey nociceptive information to higher centers for perception, then increased levels of excitability can mean that individuals experience *allodynia*, that is, a sense of pain in response to low-threshold input, e.g., tactile input as with lightly touching the injured part. They may also experience spontaneous pain, i.e., pain at rest and without pressing on the injured part. This may be part of the reason for the pain experienced in injured masticatory muscles at rest and why light pressure on the masticatory muscles or normal mandibular movements are associated with pain or worsening of pain. Another good example of allodynia is pain associated with light touch of sunburnt skin.

As indicated above, many of these 2nd order nociceptive neurons also receive convergent input, and these inputs may only become unmasked in pathophysiological conditions where the neurons undergo central sensitization. Under these circumstances, the higher centers of the brain responsible for perception may misinterpret the injury as occurring from the peripheral site innervated by one of the convergent inputs and that may have nothing to do with the original injury. This can be a reason for the spread and referral of pain that is such a characteristic of pain associated with inflammation (Sessle 2008). These processes are likely to play a significant role in the muscle and/or TMJ pain associated with TMD. In most individuals these central neuroplastic changes reverse after the peripheral injury resolves, but in some people the changes may persist and thereby may lead to persistent or chronic pain states. It is not clear why these neuroplastic changes do not reverse in all individuals, but it is thought that genetic and phenotypic (including environmental) factors may play a role in these persistent effects.

There is added complexity in that the activity of these 2nd order nociceptive neurons can be modulated by somatosensory inputs and by descending influences from higher centers. These modulatory influences have been described in terms of the gate control theory proposed by Ron Melzack and Pat Wall in the 1960s (Melzack and Wall 1965). Figure 3.6 outlines some possible pathways involved in the gate control theory. In terms of somatosensory modulation, pain can be alleviated through activation of tactile inputs by rubbing the sore area or by clinical procedures such as pressure/vibration to the lip during an intraoral injection, acupuncture, or transcutaneous electrical nerve stimulation (TENS). These procedures activate low-threshold somatosensory inputs (blue pathway, Fig. 3.6) that act, via inhibitory interneurons (black pathway, insert, Fig. 3.6) in the brainstem, to inhibit (minus sign, insert, Fig. 3.6) the activity of nociceptive 2nd order neurons, that is, to close the gate and suppress the transmission of nociceptive information to higher brain centers where the perception of pain occurs. The gate control theory also includes other modulatory factors, including those coming from higher centers of the brain (such as the periaqueductal gray (PAG), the brainstem raphe system, as well as the limbic system, e.g., amygdala, hypothalamus) and which send descending pathways to these same 2nd order nociceptive neurons and can have either inhibitory effects (minus sign, insert, Fig. 3.6) or excitatory effects (plus sign, insert, Fig. 3.6). The inhibitory effects can come into play in situations where the peripheral injury carries little emotional significance given the situation, for example, a football player injuring his/her wrist during an intense game and only becomes aware of the injury after the game. In this situation, powerful descending pathways from higher brain centers are inhibiting the activity of the 2nd order neurons that would be receiving a barrage of nociceptive activity from the injured wrist. This intrinsic pain inhibitory system also operates in more normal situations and likely contributes to our natural ability to have some control over our experience of pain. It also may contribute to the effectiveness of some pain-relieving approaches, such as acupuncture and TENS that appear capable of recruiting these

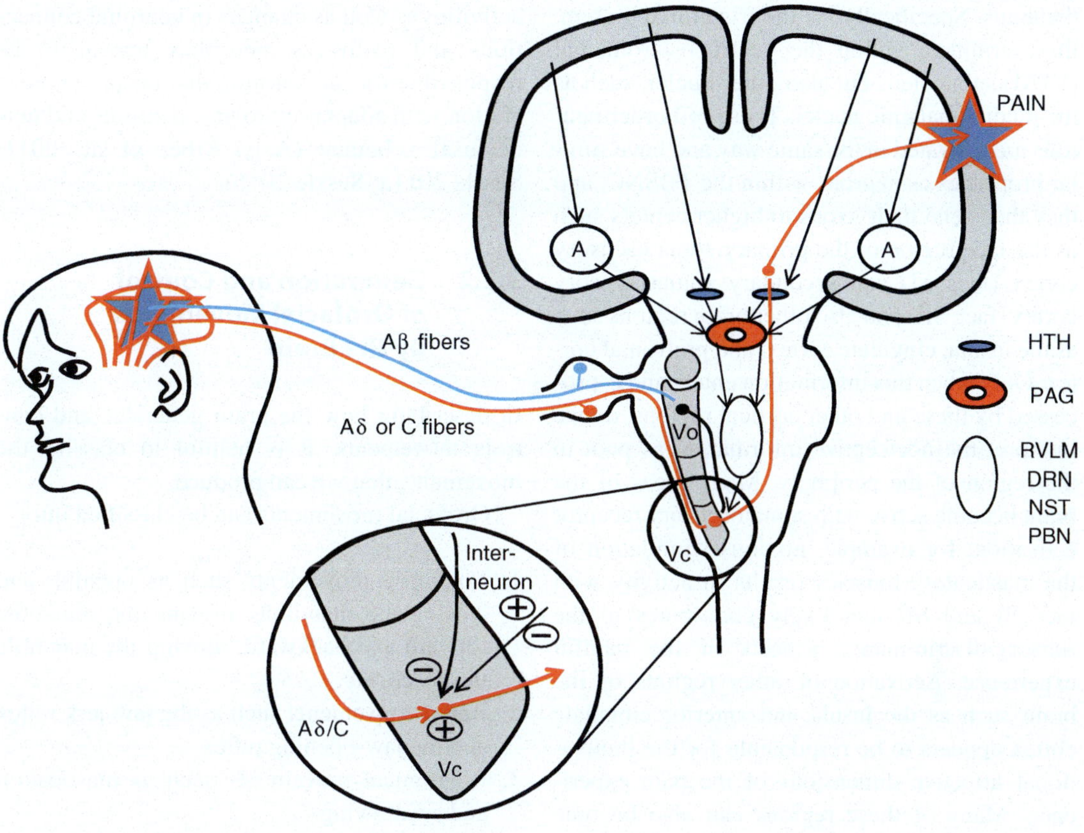

Fig. 3.6 This shows the two basic components of the gate control theory. Information about a noxious stimulus, in this case, a blow to the temporalis muscle, is conveyed by Aδ and C afferent fibers to terminate on 2nd order neurons (see *inset*) in the subnucleus caudalis of the trigeminal brainstem sensory nuclear complex. The nociceptive information is transmitted to higher centers for the conscious perception of pain (indicated by the *star*). The synaptic connections between the nociceptive afferent fibers and the 2nd order neurons are subject to powerful modulating influences from two sources. The first is from low-threshold Aβ fibers which can be activated by rubbing the sore area. The Aβ fibers activate inhibitory interneurons (black connection between Vo and Vc) that exert inhibitory effects on the synapses between the Aδ and C afferent fibers and the 2nd order neurons. The other modulatory influences come from higher centers and these can be inhibitory or excitatory. The inhibitory pathways are operative under most circumstances of acute pain and act to dampen the nociceptive transmission to higher centers. These descending pathways may be dysfunctional in certain orofacial pain states, such as some TMD. Excitatory effects can also occur and can promote the transmission to higher centers of nociceptive information, and these effects may operate in, for example, the fearful dental patient. The transmission to higher centers of nociceptive information may in fact be facilitated in these patients. *HTH* hypothalamus, *PAG* periaqueductal gray matter, *RVLM* rostroventrolateral medulla, *NST* nucleus of the solitary tract, *PBN* parabrachial nucleus, *A* amygdala, *Vo* subnucleus oralis, *Vc* subnucleus caudalis, + excitatory connection, – inhibitory connection

pathways (as well as through peripheral mechanisms as mentioned above).

Not only can the "gate" be closed, it appears that it also can be "opened up," and this may occur in fearful situations such as the highly anxious dental patient. In this situation, descending influences appear capable of reducing the threshold of firing of these nociceptive 2nd order neurons so that they more easily respond to even the slightest nociceptive stimuli or even non-nociceptive input (plus sign, insert, Fig. 3.6). This emphasizes that pain is an individualized personal sensory and emotional experience and that assessment and management need to consider these multidimensional aspects.

These axons of these 2nd order nociceptive neurons mostly cross the midline and ascend to terminate on 3rd order neurons within the thalamus. Specifically for the trigeminal system, they terminate within the ventroposteromedial (VPM) subnucleus but also other nuclei, such as the medial thalamic nuclei. These 3rd order neurons are activated in the same way and have similar properties as neurons within the TBSNC, and they then send their axons to higher centers such as the face region of the primary somatosensory cortex (face SI) and secondary somatosensory cortex (face SII) and also other brain regions such as the insula, cingulate cortex, and prefrontal cortex. Only when this information enters and is processed by these and other cortical regions, do we interpret the nociceptive information as pain in the region of the periphery. Many areas of the brain become active with somatosensory receptor activation, for example, noxious stimulation of the masticatory muscles results in activity with face SI and SII that likely contributes to the sensory-discriminative aspects of the painful experience. Activation of other regions of the brain such as the insula and anterior cingulate cortex appears to be responsible for the motivational–affective dimensions of the pain experience. Many of these regions can also become active in chronic pain states (Apkarian et al. 2011; Lin 2014).

The axons of the 2nd order neurons also pass to regions of the brainstem such as the reticular formation and other parts of the brainstem for involvement in autonomic reflex responses such as salivation in response to taste and texture of food, as well as cardiorespiratory changes to orofacial noxious and non-noxious (e.g., textures, taste of food) stimuli. Some of these axons also terminate locally around the TBSNC for the generation of reflex responses in response to nociceptive and non-nociceptive stimuli (see below) and also send their inputs to the CPGs for mastication and swallowing.

It is also worth noting that not only can neuroplastic changes occur in association with nociceptive inputs (discussed above under central sensitization) but neuroplastic changes can also occur in 2nd order and higher neurons responsible for the transmission of non-nociceptive information to higher centers. These changes can be functional changes in neuronal activities as well as changes in neuronal connections and pathways, and they appear to be responsible for the learning that occurs in association with adaptation to new dentures and new occlusal schemes (Avivi-Arber et al. 2011; Sessle 2011a; Sessle 2016).

3.2.2 Generation and Control of Orofacial Movements by the Brain

In describing how the brain generates and controls movements, it is helpful to classify the movements that we can produce.

Orofacial movements can be classified into:

1. Voluntary movements such as opening and closing the mandible, moving the mandible forward and backward, moving the mandible in speech, etc.
2. Reflex movements such as the jaw-jerk reflex and the jaw-opening reflex
3. Rhythmical movements such as mastication and swallowing

3.2.2.1 Voluntary Movements

In general terms, voluntary movements are movements that we voluntarily perform, such as playing the piano, speaking, making an alginate impression, and moving the mandible to one side or the other. All these movements are driven by the primary motor cortex (termed MI) as well as higher motor cortical areas such as the supplementary motor area (SMA) and the premotor cortex. The face MI lies just in front of the central sulcus (Fig. 3.7), and the face MI initiates and produces voluntary movements of the face, mandible, and tongue. When a person moves the tongue forward and to the right side and opens their mouth, the basal ganglia select a set of programs within the SMA and the premotor cortex (area 6) which then send signals to the face MI. These motor programs contain the details of those parts of the face MI to be activated so as to activate the correct combination of motor units within the tongue so as to generate this movement of the tongue to the

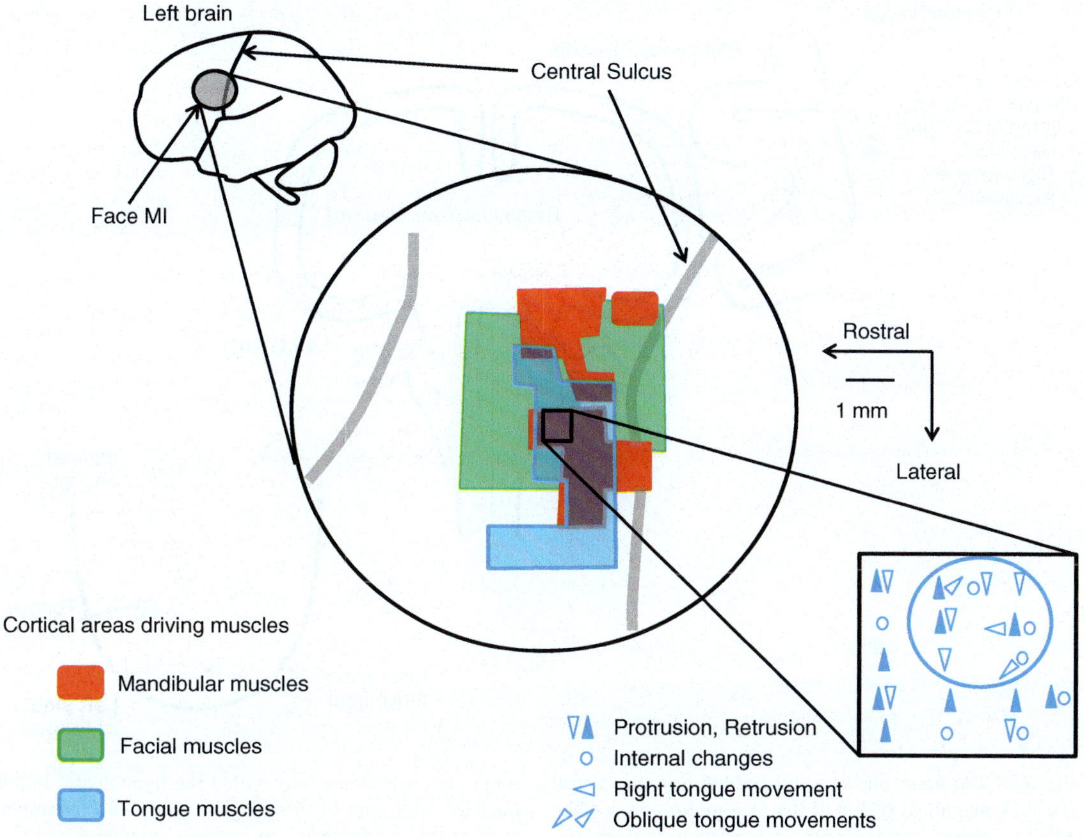

Fig. 3.7 This figure shows a two-dimensional hypothetical mapping of the organization of the motor representation within the left face primary motor cortex (MI). The diagram at the *top left* is an outline of the left brain. The overlying *circle* covers the face MI and is expanded in the central panel to show regions of the face MI that are responsible for activating α-motoneurons that drive muscle fibers within the masticatory muscles (*red areas*), facial muscles (*green areas*), and tongue muscles (*blue area*). For example, the areas of the face MI covered by the *blue outline* contain elemental cortical zones that send outputs down to hypoglossal α-motoneurons that drive motor units within the tongue. The *black square box* overlying the tongue muscle cortical region is expanded at the *bottom right* to show the fine structure of these elemental tongue zones within the face MI which, when activated, result in activation of tongue motor units leading to different types of tongue movements, as indicated by the *arrowheads* and the *circles*. Note that these elemental movements are represented multiple times in different locations in the face MI, and one particular movement can be close to other elemental movements at these different locations. It is thought that the higher centers of the brain can select different combinations of tongue output zones to allow the generation of more complex movements (similar to the generation of more complex sounds, as when playing chords on a piano). A small section of the tongue motor cortex is shown in Fig. 3.8 to show the neural connections from the face MI down to hypoglossal motoneurons. There is a similar complexity of organization for face and mandibular movements

right side. The MI is then responsible for activating the required motor units to produce this tongue movement to the right side.

The face MI consists of specific elemental zones for the production of specific elemental movements, and this organization is illustrated in Fig. 3.7. Note that there is a lot of overlap of mandibular, facial, and tongue elemental zones, and this overlap is thought to facilitate the combined activation of mandibular, facial, and tongue movements by higher centers of the brain driving the face motor cortex. For example, most mandibular movements involve not just a movement of the mandible but also there are usually associated facial and tongue muscle activations that accompany the mandibular movements.

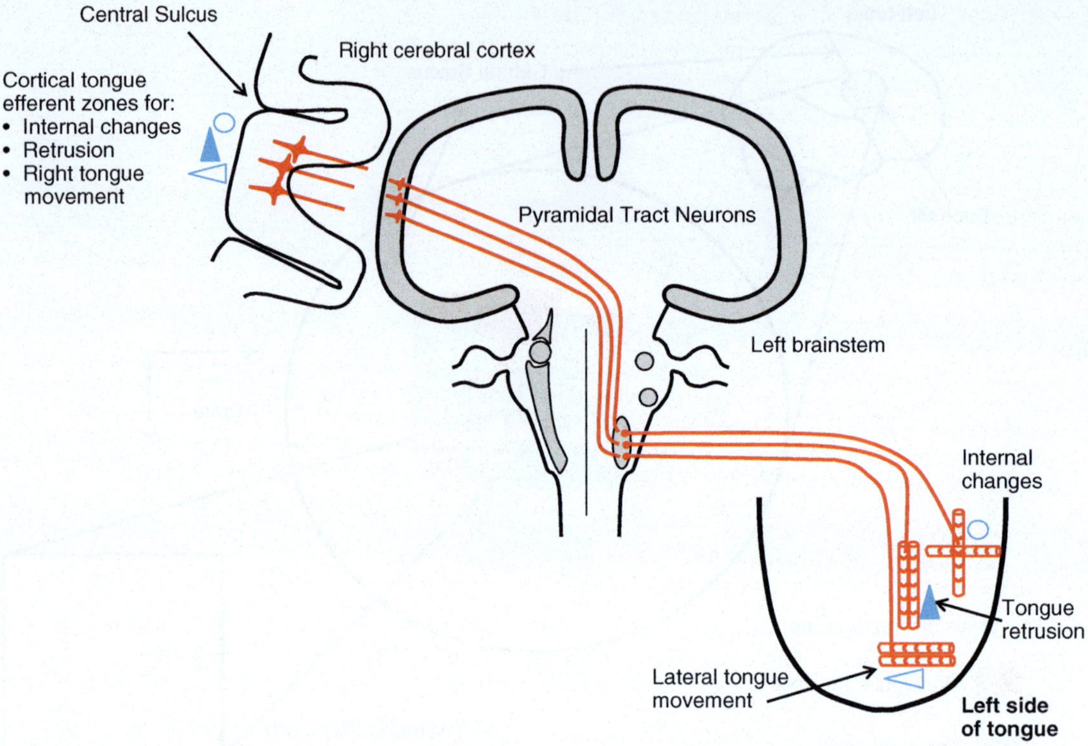

Fig. 3.8 The figure shows a stylized brain in the central panel. A magnified region of the face motor cortex (face MI) in cross-section is shown on the left with three elemental tongue zones for the generation of three elemental tongue movements, namely, internal changes to the tongue shape, tongue retrusion, and right tongue movement. Each elemental tongue movement is driven by pyramidal tract neurons (only one shown for each elemental tongue zone) that send fibers in the pyramidal tract that cross to the other side to synapse directly or indirectly (via interneurons) onto α-motoneurons within the hypoglossal motor nucleus. Note that in this diagram, only one pyramidal tract neuron is connected to one α-motoneuron and two muscle fibers for the generation of each type of elemental tongue movement, but in reality, there are many of each with extensive connections. The α-motoneurons then activate the relevant muscle fibers for the generation of the required tongue movement, in this case a tongue movement to the right, tongue retrusion, and an internal change to tongue shape

Figure 3.8 shows three selected elemental tongue zones and how they are represented by pyramidal tract neurons that send fibers in the pyramidal tract to synapse directly or indirectly (via interneurons) onto α-motoneurons within the hypoglossal motor nucleus.

The face MI therefore contains an extensive representation of elemental movements for all the muscles of the face, mandible, and tongue. The face MI therefore can be considered to be the "keys of a piano" that the higher motor centers *play* in order to allow the generation of the required voluntary movement.

As described above, Fig. 3.4 shows the somatosensory pathway conveying information to the face SI. Another complexity is that not only does the face SI receive somatosensory information from the periphery, but there is also an extensive somatosensory input to neurons in the face MI. For the tongue region of the face MI, for example, many of the neurons in the motor cortex receive low-threshold tactile inputs from the tongue dorsum. This tactile input is thought to play a role in the fine modulation of tongue movements to accommodate quickly to the particular requirements of the tongue movement; for example, with moving food around in the mouth, the motor cortical zones driving motor units in the tongue are greatly assisted by having a continual feedback of the amount of pressure, for example, being exerted by the tongue on the food bolus. There is a similar extensive somatosensory input from orofacial mechanoreceptors to the facial muscle and masticatory muscle elemental zones. This information would provide continual feedback for the refinement of these movements in voluntary movements of the mandible and face. For example, in the assessment of interdental size discrimination, periodontal feedback will play a very important role in modulating the amount of activation within the masticatory muscle region of the face MI so that the correct level of activation occurs within the masticatory muscle region of the face MI so as to drive the required combination of motor units in the various mandibular closing muscles to achieve the required mandibular closing force for assessment of thickness.

In recent years it has become apparent that the brain can undergo neuroplastic changes. Neuroplasticity refers to the structural and functional changes in the brain in association with motor skill acquisition and learning and also in adaptation to changes at the periphery that result in alterations of sensory inputs. The changes can include unmasking of existing synaptic connections that were previously silent, increases or decreases in the synaptic strengths of existing connections, and development of new neural connections. In the case of the orofacial motor system, these changes can occur following changes to the dental occlusion through loss of teeth, placement of restorations, provision of implants and dentures, and orthodontic tooth movement. It is thought that new dental occlusion leads to alterations in the somatosensory information that comes back into the brain because, for example, if some teeth have been extracted, then there will be fewer afferent neurons conveying somatosensory information from periodontal mechanoreceptors, and therefore there will be less information about the magnitude and direction of forces on teeth as artificial teeth or implants do not have an equivalent periodontal mechanoreceptor innervation. Other receptors may be relied upon more to provide the needed information about the direction and magnitude of tooth contacts, and these may include periodontal mechanoreceptors around any remaining teeth, muscle spindles, Golgi tendon organs, mucosal mechanoreceptors underneath dentures, etc. It is thought that with changes to the occlusion, the motor systems controlling voluntary and rhythmical (see below) orofacial movements will undergo changes in their neural circuitry (i.e., neuroplastic changes) to allow the required mandibular, facial, and tongue movements still to be performed. There is indeed evidence in the human for neuroplastic changes within the sensorimotor cortex following the insertion of implant-supported prostheses in edentulous individuals (Palla and Klineberg 2016). Nonetheless, there is good evidence that the efficiency of the resulting movements may not always be equivalent to the efficiency before the loss of teeth, particularly if most/all of the teeth are lost (Van der Bilt 2011). There are clearly limits therefore to the adaptability of the brain in terms of the neuroplastic changes that can occur, and genetic and age factors likely play an important role in this.

These neuroplastic changes are also thought to be important in more subtle adjustments to the motor system, for example, in allowing an individual's motor system to accommodate to new dentures. Some patients can experience difficulty in accommodating to dentures which are different from the old dentures in terms of vertical dimension, flange contours, occlusal form and position, etc. A feature of neuroplastic changes in the brain is that an older brain appears less able to undergo neuroplastic changes than a younger brain, and the elderly may have trouble adapting to their new dentures, despite being technically acceptable, because of the limited ability of their brains to undergo neuroplastic changes. As a general rule, it is best to minimize any changes to the dental status of elderly individuals to avoid stretching the limited ability of the elderly brain to undergo neuroplastic changes. For example, increases in vertical dimension, as might be recommended in a complete denture patient who has a significantly over-closed vertical dimension, should be done in a staged approach, particularly in the older patient. There is also evidence that pain interferes with the ability of the brain to undergo the neuroplastic changes occurring during skill acquisition. This probably is a reason why people in pain may not be able to adapt to new dentures or prosthetic devices (Sessle 2016).

The outline above of the neural control of voluntary movements has focused on the motor cortex. Another important component of the motor system is the cerebellum which plays a role in the refinement of movements. A classic test for a cerebellar lesion is to ask the patient to touch an object at arm's length with their finger. A normal healthy person performs this accurately and quickly. A patient with a cerebellar lesion performs this movement slowly and inaccurately and with many mid-trajectory corrections. So the movement can still be performed, but it is very inaccurate. When the motor cortex drives a voluntary movement, it sends a copy of the signal that goes to the motoneurons also to the cerebellum. As the movement is progressing, somatosensory receptors are activated as a normal part of the movement, and this information not only goes to the somatosensory and motor cortices (as mentioned above), but also a copy of the signal goes to the cerebellum. The cerebellum uses both signals, the intended drive signal from the motor cortex and the actual signal from the movement, to work out errors in the movement. Thus when the somatosensory feedback from the part of the body being moved does not match the drive signal from the motor cortex, an error signal is generated that helps to correct the movement by modifying the activity of the motor cortex. Corrections to each movement can also occur via shorter pathways that involve fewer neurons, and many of these pathways are located entirely at the brainstem level. These pathways can be demonstrated clinically by evoking reflexes.

3.2.2.2 Reflex Movements

When the word *reflex* is mentioned, we tend to think of the medical physician evoking the knee-jerk reflex by a brief tap to the knee leading to a single motor response. But this is a very artificial situation that does not usually operate as such in normal life—we do not need to tap our knees to allow us to walk! The ability to evoke a reflex simply demonstrates that there are connections between certain somatosensory afferent nerve fibers and certain α-motoneurons. These neural pathways are critically important and are continuously used to refine and modulate both voluntary and rhythmical movements. It just so happens that an artificial reflex response can be demonstrated clinically and in the research setting by selective sudden activation of some somatosensory afferents.

In general, reflex pathways are organized at the brainstem or spinal cord level and generally do not involve higher centers of the brain such as the motor cortex. Therefore information travelling along these pathways at the brainstem or spinal cord level brings about its effects very quickly, and these effects are little modified by voluntary will. In the masticatory muscle motor system, reflexes include the jaw-closing or jaw-jerk reflex and the jaw-opening reflex. These reflexes have been extensively reviewed (Türker 2002).

Role of Reflex Pathways in Masticatory Movements

Non-noxious Reflex Pathways

Reflex pathways provide a very fast neural circuit whereby somatosensory information from the oral cavity can be used to fine-tune movements (see below) so that they occur in a manner that adapts to the particular loads imposed on the mandible during movement. Of particular importance in the fine control of masticatory movements is the information provided through the activation of periodontal mechanoreceptors and muscle spindles. These mechanoreceptors allow fast feedback (in ~10 ms) that adjusts a movement to overcome small, unpredicted irregularities in an ongoing movement as can occur from unexpected changes in food bolus consistency. The information does not have to go to higher centers (which will take much longer) before the subtle refinement can be carried out. The reflex effects also add smoothness to a movement.

For example, as food is crushed between the teeth, the activation of periodontal mechanoreceptors can cause a reflex *increase* in activity in the mandibular closing muscles to assist in crushing of food. This increase in activity comes about because low levels of activation of periodontal afferents, as occurs during chewing, facilitates the activation of specific mandibular closing motor units. The effect of this is to generate the appropriately directed mandibular movements to assist, for example, the masticatory muscles in guiding the teeth to crush the food with the correct force and as the teeth slide smoothly past each other during the slow closing phase of chewing.

As described above, muscle spindles are very sensitive to changes in length of the muscle and also play a role in assisting chewing. Also as described above (Fig. 3.5), unexpected changes in length or velocity of contraction are signaled by the muscle spindles which send action potentials into the brainstem. Within about 8 ms of a slowing of closing brought about by encountering harder food (i.e., a nut) within a food bolus, α-motoneurons to the mandibular closing muscles increase their activity to help crush through the nut. This effect, which depends on these reflex pathways, does not involve higher centers (and therefore conscious perception) and therefore is very fast. There is however an awareness of the increase in food resistance, and we can also voluntarily increase the force by activating the mandibular (i.e., jaw) efferent zones in the face MI, but these perceptual and motor effects come well after the fast reflex effects. If higher centers were only involved every time we closed onto harder food within a food bolus, then our voluntary mandibular closing movements would be much slower and less efficient because the pathways to and from the higher centers are much slower than those to and from the brainstem. Therefore muscle spindles allow very fast adjustments to the forces generated by jaw-closing muscles so that these forces are appropriate for the needs of the mandibular movement or mandibular forces at the time required. This fast pathway from muscle spindle Ia afferents to jaw-closing motoneurons is shown in Fig. 3.9.

It is also likely that other mechanoreceptors such as TMJ mechanoreceptors, Golgi tendon organs, and mucosal and possibly cutaneous mechanoreceptors also provide feedback to the motor system possibly individually or in some complex combination given the convergence of this information centrally to help modulate motor unit activity and recruitment to achieve the most optimal chewing cycle.

Noxious Reflex Pathways

While many orofacial inputs can enhance or modulate muscle activity to assist in mastication as described above, noxious orofacial stimulation generally has a profound inhibitory effect on mandibular closing muscles. For example, sudden high-intensity activation of periodontal afferents results in inhibition of mandibular closing muscles and cessation of the patterned output from the masticatory CPG so that the teeth are not damaged. An immediate cessation of the output from the CPG also occurs with noxious stimulation of orofacial tissues such as when biting the lip or cheek by mistake. We all know how biting the cheek suddenly stops chewing. This occurs via, again, a very fast brainstem-based reflex, the jaw-opening reflex, and this reflex can operate in about 10 ms.

The jaw-opening reflex can be evoked by a variety of types of orofacial afferents. Activity in primary afferent nerve fibers from, for example, mucosal nociceptors, enters the brainstem to contact inhibitory interneurons that then synapse on jaw-closing α-motoneurons and reduce the activity of these motoneurons. At the same time, these same primary afferents send branches to activate other interneurons that are excitatory to mandibular opening muscles, such as the digastric. The overall effect is an opening of the mouth.

Nociceptor activation within muscles can have effects on the sensitivity of muscle spindles with both increases and decreases being noted (Capra et al. 2007). These changes to the sensitivity of muscle spindle afferents in muscle pain may contribute to the deficits in interdental size discrimination as well as the decreases in the force of contraction and irregular chewing cycles noted in TMD patients (Capra et al. 2007).

Role of Reflex Pathways in Voluntary Closing Movements

When cracking a hard nut between the teeth, there is an initial increase in force when the teeth are contacting the nut and before the nut cracks.

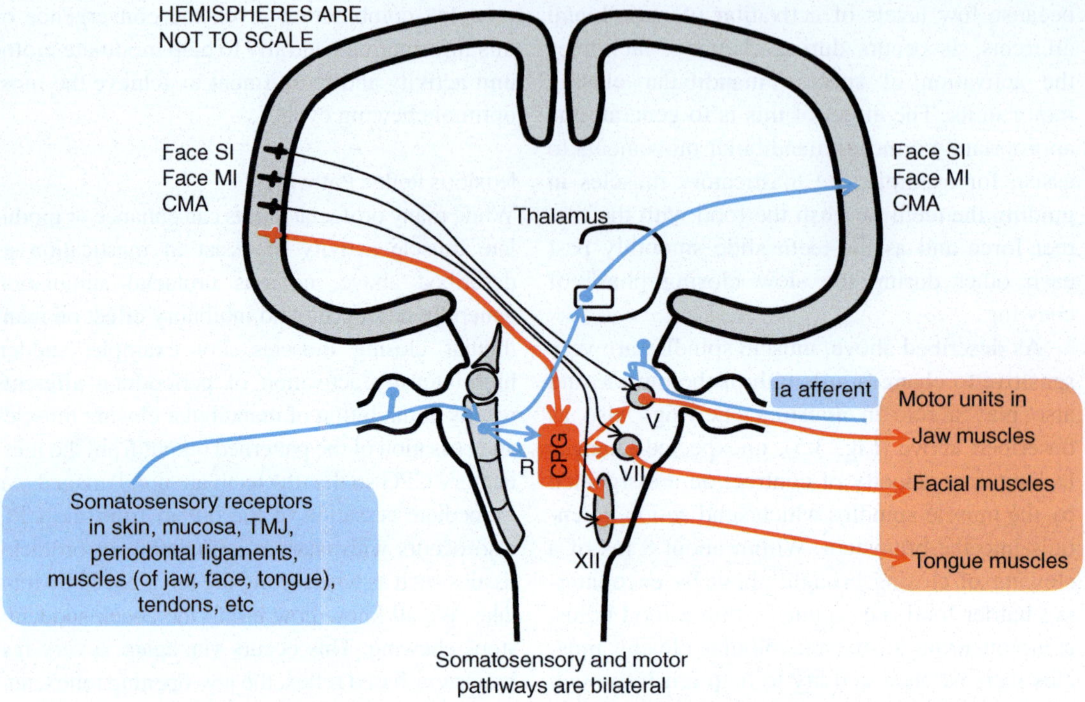

Fig. 3.9 This figure shows a stylized brain with some important pathways and nuclei for the generation of mastication. Somatosensory nuclei are shown on the left side and motor nuclei on the right side, but in reality the nuclei are on both sides. The masticatory central pattern generator (CPG) is located in the pontomedullary reticular formation and when activated sends the appropriately timed impulses to the various mandibular, facial, and tongue muscle α-motoneurons in the trigeminal (V), facial (VII), and hypoglossal (XII) motor nuclei and thereby to generate mastication. The masticatory CPG can be activated and modulated by descending inputs from higher centers as shown by the *red* pathway from the cortical masticatory area (CMA), face primary somatosensory cortex (SI), and face primary motor cortex (MI). It can also be modulated by somatosensory receptors in the skin, mucosa, TMJ, periodontal ligaments, muscles, tendons, etc., which send afferent nerve fibers to terminate on 2nd order neurons within the trigeminal brainstem sensory nuclear complex; muscle spindle afferent cell bodies lie in Mes V, Fig. 3.4. These 2nd order neurons ascend through the thalamus to higher centers for perception (face SI, face SII, etc.) and also pass to the masticatory CPG for modulation of the masticatory movements to accommodate to the texture and hardness of the food bolus. Other connections (R; Ia afferent) can modulate α-motoneuron activity within mandibular muscles to provide fast adjustments to mandibular muscle activity (e.g., see Fig. 3.5). The direct pathways from the face MI to α-motoneurons to allow voluntary activation of mandibular, facial, and tongue muscles are shown in black. *TMJ* temporomandibular joint

This increase in force is due to two factors. One is the increased α-motoneuron discharge to motor units in masticatory muscles because of voluntary activation from the motor cortex (see Fig. 3.9). The other factor that contributes to increased muscle activity comes from γ-motoneuron activation that usually keeps the intrafusal muscle fibers contracting at the same rate as the main extrafusal muscle fibers to maintain spindle sensitivity (see above). However, the mandible has stopped closing (because of the nut) and the continued γ-motoneuron activation causes the intrafusal muscle fibers to keep shortening, and this results in stretching of the Ia afferent terminals in the center of the spindle (see Fig. 3.5c). This leads to an intense discharge in the Ia afferents that feeds back within about 8 ms to the α-motoneurons so that there are further increases in α-motoneuron activity until the nut cracks. As soon as the nut cracks, however, there needs to be a mechanism that prevents the opposing teeth crashing together and possibly causing damage. This is also achieved in a number of ways. There is a very fast cessation of α-motoneuron activity to the mandibular closing muscles brought about by a sudden unloading of the muscle spindles due to the sudden mandibular closure. The unloading leads to a sudden decrease in Ia afferent input to the mandibular closing motoneurons. This decreases the activity of the mandibular closing motoneurons and thereby decreases activity in the motor units of the mandibular closing muscles. At the same time, a jaw-opening reflex is activated as described above where the mandibular openers are briefly activated and the mandibular closers are briefly further inhibited to help to prevent further mandibular closing. Furthermore there are likely other physical properties of the masticatory system such as viscoelasticity (damping) of the soft tissues and the individual's intent that contributes to limiting damage to events such as sudden unloading of the mandible (Johansson et al. 2014; Peck et al. 2002).

Role of Reflex Pathways in Mandibular Posture

We can also sense the rapid downward force applied to the mandible as the front foot hits the ground in running. The fast feedback of afferent information from the muscle spindles to the α-motoneurons of the mandibular closing muscles results in a brief contraction that minimizes the opening of the mandible that prevents the mandible flopping up and down when you are walking and running.

As mentioned above, muscle spindles are very sensitive and appear to play a role in the maintenance of the mandibular rest position or postural position. Some authors have proposed that the postural position is maintained only by the passive viscoelastic forces of the tissues supporting the mandible. While there is little evidence for muscle activity in the masseter muscles when the mandible is in the postural position, recent data have demonstrated tonic activity in the medial pterygoid and temporalis muscles while the mandible is in the postural position (Yilmaz et al. 2015; Chen, Mojaver, Whittle, Klineberg, Murray, unpublished observations). While these initial observations need further confirmation, it appears nonetheless that the rest or postural position of the mandible may be at least partly maintained by activity in some mandibular closing motor units, and these may be located in the medial pterygoid and temporalis muscles. It is likely that this tonic activity arises from the slight stretch of the muscle spindles within the medial pterygoid and temporalis muscles because of the pull of gravity on the mandible. The subsequent Ia afferent discharge then would tonically activate the lowest-threshold (i.e., most easily activated) motor units of these mandibular closing muscles to help maintain mandibular posture (see Fig. 3.9).

3.2.2.3 Rhythmical Movements

The generation and control of rhythmical orofacial movements, namely, mastication and swallowing, have been extensively reviewed (Jean 2001; Lund 1991).

Rhythmical movements are movements such as mastication, swallowing, breathing, walking, running, and swimming. They share features of both reflex and voluntary movements. We do not have to think about these movements for them to occur and in that sense they have features of reflexes. However, they also have features of voluntary movements in that we can start and stop rhythmical movements, we can usually make them go faster or slower, or we can exert more effort or less effort. For example, we can chew, breathe, and walk without thinking specifically about the task, and we can at any time stop chewing, breathing, and walking or move faster or slower or exert more force or less force during the movement.

The rhythmical movements associated with mastication are generated and controlled by a group of neurons in the pontomedullary reticular formation of the brainstem. These neurons constitute the CPG for mastication. Figure 3.9 shows some relations of the CPG for mastication in the brainstem. Swallowing is also controlled by a CPG located in the medulla oblongata and is likely associated with neural circuitry that overlaps the neural circuitry for mastication.

A CPG is a neural network (red box labelled CPG in Fig. 3.9) that is like a computer program. When it is activated, the CPG generates action potentials of the required intensity and timing to the various facial, mandibular, and tongue muscle motoneurons (red outputs from trigeminal, facial, and tongue motor nuclei, Fig. 3.9) so that the associated muscle fibers become activated in the correct sequence and magnitude to allow the rhythmical facial, mandibular, and tongue movements seen in mastication to occur.

We can also voluntarily start and stop chewing as well as change the rate and magnitude and shape of the chewing movements, and these modifications are done through descending commands to the CPG from the motor cortical regions. These descending commands are indicated by the bold red line from the face SI, face MI, and the cortical masticatory area (CMA) regions of the cortex to the CPG (Fig. 3.9). The CMA and parts of the face MI and SI are thought to be responsible for many of the voluntary changes in the chewing cycle that are possible such as voluntarily starting and stopping chewing and voluntarily chewing harder and softer.

A CPG for mastication would be of little use to us if it did not accommodate and be capable of changing its activity in accordance with the nature of the food bolus or even to changes in the occlusion. For example, and as described above (Van der Bilt 2011; Woda et al. 2006), our chewing cycle automatically adjusts to harder foods and softer foods. Also as indicated above, somatosensory feedback is crucial for proper functioning of the masticatory CPG. This feedback is provided by mechanoreceptors such as periodontal mechanoreceptors which signal the magnitude and direction of tooth contact and also mucosal mechanoreceptors which signal food contact with mucosa. In addition, muscle spindles signal muscle length and rate of change of muscle length as the mandible closes, while Golgi tendon organs signal forces generated within muscles, and TMJ mechanoreceptors signal mandibular position and joint loads.

Somatosensory information plays a crucial role in allowing the chewing cycle to modulate so as to accommodate to changes in food bolus consistency (Lund and Olsson 1983). Chewing is associated with a barrage of somatosensory information entering the CNS. Some of this information passes rapidly to the cerebral cortex (e.g., face SI and higher cortical areas, Fig. 3.9) for perception, e.g., perception of a food bolus between the teeth during chewing, and contact between tongue and a food bolus during chewing. Some of the afferent information also passes directly to the CPG (Fig. 3.9; blue arrow from TBSNC to CPG) to allow rapid modulation of the CPG to adjust the chewing cycle timing and amplitude to accommodate to the texture and hardness of the food bolus. Thus, for example, encountering hard foods in the early part of chewing means that chewing needs to start off so that forces are sufficiently high to break through the food bolus. Then, as the food is softened as chewing progresses, the forces need to be reduced rapidly in magnitude so that the teeth do not bang together. This can all be done without thinking about the changes required in the levels of muscle activity during chewing and can be controlled by the CPG aided by somatosensory input from mechanoreceptors in the oral cavity. As indicated above, periodontal mechanoreceptors can play an important role here as they signal the magnitude and direction of forces applied to the teeth, and also muscle spindles play a role (Fig. 3.9; blue arrow-labelled R indicates afferent input, e.g. periodontal, passing to modulate α-motoneuronal activity).

Many of the orofacial afferents that are activated during the mandibular closing phase of chewing can evoke a jaw-opening reflex (see above). If this occurred during chewing, then this would not be useful as closing would be prevented. Lund and Olsson carried out some elegant research in the 1970s and 1980s to show that the masticatory CPG actually depresses the responsiveness of the jaw-opening reflex during the closing phase of the chewing cycle (Lund and Olsson 1983). This means that the normal operation of the jaw-opening reflex is markedly depressed during the closing phase of the chewing cycle. If this did not happen, then we would have difficulty in chewing our food. This effect allows the mandible to close unhindered.

During the opening phase of the chewing cycle, muscle spindles in the mandibular closing muscles will be stretched, and the sensory information from them will have an excitatory effect on mandibular closing motoneurons. This could lead to activation of mandibular closing muscles with the net effect of resisting mandibular opening. However, during the opening phase of the chewing cycle, the masticatory CPG hyperpolarizes (i.e., inhibits) mandibular closing motoneurons and makes it much harder for them to become activated, and therefore the excitatory input from muscle spindles, which would normally activate the mandibular closing muscles, does not activate during mandibular opening.

The activation of nociceptive afferents during chewing, however, has a profound inhibitory effect on the entire chewing cycle and will immediately stop chewing from occurring. Take, for example, what happens when you bite your cheek during chewing. The activity in nociceptors activates inhibitory connections to the CPG to stop it from cycling.

There is also good evidence for neural changes at higher levels of the CNS in association with changes to the occlusion (Lund and Olsson 1983; Sessle 2016), and these changes are also likely to be operative at the level of the CPG. Thus, it is likely that the CPG can undergo neuroplastic changes to allow it to accommodate to changes in occlusion as would be provided by new dentures, new crown and bridgework, implants, etc.

3.2.2.4 Some Autonomic Aspects

The sympathetic nervous system plays a critical role in normal muscle function and has also been implicated in the mechanisms of muscle pain. These effects have been reviewed (Passatore and Roatta 2007) and are briefly summarized here. Thus, the use of muscles involves not only activation of α-motoneurons to muscle fibers but also a parallel set of commands to sympathetic systems to increase blood flow to the active muscle. The vasoconstrictor action of the sympathetic nervous system is overridden by the powerful vasodilator actions of muscle metabolites. An imbalance between these two forces may lead to ischemia in the working muscles, which together with the buildup of metabolites may activate muscle nociceptive terminals and result in muscle pain, or myalgia.

An interesting effect noted for the sympathetic nervous system control of muscles is that sympathetic activation depresses the sensitivity of muscle spindle afferents to be able to detect length and velocity changes. This effect is thought to be brought about through the sympathetic innervation of muscle spindles so that an increased sympathetic activation results in an impairment in the ability of the muscle spindle to detect length and velocity changes in the muscle. Therefore under stressful conditions, this effect could significantly impair the abilities, described above, of the muscle spindle in correcting for unexpected perturbations in the masticatory cycle, as well as impairing feedback from the muscle spindle to be used for refinement of the masticatory CPG during chewing. Sympathetic stimulation under stress may also have effects on postural maintenance.

As previously noted (Passatore and Roatta 2007), acute states of stress demand sympathetic activation and result in adjustments that help the organism cope with environmental changes. Prolonged stress however impacts negatively on the individual, and in terms of prolonged sympathetic effects on muscles, it may result in impaired motor control such that individuals may adopt suboptimal strategies of muscle activation that may be harmful in the long term and result in muscle pain.

A close relationship has also been noted between masticatory function and cardiac autonomic function (Hasegawa et al. 2009; Koizumi et al. 2011; Nitta et al. 2003). For example, in experimental animal models, chewing during stress exposure can reduce sympathetic hyperactivity and stress-induced arrhythmias (Koizumi et al. 2011).

3.3 The Relations Between Pain and Motor Activity

Chapter 6 describes in detail dysfunction of the masticatory muscles and includes a description of pain–motor interactions. In brief, orofacial pain clinical diagnosis and management, and even research, has been dominated by the notion that there is a simple, reflex-like association between pain and muscle activity (Stohler 1999; Svensson and Graven-Nielsen 2001; Travell et al. 1942; van

Dieën et al. 2003) These theories operate at spinal or brainstem levels and do not incorporate input from higher centers. The vicious cycle theory (Travell et al. 1942) proposes a positive interrelationship between pain and the so-called muscle "hyperactivity." Proponents argue that abnormalities in posture, structure (e.g., jaw misalignment, malocclusion), movement, or stress lead to muscle hyperactivity that leads to further abnormalities and a vicious cycle. Many management strategies based on this theory attempt to break this cycle by, e.g., irreversible and often expensive changes to the anatomy (e.g., surgery, tooth adjustments) (Mense et al. 2001; Sessle et al. 1995; Stohler 1999; Travell and Simons 1983; van Dieën et al. 2003). In contrast, the pain adaptation model (Lund 2008) proposes that pain leads to reduced agonist (the driver of an action) and increased antagonist (resists an action) muscle activity that results in slower and smaller movements so as to minimize further injury and therefore aid healing (Lund 2008; Stohler 1999; van Dieën et al. 2003). Management strategies influenced by the pain adaptation model see no need to break a vicious cycle but rather invoke pharmacological and behavioral strategies to reduce pain and minimize movement to allow the masticatory motor system to heal and recover (Fricton and Schiffman 2008).

Accumulating evidence however indicates that neither the vicious cycle theory nor the pain adaptation model provides an adequate explanation of the association between pain and muscle activity (Lund 2008; Murray and Peck 2007; Simmonds et al. 2006; Stohler 1999; Svensson and Graven-Nielsen 2001; van Dieën et al. 2003). Therefore, two recent new models have been proposed to explain how pain modifies muscle activity, the integrated pain adaptation model (Murray and Peck 2007) and a new theory of the motor adaptation to pain (Hodges and Tucker 2011). Essentially both models propose that noxious stimulation at a site results in a redistribution of activity within and between muscles, and both models incorporate changes in higher centers of the brain (e.g., psychosocial aspects) in determining the final nature of the redistributed motor activity.

3.4 Summary

This chapter has summarized the normal internal anatomy and functions of the masticatory muscles. A detailed description is provided as to how the brain controls these muscles in voluntary movements, reflex movements, and rhythmical movements. The basic functional unit of muscle, the motor unit, is described in detail in terms of physiological properties and how motor units are arranged within the masticatory muscles. The muscles have a complex internal architecture where subcompartments of the muscles can be selectively activated independently of other regions, and this is thought to contribute to the sophistication with which forces can be applied to the mandible to achieve the finely controlled forces and movements characteristic of chewing, speech, and other orofacial movements. The orofacial area is richly endowed with somatosensory receptors that not only allow us to sense textures, temperatures, and consistencies of food and liquids but also provide continual feedback that is used by the brain motor systems to refine masticatory movements. Nociceptive pathways are also described and how information along these pathways can be modulated depending on environmental influences as well as how these pathways can become sensitized and responsive even to non-noxious (non-painful) stimuli. These effects can contribute to the allodynia and hyperalgesia seen in acute and chronic pain states. The chapter concludes with a brief outline of possible relations between pain and motor activity. One of the aims of this chapter is to highlight the complexity of the masticatory muscles as well as their sensorimotor brain control systems. Advancements in knowledge will no doubt elaborate on the complexity of the muscles and their control systems that clinicians are called upon to treat. It is incumbent on the clinician to be cognizant that the masticatory system is highly complex, that a simple mechanistic approach to chronic pain management is unlikely to be successful, and that a multimodal and multidisciplinary approach is more appropriate.

References

Apkarian AV, Hashmi JA, Baliki MN. Pain and the brain: specificity and plasticity of the brain in clinical chronic pain. Pain. 2011;152:S49–64.

Avivi-Arber L, Martin RE, Lee J-C, Sessle BJ. Face sensorimotor cortex and its neuroplasticity related to orofacial sensorimotor functions. Arch Oral Biol. 2011;56:1440–65.

Blanksma NG, van Eijden TMGJ. Electromyographic heterogeneity in the human temporalis muscle. J Dent Res. 1990;69:1686–90.

Blanksma NG, van Eijden TMGJ. Electromyographic heterogeneity in the human temporalis and masseter muscles during static biting, open/close excursions, and chewing. J Dent Res. 1995;74:1318–27.

Cairns BE, Ren K, Tambeli CH. Musculoskeletal orofacial pain mechanisms: insights from animal models. In: Sessle BJ, editor. Orofacial pain: recent advances in assessment, management, and understanding of mechanisms. Washington, DC: IASP Press; 2014. p. 351–72.

Capra NF. Mechanisms of oral sensation. Dysphagia. 1995;10:235–47.

Capra NF, Hisley CK, Masri RM. The influence of pain on masseter spindle afferent discharge. Arch Oral Biol. 2007;52:387–90.

Chiang CY, Dostrovsky JO, Iwata K, Sessle BJ. Role of glia in orofacial pain. Neuroscientist. 2011;17:303–20.

Dubner R, Sessle BJ, Storey AT. The neural basis of oral and facial function. New York: Plenum Press; 1978.

Fricton JR, Schiffman E. Management of masticatory myalgia and arthralgia. In: Sessle BJ, Lavigne G, Lund JP, Dubner R, editors. Orofacial pain: from basic science to clinical management. Chicago: Quintessence Publishing Co, Inc; 2008. p. 179–85.

Goldspink G. Cellular and molecular aspects of muscle growth, adaptation and ageing. Gerodontology. 1998;15:35–43.

Greene CS. Managing the care of patients with temporomandibular disorders: a new guideline for care. J Am Dent Assoc. 2010;141:1086–8.

Haggard P, de Boer L. Oral somatosensory awareness. Neurosci Biobehav Rev. 2014;47:469–84.

Hannam AG, McMillan AS. Internal organization in the human jaw muscles. Crit Rev Oral Biol Med. 1994;5:55–89.

Hasegawa Y, Sakagami J, Ono T, Hori K, Zhang M, Maeda Y. Circulatory response and autonomic nervous activity during gum chewing. Eur J Oral Sci. 2009;117(4):470–3.

Hodges PW, Tucker KJ. Moving differently in pain: a new theory to explain the adaptation to pain. Pain. 2011;152:S90–8.

Jean A. Brainstem control of swallowing: neuronal network and cellular mechanisms. Physiol Rev. 2001;81:929–69.

Johansson AS, Pruszynski JA, Edin BE, Westberg K-G. Biting intentions modulate digastric reflex responses to sudden unloading of the jaw. J Neurophysiol. 2014;112:1067–73.

Klineberg IJ, Murray GM. Osseoperception: sensory function and proprioception. Adv Dent Res. 1999;13:120–9.

Koizumi S, Minamisawa S, Sasaguri K, Onozuka M, Sato S, Ono Y. Chewing reduces sympathetic nervous response to stress and prevents poststress arrhythmias in rats. AJP: Heart and Circulatory Physiology. 2011;301(4):H1551–8.

Korfage JAM, Koolstra JH, Langenbach GEJ, van Eijden TMGJ. Fiber-type composition of the human jaw muscles - (Part 1) origin and functional significance of fiber-type diversity. J Dent Res. 2005a;84:774–83.

Korfage JAM, Koolstra JH, Langenbach GEJ, van Eijden TMGJ. Fiber-type composition of the human jaw muscles - (Part 2) Role of hybrid fibers and factors responsible for inter-individual variation. J Dent Res. 2005b;84:784–93.

Lin C. Brain signature of chronic orofacial pain: a systematic review and meta-analysis on neuroimaging research of trigeminal neuropathic pain and temporomandibular joint disorders. PLoS One. 2014;9(4):e94300. doi:10.1371/journal.pone.0094300.

Lund JP. Mastication and its control by the brain stem. Crit Rev Oral Biol Med. 1991;2:33–64.

Lund JP. Persistent pain and motor dysfunction. In: Sessle BJ, Lavigne G, Lund JP, Dubner R, editors. Orofacial pain: from basic science to clinical management. Chicago: Quintessence; 2008. p. 117–24.

Lund JP, Olsson KA. The importance of reflexes and their control during jaw movement. Trends Neurosci. 1983;6:458–63.

Melzack R, Wall PD. Pain mechanisms: a new theory. Science (Washington, DC). 1965;150:971–9.

Mense S, Hoheisel U. Mechanisms of central nervous hyperexcitability due to activation of muscle nociceptors. In: Graven-Nielsen T, Arendt-Nielsen L, Mense S, editors. Fundamentals of musculoskeletal pain. Seattle: IASP Press; 2008. p. 61–73.

Mense S, Simons DG, Russell IJ. Muscle pain: understanding its nature, diagnosis, and treatment. Philadelphia: Lippincott Williams & Wilkins; 2001.

Miller AJ. Craniomandibular muscles: their role in function and form. Boca Raton: CRC Press; 1991.

Murray GM. The lateral pterygoid muscle: function and dysfunction. Semin Orthod. 2012;18:44–50.

Murray GM, Bhutada MK, Peck CC, Phanachet I, Sae-Lee D, Whittle T. The human lateral pterygoid muscle. Arch Oral Biol. 2007;52:377–80.

Murray GM, Peck CC. Orofacial pain and jaw muscle activity: a new model. J Orofac Pain. 2007;21:263–78.

Nitta E, Iwasa Y, Sugita M, Hirono C, Shiba Y. Role of mastication and swallowing in the control of autonomic nervous activity for heart rate in different postures. J Oral Rehabil. 30(12):1209–15.

Palla S, Klineberg IJ. Occlusion and adaptation to change: neuroplasticity and its implications for cognition. In:

Klineberg IJ, Eckert SE, editors. Functional occlusion in restorative dentistry and prosthodontics. Edinburgh: Elsevier Mosby; 2016. p. 43–53.

Passatore M, Roatta S. Modulation operated by the sympathetic nervous system on jaw reflexes and masticatory movement. Arch Oral Biol. 2007;52:343–6.

Peck CC, Sooch AS, Hannam AG. Forces resisting jaw displacement in relaxed humans: a predominantly viscous phenomenon. J Oral Rehabil. 2002;29:151–0.

Phanachet I, Whittle T, Wanigaratne K, Klineberg IJ, Sessle BJ, Murray GM. Functional heterogeneity in the superior head of the human lateral pterygoid. J Dent Res 2003;82:106–111.

Phanachet I, Whittle T, Wanigaratne K, Murray GM. Functional properties of single motor units in inferior head of human lateral pterygoid muscle: task relations and thresholds. J Neurophysiol. 2001;86:2204–18.

Sessle BJ. Mechanisms of oral somatosensory and motor functions and their clinical correlates. J Oral Rehabil. 2006;33:243–61.

Sessle BJ. Central mechanisms of craniofacial musculoskeletal pain: a review. In: Graven-Nielsen T, Arendt-Nielsen L, Mense S, editors. Fundamentals of Musculoskeletal Pain. Seattle: IASP Press; 2008. p. 87–103.

Sessle BJ. Face sensorimotor cortex: its role and neuroplasticity in the control of orofacial movements. Prog Brain Res. 2011a;188:71–82.

Sessle BJ. Peripheral and central mechanisms of orofacial inflammatory pain. Int Rev Neurobiol. 2011b;97:179–206.

Sessle BJ. The biological basis of a functional occlusion: the neural framework. In: Klineberg IJ, Eckert SE, editors. Functional occlusion in restorative dentistry and prosthodontics. St. Louis: Elsevier Mosby; 2016. p. 3–22.

Sessle BJ, Bryant PS, Dionne RA. Temporomandibular disorders and related pain conditions. Seattle: IASP Press; 1995.

Sheppard IM, Markus N. Total time of tooth contacts during mastication. J Prosthet Dent. 1962;12:460–3.

Simmonds MJ, Goubert L, Moseley GL, Verbunt JA. Moving with pain. In: Flor H, Dostrovsky JO, editors. Proceedings of the 11th World Congress on Pain. Seattle: IASP Press; 2006. p. 799–811.

Stohler CS. Craniofacial pain and motor function: pathogenesis, clinical correlates, and implications. Crit Rev Oral Biol Med. 1999;10:504–18.

Svensson P, Graven-Nielsen T. Craniofacial muscle pain: review of mechanisms and clinical manifestations. J Orofac Pain. 2001;15:117–45.

Travell JG, Rinzler S, Herman M. Pain and disability of the shoulder and arm. Treatment by intramuscular infiltration with procaine hydrochloride. J Am Med Assoc. 1942;120:417–22.

Travell JG, Simons DG. Myofascial pain and dysfunction: the trigger point manual. Baltimore: Williams and Wilkins; 1983.

Trulsson M. Force encoding by human periodontal mechanoreceptors during mastication. Arch Oral Biol. 2007;52:357–60.

Trulsson M, Van der Bilt A, Carlsson GE, Gotfredsen K, Larsson P, Müller F, et al. From brain to bridge: masticatory function and dental implants. J Oral Rehabil. 2012;39:858–77.

Türker KS. Reflex control of human jaw muscles. Crit Rev Oral Biol Med. 2002;13:85–104.

Van der Bilt A. Assessment of mastication with implications for oral rehabilitation: a review. J Oral Rehabil. 2011;38:754–80.

van Dieën J, Selen LPJ, Cholewicki J. Trunk muscle activation in low-back pain patients, an analysis of the literature. J Electromyogr Kines. 2003;13:333–51.

van Eijden TMGJ, Turkawski SJJ. Morphology and physiology of masticatory muscle motor units. Crit Rev Oral Biol Med. 2001;12:76–91.

Weijs WA, Kwa SHS. The rabbit masseter: organization and function of a heterogeneous muscle. In: Morimoto T, Matsuya T, Takada K, editors. Brain and oral functions. Amsterdam: Elsevier Science B.V; 1995. p. 11–8.

Woda A, Foster K, Mishellany A, Peyron MA. Adaptation of healthy mastication to factors pertaining to the individual or to the food. Physiol Behav. 2006; 89:28–35.

Yilmaz G, Ugincius P, Sebik O, Türker KS. Tonic activity of the human temporalis muscle at mandibular rest position. Arch Oral Biol. 2015;60:1645–9.

Part II

Normal Function of the Masticatory System

Musculature

4

James M. Hawkins, Istvan A. Hargitai,
and A. Dale Ehrlich

Abstract

The masticatory and cervical muscles are unique and complex structures that work synergistically to perform such multifaceted behaviors as chewing, swallowing, and talking. Functional observation, dissection, and basic research related to the masticatory muscles have provided most of the knowledge regarding masticatory muscle function and dysfunction and dictated many therapies that are provided today. However, recent technological advances have allowed rigorous testing of the scientific validity of these previous assumptions and provided a greater understanding of individual masticatory muscle function, as well as the functional behaviors they enable.

4.1 Introduction

This chapter presents current information on normal function of the masticatory muscles, which will help provide a solid foundation for assessing function and addressing dysfunction of this complex system. It will begin with a discussion of the individual muscles and their unique features, followed by a description of how these muscles work together to accomplish functional behaviors. It will conclude with important considerations a clinician must take into account when evaluating this complex system.

4.1.1 Masticatory Muscle Biomechanics

The masticatory muscles consist of four paired muscle groups, to include the masseter, temporalis, medial pterygoid, and lateral pterygoid muscles. These unique muscle groups work synergistically to determine position and movement of the mandible, as well as create force at

J.M. Hawkins (✉)
Naval Medical Center San Diego,
San Diego, CA, USA
e-mail: James.m.hawkins77.mil@mail.mil

I.A. Hargitai
Naval Postgraduate Dental School,
Bethesda, MD, USA
e-mail: Istvan.a.hargitai.mil@mail.mil

A. Dale Ehrlich
Louisiana State University School of Dentistry,
New Orleans, LA, USA
e-mail: aehrli@lsuhsc.edu

© Springer International Publishing AG 2018
H.A. Gremillion, G.D. Klasser (eds.), *Temporomandibular Disorders*,
https://doi.org/10.1007/978-3-319-57247-5_4

the tooth to tooth interface and temporomandibular joints. The internal organization of these muscles is unique from other skeletal muscle, enabling them to perform a much larger variety of motor tasks and adapt to the complex functional demands placed on the masticatory system. This unique structure makes these muscles the most complex and powerful in the human body (Grunheid et al. 2009), and allows them to perform such complex behaviors as chewing, swallowing, and speaking.

In order to appreciate the complexities of normal masticatory behavior, as well as comprehend what may be causing dysfunction within this system, an understanding of the individual components of the masticatory system is essential. The previous chapters provided a foundational understanding of this system at a developmental, anatomical, and physiologic level. This chapter will seek to expand upon that foundation and provide a description of normal masticatory and cervical muscle function, as well as the functional behaviors these muscles enable. This chapter will be separated into four main sections that will facilitate a translational understanding from the basic science of these muscles to the clinically applicable presentation of the behaviors they produce. The first section discusses microscopic characteristics of the masticatory and cervical muscles that distinguish them from other skeletal muscles and enable them to perform the complex demands placed on them. The second section will provide a comprehensive review of the unique structural and functional characteristics of each individual masticatory muscle, tendon, and ligament. The third section will provide an overview of the upper cervical muscles and discuss the bidirectional influence the masticatory and cervical muscles have on one another. The fourth section will provide a synthesis of the aforementioned information to provide a macroscopic overview of how the function of these muscles translates into the complex masticatory functions of chewing, swallowing, and speaking. The chapter will conclude with a brief discussion of other lesser known factors that may play a major role in masticatory function.

4.1.1.1 Translation from Microscopic Function to Macroscopic Movement

Multiple masticatory and cervical muscles work synergistically to open, close, and move the mandible laterally and protrusively. Despite the varied functional demands placed on these muscles, they are able to perform efficiently because of their unique microscopic architecture. The general concepts of these microscopic features will be discussed first, followed by a specific description of how these characteristics suit the individual muscles for their primary functions.

4.1.1.2 Functional Heterogeneity

Many texts present the muscles of mastication from a macroscopic viewpoint as being homogenous in nature. That is, they contract as one unit with a single force vector and magnitude. This view, while simple to comprehend, is inappropriate for such complex muscles (Herring et al. 1979). In reality, the masticatory muscles are highly complex and functionally heterogeneous. Heterogeneity can be conceptualized as an intramuscular compartmentalization that permits selective activation of specific regions within the muscle. This compartmentalization gives the nervous system the ability to utilize a single muscle to produce a range of forces with varying magnitudes and orientations in an energy-efficient manner (Bhutada et al. 2008). Therefore, complex and precise mandibular function is not only created by synchronized activity between the masticatory muscles but also by activation of appropriate compartments within the masticatory muscles themselves (Johansson et al. 2014). These intramuscular compartments are formed anatomically by a complex internal tendinous architecture and further subdivided into neuromuscular compartments controlled by individual motor units (Widmer et al. 2007).

4.1.1.3 Anatomical Compartmentalization

The muscles of mastication, in particular the mandibular closing (elevator) muscles and lateral pterygoids, have numerous intramuscular partitions formed by aponeuroses. An aponeurosis is composed of layers of flat broad tendons, and will often be referred to as a tendon in the literature. The amount of tendinous structure within the muscle varies but can be significant, with some masticatory muscles having up to 18% of its total mass being tendinous (Van Eijden et al. 1997). These tendons often differ in orientation and size within the same muscle. Muscle fibers may lie parallel to these tendons or attach to the tendons at multiple angles. Fibers that lie in parallel produce a force linear to the direction of the fiber. Fiber groups that attach at an angle on both sides of the tendon are termed pennate (penna is Latin for feather). These fibers often differ from each other in both length and angle of attachment. During contraction pennate muscle fibers rotate about their origin, and the attached tendon is pulled in the desired direction. The masticatory muscles can be categorized as unipennate, bipennate, or multipennate muscles. Examples are the bipennate temporalis muscle and the multipennate masseter muscle, which will be discussed below. The various fiber directions and attachments within a muscle allow numerous force vectors and large force magnitudes to be created within a confined space, which is ideal for masticatory muscle biomechanics (Hannam and Mcmillan 1994).

4.1.1.4 Neurophysiologic Compartmentalization

Heterogeneous activation of a muscle is also facilitated at a neurophysiologic level. A motor unit, which was discussed in detail in the previous chapter, facilitates this process. As one or more approximated motor units are activated together, the activated group effectively compartmentalizes the muscle.

There is a large variation in motor unit morphology and physiology (Van Eijden and Turkawski 2001). Motor unit recruitment depends on the magnitude and orientation of muscle contraction (Ogawa et al. 2006). The fewer muscle fibers innervated by a single motor neuron, the more precise the movement that can be performed. The masticatory muscles have a relatively low ratio of motor units to muscle fibers, allowing for fine motor control to take place. When comparing the masseter muscle to arm and leg muscles, the motor unit territories of the masseter muscle are small and restricted, and a majority of the territories are located within discrete tendon-bound compartments. This organization permits greater differential control of separate muscle portions with various internal force vectors and magnitudes compared to limb muscles. This suggests more localized organization of motor control in the masticatory muscles (Van Eijden and Turkawski 2001).

Compartmentalization has other distinct advantages as well. During continuous low-level contraction, it has been shown that there is an increase in the number of active motor unit compartments as the contraction continues. This additional recruitment of new motor units may assist in counteracting the effects of fatigue (Farella et al. 2011). Additionally, when pain is present, there is a reorganization of motor unit activity within the muscle that allows continued function with minimal damage (Minami et al. 2013). Neuromuscular motor control strategies vary intra- and intermuscularly, as well as between individuals. This strategy may provide an individualized protective mechanism to minimize the chance of potential negative consequences of the maladaptive behaviors (Farella et al. 2009).

4.1.1.5 Fiber Type

Masticatory muscles also are composed of a heterogeneous fiber makeup (Van Eijden and Turkawski 2001). These fibers are diverse and adaptable, which allow them to meet the functional demands placed on these muscles while minimizing energy expenditure (Korfage et al. 2005a). As in the rest of the body, masticatory muscle fibers are classified according to the isoforms of the myosin heavy chain (MyHC). These isoforms are differentiated by histochemical staining and classified by the rate at which they convert adenosine triphosphate (ATP) into energy (Korfage et al. 2005a). This rate correlates well with the speed of force generating power strokes, as well as fatigability (Neunhauserer et al. 2011). Pure isoforms include MyHC-I and MyHC-II fibers. MyHC-I fibers are aerobic, have a slow contraction velocity, are slow to fatigue, and are typically activated for sustained (tonic) contractions. Type-II fibers are fast contracting, anaerobic, and quick to fatigue. They are typically involved in short, powerful (phasic) contractions. MyHC-II fibers have two chief isoforms, IIA (slower) and IID (faster). The shortening velocity of MyHC-IID fibers is approximately ten times faster than MyHC-I fibers (Bottinelli et al. 1994). MyHC-I fibers use less energy when contracting compared to MyHC-II fibers, with fast fibers utilizing approximately four times more ATP than slow fibers (He et al. 2000; Stienen et al. 1996). A third type of fiber, termed a hybrid fiber, contains multiple MyHC isoforms in varying ratios. These fibers allow intermediate contractile properties and provide a mechanism that produces a very fine gradation of force magnitude and orientation (Korfage et al. 2005b).

Fiber type varies based on the location and function of the muscle. Muscles of the head and neck have a much higher proportion of hybrid fibers compared to limb muscles, with the masseter, anterior digastric, and mylohyoid muscles composed of between five and seven MyHC isoforms (Cvetko et al. 2012). The variety of isoforms may reflect the diverse functional requirements of the masticatory system. Additionally, the masticatory muscles express small amounts of MyHC-fetal and MyHC-cardiac α fibers, which are not found in the limb or trunk muscles. The purpose of these fibers is currently unknown but may provide additional adaptability to the masticatory muscles (Korfage et al. 2005a). The masticatory muscles are also unusual regarding fiber size. MyHC-II fibers have a smaller cross-sectional area than MyHC-I fibers in the masticatory muscles, which is opposite to limb and trunk muscles. This may facilitate an increase exchange of oxygen and nutrients, facilitating improved resistance to fatigue in the masticatory muscles (Korfage et al. 2005b).

A distinct difference in fiber composition has also been noted between the jaw-closing muscles (along with the superior belly of the lateral pterygoid muscle) and the jaw-opening muscles. The closing muscles and inferior belly of the lateral pterygoid muscle are made up of approximately 40% hybrid fibers, with both pure and hybrid fibers composed of 70% type-I fibers. The opening muscles only expressed 10% hybrid fibers, with both pure and hybrid fibers composed of approximately 45% type-I fibers. These differences may allow the closer muscles to perform prolonged activity, such as maintenance of the mandibular rest position or prolonged chewing. Differences also exist intramuscularly, particularly within the closing muscles, as deep and anterior portions generally containing more MyHC-I fibers are suited for prolonged use (Korfage et al. 2005a).

Changes in fiber phenotype can occur for a variety of reasons and can be temporary or permanent. Reasons include activity, age, gender, diet, and sleep. Genetic influences also play a major role, although its impact has not been clarified at this time (Korfage et al. 2005b). These changes may occur as follows:

1. Activity: Muscle activity tends to cause an increase in MyHC-I fibers, whereas prolonged deactivation tends to cause an increased amount of MyHC-II fibers. An example of this may be the anterior aspect of the superficial masseter and anterior temporalis muscles, which both have a high rate of activation and contain predominantly MyHC-I fibers (Korfage et al. 2005a). These changes promote muscle efficiency and optimization of energy use.
2. Age: Aging tends to increase the proportion of pure MyHC-II and hybrid fibers, with a noted decrease in MyHC-I fibers. This may impact masticatory performance as a person ages (Korfage et al. 2005b).
3. Gender: Females have a higher percentage of MyHC-I fibers than males, with males tending to have a higher number of MyHC-II fibers (Arima et al. 2013). This may be due to the influence of testosterone causing a phenotypic transition between fiber types (Widmer et al. 2007).
4. Diet: Although no human studies exist, rats with a long-term diet of easily chewable food demonstrated decreased MyHC-I fibers with a decreased cross-sectional area of the fibers (Korfage et al. 2005b).

5. Sleep: Chronic sleep deprivation in rats has been shown to increase MyHC-I and decrease MyHC-II expression in both the superficial and deep masseter (Cao et al. 2015).

4.1.1.6 Muscle Spindle Content

Muscle spindles provide proprioceptive feedback to the central nervous system (CNS) and allow the muscle to react appropriately to opposing forces. Jaw-closing muscles (e.g., masseter and anterior temporalis muscles) contain a high number of muscle spindles, while the jaw-opening muscles (e.g., digastric muscles and lateral pterygoid muscles) contain little to no spindles (Saverino et al. 2014). This enables the jaw-closing muscles to react quickly and appropriately to opposing forces that are encountered regularly while chewing. Meanwhile, jaw-opening muscles rarely encounter any opposition and therefore have minimal need to have continuous sensory feedback (Abbink et al. 1998). Spindle activity also assists in modulating antagonist muscle activity. When movement occurs, the opposing muscle has very little activity. For example, during mouth opening, the jaw-closing muscles showed little activity, and during jaw closing, the jaw-opening muscles showed little activity (Abbink et al. 1998). Lastly, unlike anywhere else in the body, the jaw-closing muscles have a very large amount of intrafusal fibers per spindle. This facilitates a strong proprioceptive impact on masticatory control (Turker 2002).

4.1.2 Mandibular Movement

Normal masticatory muscle function and dysfunction have been described over the years based on observation, dissection, and basic science research. These descriptions have dictated many therapies that are provided today. However, recent technological advancements in image-guided EMG studies have allowed rigorous testing of the scientific validity of these past assumptions and provided a greater understanding of individual masticatory muscle function (Salame et al. 2007). This section presents the current information on normal function of the individual masticatory muscles.

Table 4.1 Muscles contributing to mandibular movement

Opening	Digastric (rotation) Bilateral lateral pterygoid (translation) – Superior and inferior bellies
Closing	Masseter Medial pterygoid Temporalis Lateral pterygoid superior belly (minimally)
Protrusion	Bilateral lateral pterygoids – Superior and inferior bellies Superficial masseter Medial pterygoid (possibly)
Retrusion	Deep masseter Middle and posterior aspect of temporalis Lateral pterygoid superior belly (minimally)
Lateral	Contralateral lateral pterygoid – Superior and inferior bellies Ipsilateral masseter Ipsilateral temporalis Contralateral medial pterygoid

Movement of the mandible is often discussed in the literature two-dimensionally. For simplicity, the mandibular movements discussed below will be described in this context also and are summarized in Table 4.1. However, clinical reality demands a three-dimensional understanding of these movements, and the reader is encouraged to apply the structure and function of the muscles described below to real-life situations (Hannam and Mcmillan 1994). An understanding of both the two- and three-dimensional nature of these movements will better equip the clinician to interpret clinical presentations of masticatory dysfunction when encountered.

4.1.2.1 Mandibular Opening and Closing Muscles

Major architectural differences have been noted when comparing the mandibular opening muscles and mandibular closing muscles. These differences include a larger cross-sectional area, a larger percentage of tendinous tissue, shorter fiber length, and larger pennation angles for the mandibular closing muscles. The sum of these differences suits the mandibular closing muscles for greater force production (approximately 3.7 times that of openers), with the ability to sustain active force throughout a large range of motion. Meanwhile, the mandibular opening muscles are able to achieve higher shortening velocities and produce larger excursions, but their power decreases as opening distance increases and the muscle is shortened (Koolstra and Van Eijden 1997; Van Eijden et al. 1997). Similar differences have been noted between antagonist muscles in other areas of the body. For example, the quadriceps has the ability to produce high forces, while the hamstrings have a tendency for production of excursion (Van Eijden et al. 1997). The individual mandibular closing and opening muscles, with their unique characteristics that contribute to normal function, will be discussed in the sections below. A discussion of the muscles involved in mandibular excursive movements will follow.

4.1.2.2 Mandibular Closing Muscles

The primary role of the masseter, medial pterygoid, and temporalis muscles is to close (elevate) the mandible. These are powerful muscles that play a significant role in chewing food. Each muscle will be detailed in this section.

Masseter

The masseter muscle is a heterogeneous, multipennate structure with multiple compartments and fibers running in many directions. It has a superficial and deep head, with some authors distinguishing an intermediate head as well (Widmer et al. 2007). These muscular heads, which are separated by tendinous septa, are oriented at different angles to the occlusal plane. In general, the superficial masseter is oriented at 60° to the occlusal plane, the intermediate masseter is oriented 90° to the occlusal plane, and the deep masseter is oriented 90° for the inner layer and 110° for the outer layer (Gaudy et al. 2000). As demonstrated in Fig. 4.1, each muscular head is further divided into functional compartments by a complex intramuscular tendinous architecture (superficial, two layers; intermediate, one layer; and deep, three layers). In general, the tendons exhibit a fan-shaped arrangement both anteroposteriorly and mediolaterally with greater density in the superior and deeper portions of the masseter muscle, with some tendinous portions exhibiting a thickness of up to 5 mm (Minowa et al. 1998; Cioffi et al. 2012; Brunel et al. 2003). The compartments vary in location, number, and size between individuals, but they do not differ between genders once height and weight are considered (Cioffi et al. 2012).

Motor unit territories within the masseter muscle are very small (approx. 3.7 mm), with most confined to specific compartments within the tendinous layers (Farella et al. 2011). Approximately half of the masseters' motor units are unimodal and solely activated by contracting in one direction. There is a decreasing percentage of motor units that are activated by contraction in multiple directions, with only 5% being activated with contraction in four or more directions (Schindler et al. 2014). Motor unit activation depends on both the bite force magnitude and orientation, and individual motor units have specific ranges of magnitude and orientation for optimum recruitment. Motor units with a lower threshold (more easily activated) tend to participate in more oral functions and contribute to a wider range of bite force directions. Diverse recruitment of motor units enables the masseter muscle to contract effectively in various directions (Ogawa et al. 2006).

For example, based on motor unit activation patterns, the superficial masseter muscle can be separated in three functional areas (anterior, middle, and posterior). During low bite force, the anterior is much more activated, whereas progressive posterior activation occurs as the bite force is increased above 60% maximum voluntary contraction. This may correspond to the anterior area being more active during fine motor control, as it is recruited first, whereas the posterior superficial masseter may be more concerned with force generation (Guzman-Venegas et al. 2015). Distinction has also been made between activation patterns of the anterior and posterior deep masseter muscle based on task (Blanksma et al. 1992). Masseter muscle

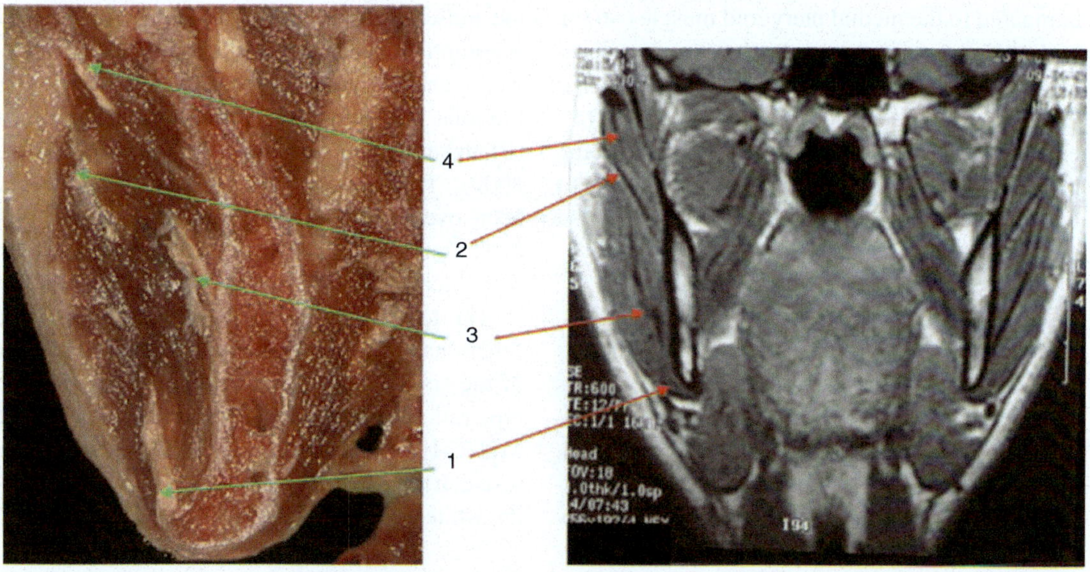

Fig. 4.1 Coronal anatomical and MRI section of the human masseter muscle with noted aponeuroses. **1** Superficial masseter, deep layer, **2** intermediate masseter, **3** deep masseter, superficial layer, **4** deep masseter, intermediate layer. (Reproduced from Brunel et al. 2003)

activation also varies between the muscular heads, with each producing different force vectors. For example, the superficial masseter muscle is more active during incisal biting, and the deep masseter muscle is more active during posterior chewing tasks (Ogawa et al. 2006). These patterns correspond well with its overall fiber directions, as the superficial masseter muscle fibers are oriented more anteroposteriorly than the vertical deep fibers (Blanksma and Van Eijden 1995). During prolonged low-level masseter muscle contraction, such as when the teeth are kept in contact, the majority of motor units are activated sporadically (<50% of the time), although some were found to be continuously active (Farella et al. 2011).

To summarize, the masseter is an incredibly complex muscle. The complex architecture and regional selective activation within this muscle provide subtle control mechanisms that enable the muscle to adjust its activity (both force magnitude and orientation) in a very flexible and efficient manner in response to complex biomechanical needs, such as those which occur during mastication (Schindler et al. 2014).

Medial Pterygoid

The medial pterygoid is a heterogeneous, multipennate muscle composed of seven alternating muscular/aponeurotic layers that allow it to perform its primary function of mandibular elevation, with a minor contribution to mandibular protrusion and contralateral excursion (El Haddioui et al. 2007; Van Eijden et al. 1995). The functionality of the individual compartments of this muscle has proved challenging to study due to its lack of accessibility. Current research attempting to address this challenge is underway, but no conclusive results are currently available (G. Murray, personal communication, 2016). Research so far has divided this muscle into two heads, anterior and posterior, both anatomically and functionally (El Haddioui et al. 2007). The heads have different activation patterns based on bite direction (Schindler et al. 2006). Along with the masseter muscle, it forms a sling around the mandible to help elevate the jaw. The medial pterygoid muscle is about 1/3 the volume of the masseter muscle. When comparing the axis of the two muscles, the masseter muscle is more vertically oriented to the palatal plane (~75°)

compared to the medial pterygoid muscle (~67°), with the masseter muscle also being more parallel to the sagittal plane (~3°) compared to the medial pterygoid muscle (~21°). These differences make a case for the masseter muscle being better suited to apply a greater magnitude of force to food products during mastication (Hsu et al. 2001).

Temporalis

The fan-shaped temporalis muscle is heterogeneous in nature and composed of three layers mediolaterally (superficial, deep, and zygomatic), as noted in Fig. 4.2 (Sedlmayr et al. 2009). These multiple layers, as well as the heterogeneous nature expounded on below, allow the muscle to precisely control the mandible to accomplish its primary movements, namely, elevation and retrusion, as well as facilitate chewing motions in multiple directions and magnitudes (Blanksma and Van Eijden 1995; Sedlmayr et al. 2009). The superficial layer, which has often been overlooked in anatomy texts, has the primary function of creating ipsilateral mandibular movement (Lee et al. 2012).

The temporalis is also been divided into six functional regions anteriorly to posteriorly. Each of the six regions is composed of different fiber type ratios, with the anterior containing the most MyHC-I fibers (slow contracting, fatigue resistant) capable of producing prolonged activity, while there is a progressive increase in type-II

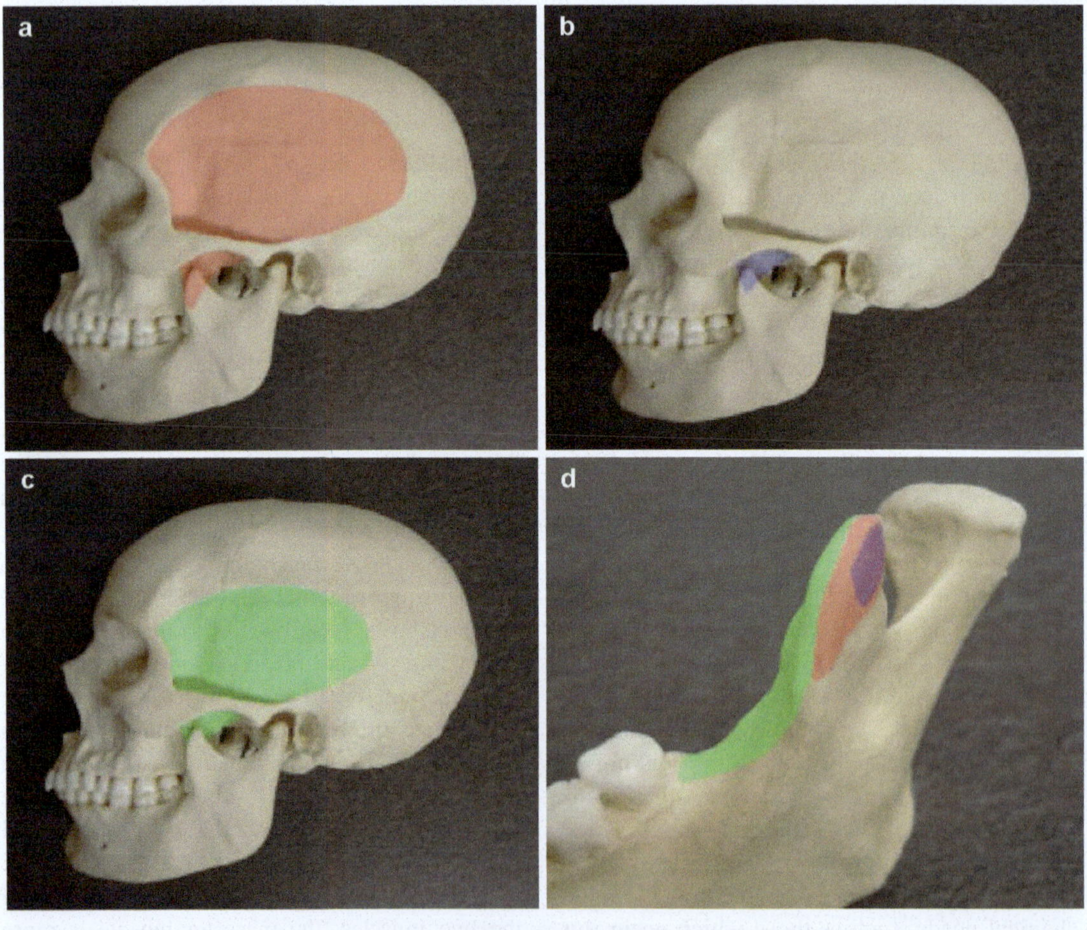

Fig. 4.2 Temporalis muscle attachments demonstrating the three muscular layers. (**a**) Superficial part, (**b**) zygomatic part, (**c**) deep part, and (**d**) anterolateral view demonstrating all three attachments. (Reproduced from Sedlmayr et al. 2009)

(fast contracting, fatigable) fibers moving posteriorly. The amount of regional activity in the temporalis muscle depends on both the bite force direction and magnitude. Directionally, all regions display at least mild activity regardless of the bite direction. The anterior region is most active in all directions, while the adjacent regions become increasingly activated with directional variation. All regions are maximally activated when the bite is directed in a posterolateral direction. The amount of activity in each region also depends on bite force magnitude, displaying a linear increase in EMG activity as bite force increases (Blanksma and Van Eijden 1990). Functionally, the fatigue-resistant anterior temporalis muscle exhibits the highest activation during masticatory endurance tasks such as gum chewing (Blanksma and Van Eijden 1995).

The temporalis fibers have the largest cross-sectional areas and contain less hybrid fibers than the other mandibular closing muscles. The temporalis muscle also has the greatest number of muscle spindles among any of the mandibular closing muscles at 342 (66%). This population is greatest in the posterior horizontal fibers (Korfage et al. 2005a).

The temporalis muscle attaches to the mandible via the temporal tendon. This tendon inserts onto the apex, anterior, posterior, medial, and lateral surfaces of the coronoid process and continues downward onto the anterior border of the mandibular ramus. The distal portion of the tendon bifurcates and attaches to the medial and lateral borders of the retromolar fossa, which is posterior to the mandibular third molar (Fig. 4.3). This large attachment of the tendon, in addition to the bifurcation, may allow significant force to be generated onto the mandible while still attaining balance at the narrow insertion (Benninger and Lee 2012).

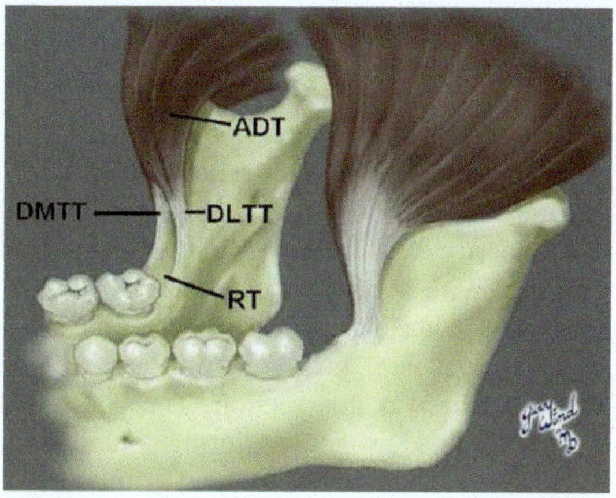

Fig. 4.3 Temporalis tendon attachment with noted bifurcation at the retromolar pad. *ADT*, anterior distal fibers of temporalis; *DMTT*, distal medial tendon of temporalis; *DLTT*, distal lateral tendon of temporalis; *RT*, retromolar triangle of mandible. (Reproduced by Benninger and Lee 2012)

4.1.2.3 Mandibular Opening Muscles

When opening the mandible, the harmonious contraction of both the right and left lateral pterygoid muscles and the digastric muscles causes translation and depression of the mandible, respectively. The lateral pterygoid muscles also play a significant role in excursive movements of the mandible. This section will briefly discuss the digastric muscles, while the lateral pterygoid muscles will be further discussed under the mandibular excursion section.

Digastric Muscles

The digastric muscles are among multiple muscles that work synergistically to rotate the mandible inferiorly and posteriorly during mandibular opening or to elevate the hyoid bone during swallowing. Although only separated by a muscle sling, the anterior and posterior digastric muscles receive innervation via different cranial nerves, the anterior belly receiving innervation from cranial nerve V via the mylohyoid nerve branch, and the posterior belly receiving innervation from cranial nerve VII via the digastric branch. The two muscles also differ from each other in fiber type, with the anterior belly containing more MyHC-IIX fibers and the posterior belly containing more MyHC-IIA fibers. This difference may suggest that the bellies can act independently (Korfage et al. 2005a). These muscles are activated to approximately twice their resting level during maximum voluntary clenching, which may be due to an anatomic link between the masticatory muscles and digastric muscles by tendons, ligaments, and fascia (Ciuffolo et al. 2005).

4.1.2.4 Mandibular Excursive Muscles

Lateral and protrusive mandibular movements are primarily controlled by the lateral pterygoid muscles, with additional modulation by other masticatory muscles. The structure and function of the lateral pterygoid muscles will be described first in this section. The additional muscles that are active during mandibular excursion will then be discussed at the end of the section.

Lateral Pterygoid

The lateral pterygoid muscle is a heterogeneous, multipennate muscle composed of eight alternating muscular/aponeurotic layers which can be selectively recruited to allow fine horizontal control of the mandible (Foucart et al. 1998). Anatomic studies have divided this muscle into two heads, superior and inferior, with different origins and insertions. The fibers of both heads run in an anterior and medial direction from the condyle at an angle of approximately 45° (El Haddioui et al. 2005). Both heads are composed primarily of aerobic, fatigue-resistant MyHC-I (80%) fibers that are capable of prolonged contraction and fine movement. Twenty percent of the muscle is composed of MyHC-II fibers that are active for quick, forceful contractions during function and parafunction (Hannam and Mcmillan 1994; Murray et al. 2001).

The function of the lateral pterygoid muscles has proven challenging to study in vivo due to its deep location, as well as its multiple anatomical and neurophysiological compartments. Past attempts to understand activation patterns of the lateral pterygoid muscles have utilized either surface EMG or unguided wire electrode EMG experiments to monitor muscle activity during movement. However, data from these studies need to be interpreted with caution due to questionable recording accuracy. Studies utilizing surface electrodes may have unintentionally recorded activity from muscles that are adjacent to or overlie the lateral pterygoid muscles, making these readings potentially inaccurate. Studies utilizing unguided wire electrode EMG based the electrode placement on anatomic landmarks. The electrode was presumed to be in the correct location of the superior or inferior head based on the assumed activation pattern of each head. Data from these studies further reinforced the assumption that each head contracts at opposite times, the superior head during closing, clenching, retrusion, and ipsilateral movements and the inferior head during opening, protrusive, and contralateral movements. These assumptions dictated many of the hypotheses and treatment recommendations for temporomandibular disorders (Bhutada et al. 2008). However, when considering the possibility of inaccurate EMG data, as well as taking into account the complex heterogeneity of the lateral pterygoid muscles, the simplistic activation model does not adequately suffice (Foucart et al. 1998; Bhutada et al. 2008). Therefore, assumptions of lateral pterygoid muscle function and dysfunction based on these methodologies should be interpreted with caution.

Recently, advances using computed tomography (CT) imaging have provided the ability to confirm placement of the wire electrodes into multiple areas of both the superior and inferior lateral pterygoid muscles (Salame et al. 2007). The results from studies using this methodology have provided a more accurate and complete understanding of lateral pterygoid muscle function, which has brought into question the role of the lateral pterygoid muscle in temporomandibular disorders (Bhutada et al. 2008). The function of each head of the lateral pterygoid muscle will be discussed below.

Superior Lateral Pterygoid

The superior lateral pterygoid muscle is a functionally heterogeneous unit. Its compartments are preferentially activated to produce the greatest mechanical advantage during its primary functions of contralateral and protrusive mandibular movements. Innervation of the muscle is complex. Neuroanatomically, the superior portion of superior lateral pterygoid muscle can be divided into four parts, each receiving indepen-

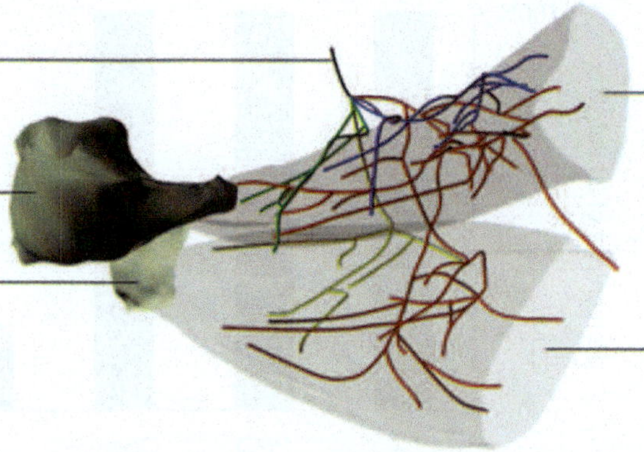

Fig. 4.4 Broad innervation pattern of the superior and inferior lateral pterygoid muscle bellies. *Red*, buccal nerve; *green*, masseteric nerve; *blue*, middle deep temporal nerve; *yellow*, muscular branches directly from the mandibular nerve (V3). (Reproduced from Davies et al. 2012)

dent innervation by a different nerve source. This includes the masseteric, posterior deep temporal, middle deep temporal, and buccal nerves. The entire inferior portion of the superior lateral pterygoid muscle receives a single source of innervation by the buccal nerve (Fig. 4.4). Considering the superior region of this muscle attaches to the disc-capsule complex in some individuals, whereas the inferior region often attaches to the condyle, this innervation may allow independent movement between the disc-capsule complex and the condyle (Davies et al. 2012).

The insertion of the superior lateral pterygoid muscle has much interindividual variation, with only a small portion of the superior lateral pterygoid muscle attaching to the temporomandibular joint disc in some patients. It has been noted that the muscle may insert into both the condyle and the disc-capsule complex (55.5%), only into the condyle (27.8%), or only into the disc-capsule complex (16.7%) (Antonopoulou et al. 2013). When it does insert into the disc-capsule complex, approximately 29.5% of the fibers still insert into the condyle (Naidoo and Juniper 1997). When considering the anatomy of the superior lateral pterygoid muscle with its origin on the roof of the infratemporal fossa and lateral pterygoid plate and narrow insertion onto the condylar fovea, capsule, and disc, its functionally heterogeneous composition offers a biomechanical advantage by allowing a range of force vectors on the condyle during mandibular movement (Bhutada et al. 2008).

Activity of the superior lateral pterygoid muscle begins almost immediately upon horizontal movement (<0.2 mm), which indicates its importance in initiating contralateral movements (Bhutada et al. 2007). During contralateral movement, activity of this muscle begins in the medial region. As the motion continues, a graded activation from the medial to the lateral region of the muscle occurs. Overall, the medial and middle regions of the muscle are most active during contralateral movement. During protrusion, the medial region is again activated first, but as the movement continues, the middle region generates the majority of the movement. Overall, the superior, middle, and insertion regions are most active during protrusion (Bhutada et al. 2008). The speed of the contraction can impact the activation pattern for both movements, with the medial region showing the greatest activation as the speed of the contraction increases (Bhutada et al. 2007).

There has been some inconsistent activity noted in the lateral region of this muscle during jaw closing, clenching, and ipsilateral movement. The lack of consistent activation suggests these movements, particularly ipsilateral movement, are not a primary function of the superior lateral pterygoid muscle (Fig. 4.5). It may be that this

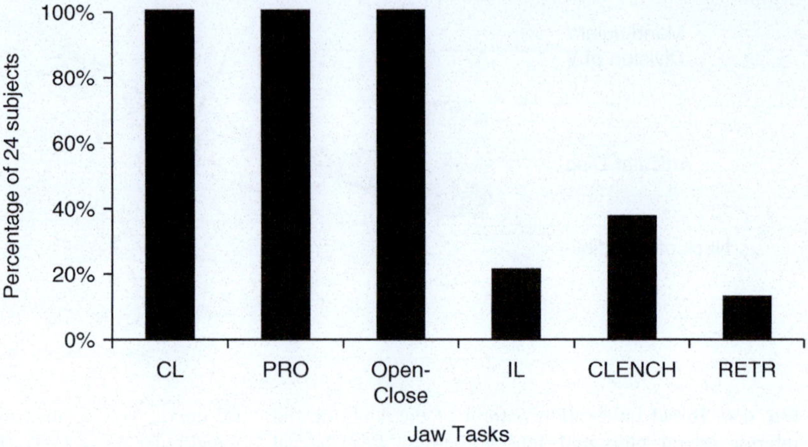

Fig. 4.5 Proportion of subjects showing activation of the superior belly of the lateral pterygoid muscle during specific mandibular movements ($n = 24$). *CL* – contralateral, *PRO* – protrusive, *IL* – ipsilateral, *RETR* – retrusion. (Reproduced from Bhutada et al. 2007)

muscle acts to stabilize the condyle and disc during the extreme of an ipsilateral movement, rather than participate in generating the motion (Bhutada et al. 2008). When the mandible is in the rest position, there is no activity in the superior lateral pterygoid muscle. This suggests a lack of anteriorly and medially directed forces on the disc and/or condyle, which would question the concept that superior lateral pterygoid muscle hyperactivity is a cause for disc displacement (Bhutada et al. 2007).

Inferior Lateral Pterygoid

The inferior lateral pterygoid muscle is approximately two to six times larger in cross section than the superior head and is also active primarily during contralateral, protrusive, and opening movement, with the lateral portion of this muscle being most active during these movements (Phanachet et al. 2002). The superomedial part of the muscle is important in initiating contralateral jaw movement, while the inferomedial part maintains fine motor control once the movement has begun. Regarding the direction of force, activity of this muscle is highest when the force is directed contralaterally, will decrease slightly as the force is directed more anteriorly, and is minimal as the force is directed ipsilaterally (Fig. 4.6) (Murray et al. 2004).

Innervation of the inferior lateral pterygoid muscle also emphasizes its heterogeneity, though it has fewer neuromuscular partitions than the superior lateral pterygoid muscle. Neuroanatomically, this muscle can be divided into two parts, lateral and medial. The lateral portion is innervated by the buccal nerve only, whereas the medial portion is innervated by the buccal nerve and muscular branches from the mandibular branch of the trigeminal nerve (V3) (Davies et al. 2012).

Summary: Data indicate that both the superior and inferior lateral pterygoid muscles play an important role in contralateral, protrusive, and jaw-opening movements (Murray et al. 2007). Neural activation within the muscle suggests that the lateral pterygoid muscles should be considered as a single functional structure with varied regional activity that allows it to respond appropriately to the functional demands encountered (Foucart et al. 1998). The buccal nerve supplies both muscles and may be the source that facilitates coordinated activity between the two muscles when performing contralateral or protrusive movement (Davies et al. 2012). This is demonstrated when noting that the medial region of the superior lateral pterygoid muscle and the anatomically adjacent superomedial region of the inferior lateral pterygoid muscle are both active at the initiation of contralateral and protrusive jaw movement, suggesting a synergistic relationship (Bhutada et al. 2007). Overall, activation of the various regions in these muscles during mastication, as well as other functions, may allow for initiation and precise control of a wide range of force directions and magnitudes on both the condyle and

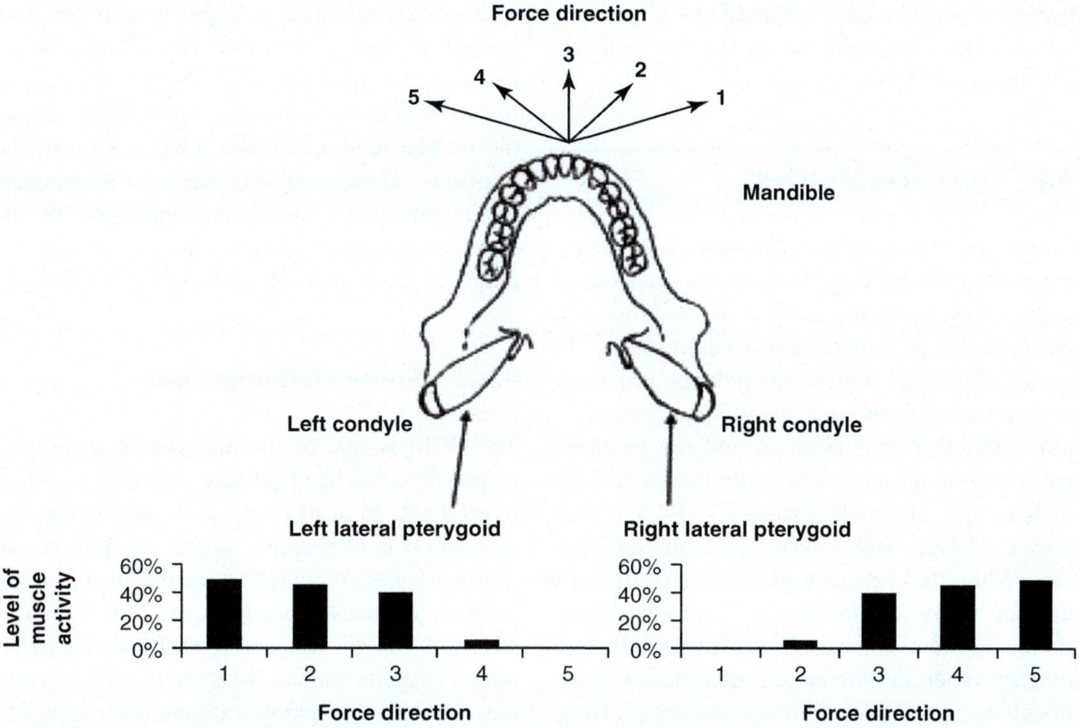

Fig. 4.6 Lateral pterygoid inferior belly activity level is based on the direction of force. The greatest amount of activity is produced during contralateral movement. (Reproduced from Murray et al. 2004)

disc-capsule complex, ensuring coordinated activity and minimized stress to these structures (Davies et al. 2012).

4.1.2.5 Lateral Movement

As noted above, the contralateral superior and inferior lateral pterygoid muscles are the primary driver behind lateral movement of the mandible. The ipsilateral temporalis, ipsilateral masseter, and contralateral medial pterygoid may also play a minor role in this movement (Hannam and Mcmillan 1994).

4.1.2.6 Protrusion

The lateral pterygoid muscles are also the primary driver behind mandibular protrusion. Additionally, the superficial masseter muscle is also active during protrusion. It has also been speculated that the medial pterygoid muscle participates in this action, but difficulty monitoring the activity of this muscle has not allowed for confirmation of this hypothesis (Hannam and Mcmillan 1994).

4.1.2.7 Retrusion

Both the deep masseter and the temporalis muscles are active during jaw retrusion (Hannam and Mcmillan 1994).

4.1.2.8 The Role of Tendons and Ligaments

Ligaments have no active role in movement of the masticatory structures. Their primarily purpose is to limit overextension of the mandible (Alomar et al. 2007).

Sphenomandibular Ligament

This ligament is a vestigial remnant of Meckel's cartilage which has a neutral role and maintains the same degree of tension in both opening and closing movements (Alomar et al. 2007).

Stylomandibular Ligament

This ligament is lax when the mouth is closed and increases in laxity with opening, as the insertion of the ligament moves superiorly and posteriorly toward its origin at the styloid process. This ligament becomes more taut during mandibular protrusion, although its functional role is still questionable (Alomar et al. 2007).

4.2 Cervical Muscles

More than 20 pairs of cervical muscles work synchronously to stabilize and control head movement. These muscles can be divided into the posterior and anterolateral cervical muscles. The posterior cervical muscles include the trapezius, semispinalis capitis, semispinalis cervicis, splenius capitis, levator scapula, and the posterior paravertebral muscles. The anterolateral muscles include the sternocleidomastoid (SCM), platysma, scalene, and anterior prevertebral muscles. While the cervical muscle are anatomically distinct from the masticatory muscles, these groups of muscles have a bidirectional influence on each other and are co-activated during functional tasks such as chewing and swallowing. One primary reason for this interaction is the need for the head to be stabilized against the shoulder girdle during forceful kinetic motor tasks, such as chewing (Giannakopoulos et al. 2013a). This section will describe the function of the major cervical muscles, followed by a discussion of the bidirectional influence between the cervical and masticatory muscles.

4.2.1 Trapezius

The trapezius muscle has the most extensive origin of any muscle in the human body and contains a wide array of fibers running in different directions, which reflect the various functional demands placed on this muscle. The trapezius is commonly divided into three regions: (1) the upper, (2) the middle, and (3) the lower. Each region has a different fiber type composition based on its function, and the regions are preferentially activated depending on the type of movement. The most superior part of the upper region is composed of MyHC-II fibers. This segment is most responsible for quick movements involved in head control, such as rapid head orientation toward an object. This suits the fast contractile properties of these fibers. MyHC-I fibers are primary found in the lower third of the upper region, the middle region, and the lower region of the trapezius. These segments are most responsible for postural and stabilizing functions in the shoulder and arm, which suit the fatigue resistant nature of these fibers (Lindman et al. 1990).

4.2.2 Sternocleidomastoid

The SCM is one of the primary neck muscles responsible for head posture and movement. It plays a role in head rotation, flexion, extension, and tilt. It is also active during respiration and mastication. Sternocleidomastoid fiber type composition includes a nearly equal distribution of MyHC-I, MyHC-IIA, and hybrid fiber (IIA/IIX) types. This mix enables the SCM to meet its complex functional demands, ranging from sustained head posture to quick orienting head movements (Cvetko et al. 2012).

4.2.3 Posterior Cervical Muscles

Aside from the trapezius, the semispinalis capitis and splenius capitis muscles reside in the posterior cervical region and assist in maintaining head position, with the splenius capitis also active during head rotation and tilt. These muscles are activated when the head is held flexed, such as during forward head posture, and have reduced activity when the head is extended (Forsberg et al. 1985).

4.2.4 Supra- and Infrahyoids

The hyoid muscles are activated during head flexion and head extension, and help to stabilize the hyoid bone and maintain the airway during activities such as swallowing. They also can play a role in stabilizing the mandible during swallowing (Forsberg et al. 1985).

4.2.5 Cervical and Masticatory Muscle Interaction

Neurophysiologically, the cervical and masticatory muscles interact at both motor and sensory level. The sensory interaction between the two areas has been discussed in the previous chapter. Therefore, the motor interaction will be the primary focus of this section, as each individual system (cervical and masticatory) can significantly impact the function of the other.

4.2.5.1 Cranial and Mandibular Positioning

The masticatory and cervical muscles work together in a coordinated manner to open and close the mouth. When preparing to open the mouth, the head will extend. This cervical extension precedes the initiation of mandibular movement, and it concludes after mandibular movement ends. The amplitude of the initial cervical extension is proportional to the amplitude of mandibular opening. This may provide a biomechanical advantage for masticatory force production, as maximal bite force increases with greater head extension (Ballenberger et al. 2012). During chewing, a cervical flexion-extension pattern will proceed with the mandibular closing-opening pattern, although the head remains slightly extended for the entire duration of a chewing cycle. The precision and timing of these mandibular and cervical movements indicate coordinated control of these two systems by the central nervous system (Ballenberger et al. 2012; Eriksson et al. 2000).

The pathway of mandibular movement is also significantly influenced by the position of the head. As the neck is flexed, the mandible moves forward and teeth occlude anteriorly. Conversely, as the head is extended, the mandible retrudes and the teeth occlude posteriorly. Clinically, this may be significant when performing a dental restoration. For example, if a restoration is placed and the occlusion is verified only with the patient lying supine in the dental chair, the cervical posture may alter the patient's functional occlusion and cause the restoration to contact prematurely during normal upright function, which is considered the alert feeding position (Haralur et al. 2014). This oversight could lead to localized pain via occlusal trauma, and possibly muscular pain due to protective co-contraction in an effort to avoid contacting the high restoration. Therefore, it is important for the restorative dentist to verify the patient's occlusion both in a supine and upright (functional) position. Additionally, in the assessment of the orofacial pain patient, it is important to note whether the patient had any dental work performed approximating the onset of the pain complaint.

Different head postures also impact EMG activity of the masseter muscle during maximal voluntary contraction. For example, cervical flexion, ipsilateral lateral flexion, and contralateral rotation significantly reduced masseter EMG activity, whereas the opposite movements tended to increase activity. This effect was not demonstrated in the anterior temporalis muscle. Clinically, patients may therefore masticate with their head in alternative postures in order to gain a biomechanical chewing advantage (Ballenberger et al. 2012).

4.2.5.2 Jaw Clenching

Maximum voluntary clenching (MVC), submaximal clenching, and chewing in both seated and supine positions can cause co-activation of the masticatory and cervical muscles. For example, MVC causes bilateral activation of the anterior neck muscles (SCM and digastric muscles) (Ciuffolo et al. 2005), with the SCM being activated up to 30% of its maximum capability (Clark et al. 1993). Activity of the trapezius muscle may also be increased during MVC up to 17% (Ehrlich et al. 1999). Submaximal clenching in a sitting and supine position also causes activation of multiple cervical muscles, including the trapezius, splenius capitis, levator scapula, and SCM. This co-activation occurs regardless of the direction of the biting force, although changing the bite direction can modify the level of activity. Chewing can also cause a co-activation of cervical muscles, particularly the SCM and levator scapula (Giannakopoulos et al. 2013a, b). An important finding from these studies is that low-level masticatory muscle activity such as gum chewing can initiate a prolonged action potential train in a cervical motor unit(s) that outlasts the masticatory muscle function by more than 30 min. In susceptible individuals, this may lead to local cervical muscle overload and injury (Giannakopoulos et al. 2013a, b).

4.2.5.3 Noxious Input

A functional connection between the masticatory and cervical muscles has also been demonstrated by applying a painful electrical and mechanical stimulus intraorally. In humans, both stimuli caused co-inhibition of the masseter, SCM, and dorsal neck muscles, with the cervical muscles being inhibited up to 80% of baseline (Browne et al. 1993; Torisu et al. 2014). On the other hand, a study in rodents showed a co-activation of masticatory and cervical muscles after injection of a noxious substance into the deep paracervical muscles (Hu et al. 1993). Clinically, these findings should prompt the clinician to assess for painful areas in both the masticatory and cervical systems, as this may lead not only to pain referral but also manifest as the source of dysfunction.

4.2.6 Conclusion

Considering this anatomical, physiological, and functional overlap and impact the masticatory and cervical muscles have on one another, it could be argued that both the traditional masticatory muscles and cervical muscles should be grouped under the term "muscles of mastication" and should be a standard part of any orofacial pain evaluation.

4.3 Functional Behaviors

The individual masticatory and cervical muscles each perform the individual functions as reviewed above, but it is the coordination of these muscles, as well as structures such as the lips, tongue, pharynx, and larynx that enable the body to perform incredibly complex functional behaviors that are essential to everyday life such as mastication (chewing), deglutition (swallowing), and vocalization (speech). The coordination needed to accomplish these functions is often subconscious and mediated by the central nervous system. Although ethical standards will not allow for detailed study in humans, animal research has demonstrated compelling evidence of a feedback loop that allows for coordinated movement of these structures. For example, studies have shown that jaw muscle spindle afferents and apical periodontal ligament receptors, with their cell bodies in the trigeminal mesencephalic nucleus, project to the parvocellular reticular nucleus (considered a common premotor neuron pool) and dorsomedial spinal trigeminal nucleus within the brainstem. Premotor neurons located in these structures project to the trigeminal motor nucleus, facial motor nucleus, hypoglossal nucleus, and the nucleus ambiguous. This therefore suggests multiple orofacial motor neurons receive continuous input from the jaw muscle spindle afferents (e.g., the masseter muscle) during chewing/speaking/swallowing and are able to respond with appropriately coordinated jaw-lip-face-tongue-airway motor behavior to carry out the function (Fig. 4.7) (Zhang et al. 2012). A detailed description of each function and the primary muscles involved is described below.

4.3.1 Chewing

Chewing involves a coordination of multiple head and neck muscles to produce complex opening-closing, protrusive-retrusive, and excursive mandibular movements simultaneously in order to break down food particles in preparation for swallowing. The average chewing cycle lasts approximately 0.7 s, with the inter-incisal distance reaching 17–20 mm (Hannam et al. 2008). Muscle activation and the pattern of chewing movements vary based on the consistency of the food being chewed but typically open toward the non-chewing side and close from the chewing side, as seen in A–D in Fig. 4.8. While the motion of the mandible is three-dimensional, it is easiest to conceptualize this motion two-dimensionally.

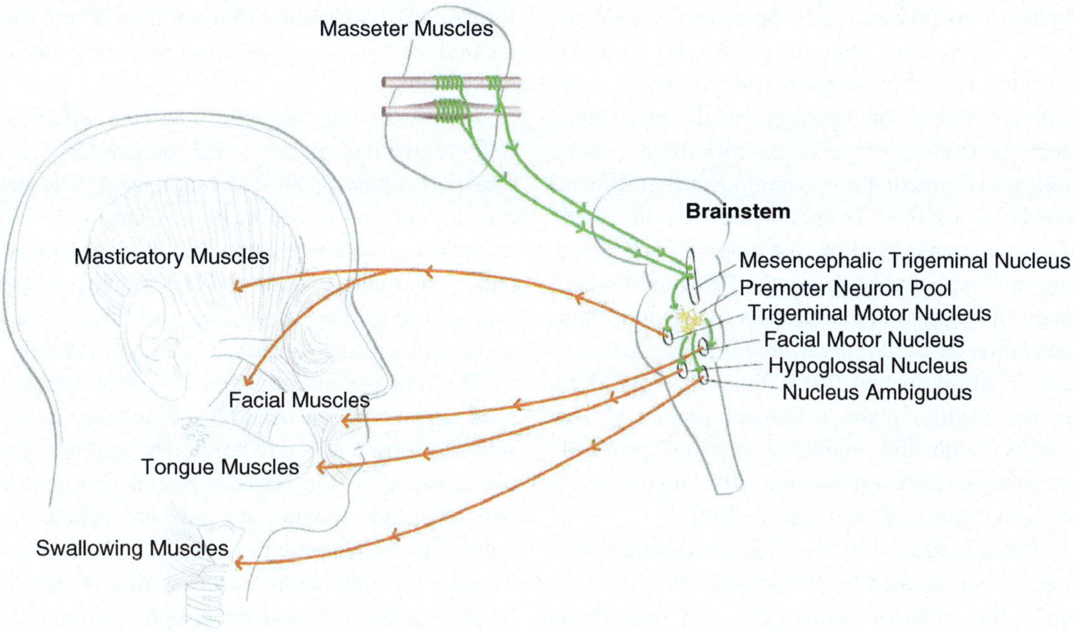

Fig. 4.7 Afferent proprioceptive input from masseter muscle spindles is transmitted to a premotor neuron pool (parvocellular reticular nucleus and dorsomedial spinal trigeminal nucleus) via the mesencephalic nucleus. These interneurons project to the trigeminal motor nucleus, facial motor nucleus, hypoglossal nucleus, and nucleus ambiguous, allowing coordinated reactions/reflexes of the masticatory, facial, tongue, airway and swallowing muscles

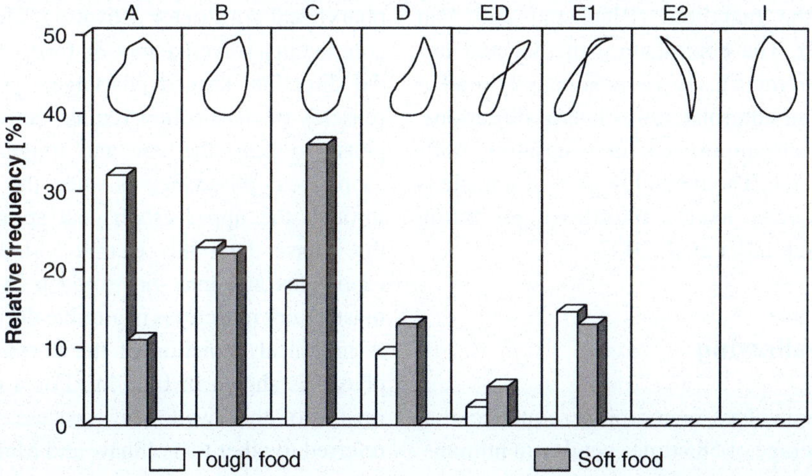

Fig. 4.8 Chewing pattern frequency distribution during mastication of tough and soft foods in 159 individuals with normal class one occlusion. **A–D** are considered within the range of a normal chewing sequence and were most frequently used during mastication of tough and soft food. Opening occurs toward the non-chewing side (*left in this diagram*), while closing occurs toward the chewing side (*right in this diagram*). **ED**, **E1**, and **E2** are mixed sequence chewing and used less frequently. **I** is a reversed chewing sequence and was not used during the mastication of tough or soft food. (Reproduced from Proeschel. 2006)

In the frontal plane, a teardrop-shaped incisal and molar movement pattern occurs (toward the working side). This shape is formed by minor lateral movement on opening, while on closing approximately 5 mm of lateral movement occurs, followed by medial movement toward midline as the bolus of food is encountered by the teeth. These movements allow for crushing and grinding of food between the teeth. The lateral movement of the mandible is caused by asynchronous activation of the bilateral lateral pterygoid muscles (Commisso et al. 2015; Hannam et al. 2008). In the sagittal plane a banana shaped pattern occurs, with the mandible moving primarily inferoposteriorly on opening and superoanteriorly on closing (Koolstra et al. 2001).

Force produced by the muscles during chewing is also dictated by food consistency. In general, the anterior temporalis and superficial masseter muscles display higher activity on the working side. Tougher foods require a near equal activation of the masseter muscles on the working and balancing side, whereas the temporalis muscle is activated only on the working side. This suggests that the masseter muscle is more suited for force production, whereas the temporalis muscle may be more concerned with laterodeviation of the mandible (Blanksma and Van Eijden 1995). The contralateral medial and lateral pterygoid muscles were most heavily loaded when biting in anterolateral to lateral directions, indicating their importance in generating horizontal bite force. The medial pterygoid muscle is the most heavily loaded muscle in all biting directions (Schindler et al. 2007).

4.3.2 Swallowing

Swallowing involves a complex sequence that occurs an average of 585 times per day in humans. Swallowing occurs most frequently while eating and least frequently during sleep, with an average of 20 min of swallow-free intervals while asleep (Lear et al. 1965). The sequence of activity is coordinated centrally within the brainstem and carried out by five cranial nerves (CN V, VII, IX, X, and XII) and three peripheral nerves (C1–C3). It involves coordination of more than 30 muscles located within the oral cavity, pharynx, larynx, and esophagus.

The swallowing sequence can be divided into four sequential phases: oral preparatory, oral transport, pharyngeal, and esophageal. The oral preparatory and transport phases are under voluntarily control, while the last two phases are under involuntary control. The activity within each phase is modifiable based on the size and consistency of the substance being swallowed.

The oral preparatory phase involves breaking food down via mastication and mixing it with saliva to form a cohesive bolus. The oral transport phase begins as the bolus is placed between the dorsum of the tongue and the hard palate. The bolus is propelled posteriorly through the oral cavity into the oropharynx. During this phase, the muscles of mastication and the suprahyoid muscles remain active and serve to stabilize the jaw and tongue during transport. The pharyngeal phase involves coordination of numerous muscles and lasts approximately 1 s. During this phase the bolus enters the area of the anterior faucial pillars. This contact initiates an involuntary response to include cessation of respiration with airway protection, rising of the pharynx and retraction of the tongue, and pharyngeal constrictor activation. The constrictors contract in a wavelike motion from a rostral to caudal direction, termed pharyngeal peristalsis. The muscles of mastication remain active during this phase to keep the jaw and tongue stable. The esophageal phase begins once the bolus passes through the upper esophageal sphincter. During this phase the bolus is transported through the esophagus and into the stomach. Activity of the masticatory muscles is negligible during this phase. A graphical depiction of the normal swallowing phases is shown in Fig. 4.9. For a more detailed review of the swallowing process, the reader is referred to other texts (Shaw and Martino 2013).

4.3.3 Speaking

Speech is one of the most precise and rapid human motor behaviors. The motor system involved in speech is incredibly complex,

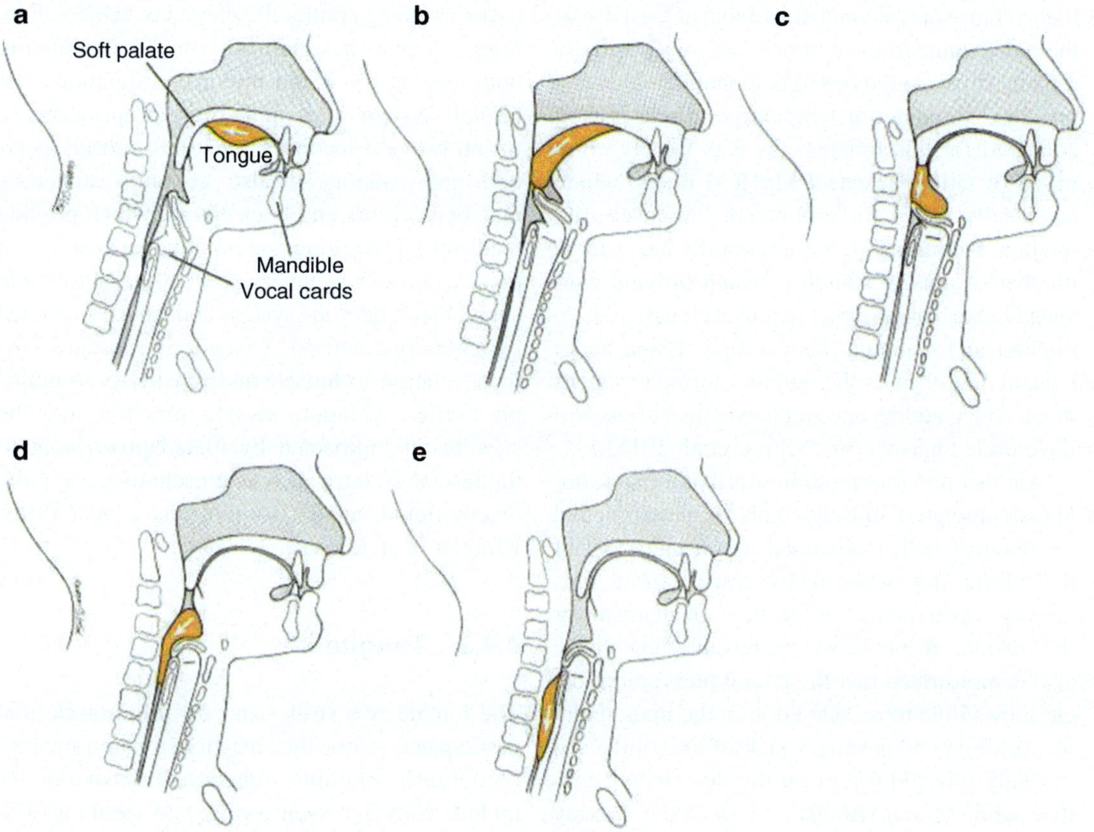

Fig. 4.9 Phases of normal swallowing beginning with (**a–b**) the oral transport phase, (**c–d**) the pharyngeal phase, and ending with (**e**) the esophageal phase. (Reproduced from Cumming Otolaryngology 6th ed. 2015)

coordinating more than 100 muscles to produce speech. These muscles contain diverse fiber types with fast contractile properties (with the exception of the mandibular closing muscles, which are primarily composed of slow contractile fibers) and are generally fatigue resistant. The speech-producing muscles can be clustered into five structural-functional groups. The first are the muscles of mastication. The second is the sphincteric muscles, to include the orbicularis oris for lip closure, as well as the pharyngeal constrictors. The third is the intrinsic muscles of the tongue. The fourth is the intrinsic muscles of the larynx, which are involved in vibration and airway valving. The fifth are the respiratory muscles. For a more detailed review of the process of speaking, the reader is referred to other texts (Kent 2004).

4.3.4 Mandibular Rest Position

The mandibular rest position is a physiologic jaw position that continuously fluctuates in humans by very small amounts. This position can be modulated by multiple factors, to include a person's body position (upright vs supine) and mood (Tingey et al. 2001; Yilmaz et al. 2015). Two main theories exist on how this position is maintained, to include the visco-elastic theory and the muscle tonus theory. The visco-elastic theory states that the passive elasticity of the muscles and connective tissue maintain this physiologic mandibular posture (Miles 2007). The muscle tonus theory dictates that there is an active low-level muscle tonus in the jaw-closing muscles that maintain the resting posture. While there is no evidence to contradict the visco-elastic theory, recent research has provided greater support for the muscle tonus theory. One study demonstrated that at least 3% of the motor units in the anterior temporalis muscle remain active at all times to help maintain this rest position. The anterior temporalis muscle is well equipped for this function, as it is largely composed of fatigue-resistant MyHC-I fibers, which are ideally suited for prolonged, low-level contraction. Additionally, the temporalis has a large number of muscle spindles, which provide constant feedback regarding the muscle length to help monitor and maintain this position. When under general anesthesia, the mouth normally opens much wider, adding anecdotal evidence to support the muscle tonus theory (Yilmaz et al. 2015).

Another previous thought was that the superior lateral pterygoid muscle, with its anteromedial direction of pull, maintained a constant state of pull on the disc while in the rest position. This activity was hypothesized to be a mechanism for disc displacement. However, recent studies have also demonstrated that the lateral pterygoid muscle shows little to no activation in the mandibular rest position, suggesting a lack of anteriorly and medially directed forces on the disc and/or condyle while at rest (Bhutada et al. 2007; Murray et al. 2004).

4.4 Other Considerations in Muscle Function

While it is tempting to consider the masticatory system in isolation due to the ease in which it would allow comprehension of dysfunction and treatment, it is impossible to ignore the complex interplay that various modulatory influences have on this system. A few of these influences will be noted below.

4.4.1 Fascia

Fascia is a connective tissue that envelops and interacts with every body structure, to include muscle, nerve, blood vessel, viscera, meninges, and bone. Muscle fibers can attach to fascia at multiple angles, and the fascia provides structure to give form and function to the muscle. Fascial tissue contains contractile elements, which allow fascia to play a significant role in modulating both muscle force and motor coordination. The fascial system has numerous proprioceptors, which provide feedback regarding muscle position and tension. It also contains numerous metaboreceptors and nociceptors, which provide feedback of fatiguing and noxious input from the muscle. Fascia is innervated by the autonomic sympathetic nervous system and can be impacted by adrenergic activity. Considering fascia's intimate relation to muscle and sensitivity to multiple forms of input, muscle function may be significantly impacted by maladaptive input to the fascial system, such as muscle overuse, pain, or emotional stress (Bordoni and Zanier 2014; Klingler et al. 2014).

4.4.2 Tongue

The tongue is a strong and flexible muscle that participates with the masticatory muscles to accomplish multiple functional behaviors, to include chewing, swallowing, and speaking. The tongue shares premotor neurons with the masticatory muscles to help coordinate function. For example, the muscles that retrude the tongue and the muscles that close the mandible share one set of premotor neurons, while the muscles that protrude the tongue and the muscles that open the mouth share a different set of premotor neurons. This allows for functional coordination of the muscles with minimal chance of injury, such as biting the tongue (Morquette and Kolta 2014). Fiber type distribution within the tongue is heterogeneous, with predominantly MyHC-IIA fibers in the anterior portion and MyHC-I fibers in the posterior portion. This distribution allows for the fast and flexible movements that are needed during speaking, chewing, and swallowing (Kent 2004).

Tongue placement can impact the activity of other masticatory muscles. When the tongue is placed on the palate, a significant increase in EMG activity was noted in the masseter, temporalis, and suprahyoid muscles, both when the teeth were separated and during MVC (Schmidt et al. 2009; Valdes et al. 2014). Additionally, heart rate variability, which is a measure of autonomic function, showed a significant decrease (less autonomic flexibility and potentially poorer health) when the tongue was braced against the palate compared with resting the tongue on the floor of the mouth (Schmidt et al. 2009).

4.4.3 Metaboreception: From Muscle Fatigue to Muscle Pain

Skeletal muscles are innervated by numerous afferent neurons that provide input about the state of the muscle to the CNS. Group III and IV neurons, which are thinly myelinated and unmyelinated respectively, are part of this afferent innervation. These neurons correspond in conduction velocity to A-delta and C fibers that innervate cutaneous tissues. Group III and IV neurons contain both metaboreceptors and nociceptors. Metaboreceptors sense metabolites produced by the muscle and provide feedback on muscle use, with a person having an increased sensation of muscle fatigue as more metaboreceptors are activated. Three receptors that have received much attention for monitoring muscle metabolites are the acid-sensing ion channel (ASIC) receptor, the purinergic (PX2) receptor, and the transient receptor potential cation channel subfamily V member 1 (TRPV1) receptor. These receptors are densely localized near blood vessels immediately below the muscle fascia and sense metabolites produced by the muscle to include protons, adenosine triphosphate (ATP), and lactate, respectively. No single metabolite, even at supraphysiologic levels, has been shown to produce the sensation of fatigue or pain in isolation nor has a combination of the three metabolites at the level of a resting muscle. As the concentration of these metabolites increase to the level found during moderate endurance exercise, the combination of the three metabolites evokes a sensation of significant muscle fatigue. As the concentrations continue to be increased, as in vigorous exercise, greater sensations of fatigue and muscle pain are produced (Pollak et al. 2014).

Masticatory muscle fatigue is a common symptom in TMD patients. The findings noted above were from a recent innovative study performed to a thumb muscle (abductor pollicis brevis) in human subjects (Pollak et al. 2014). While it is important to be cautious when translating research findings into clinical scenarios, this research may suggest that masticatory muscle overuse (similar to moderate endurance exercise) can lead to fatigue and eventually pain in the susceptible individual, with the combination of the three noted metabolites playing a role. Therefore, attempting to modify muscle overuse should be a goal of the provider.

4.4.4 Cortical Plasticity

It has been long understood that the CNS drives muscle function, but recent studies also suggest that muscle function can drive neuroplastic change in the CNS. Within the masticatory system, two studies have demonstrated that repetitive, standardized movement of masticatory and tongue muscles can prompt neuroplastic changes to multiple corticomotor areas. These studies showed that repeated tooth clenching caused an increase in excitability to the corticomotor control areas of the jaw-closing muscles (Iida et al. 2014), and repeated tongue lifts caused an increased excitability to the corticomotor control areas of both the tongue muscles and the jaw-closing muscles (Komoda et al. 2015). While further research is needed to gain a greater understanding of this process and how it applies clinically, it has been hypothesized that these changes may contribute to the mechanism underlying tooth clenching (Iida et al. 2014).

4.5 Summary

Chewing, swallowing, and speaking are important functional behaviors that provide physical sustenance to the body and intellectual sustenance to the mind. These behaviors are performed daily in most individuals with little thought or effort, yet each require a complex synchrony of numerous muscles for completion. An appreciation of these complex behaviors involves a foundational understanding of the anatomy and physiology of these muscles, as well as a translation of the basic science of masticatory muscle composition into the intricacies of individual masticatory muscle function. This understanding will enable the clinician to not only understand normal function but also interpret potential causes of dysfunction.

Disclaimer The views expressed in this presentation are those of the authors and do not necessarily reflect the official policy or position of the Department of the Navy, Department of Defense, or the US Government.

References

Abbink JH, Van der Bilt A, Bosman F, Van Der Glas HW. A comparison of jaw-opener and jaw-closer muscle activity in humans to overcome an external force counteracting jaw movement. Exp Brain Res. 1998;118:269–78.

Alomar X, Medrano J, Cabratosa J, Clavero JA, Lorente M, Serra I, Monill JM, Salvador A. Anatomy of the temporomandibular joint. Semin Ultrasound CT MR. 2007;28:170–83.

Antonopoulou M, Iatrou I, Paraschos A, Anagnostopoulou S. Variations of the attachment of the superior head of human lateral pterygoid muscle. J Craniomaxillofac Surg. 2013;41:E91–7.

Arima T, Takeuchi T, Honda K, Tomonaga A, Tanosoto T, Ohata N, Svensson P. Effects of interocclusal distance on bite force and masseter emg in healthy participants. J Oral Rehabil. 2013;40:900–8.

Ballenberger N, Von Piekartz H, Paris-Alemany A, La Touche R, Angulo-Diaz-Parreno S. Influence of different upper cervical positions on electromyography activity of the masticatory muscles. J Manip Physiol Ther. 2012;35:308–18.

Benninger B, Lee BI. Clinical importance of morphology and nomenclature of distal attachment of temporalis tendon. J Oral Maxillofac Surg. 2012;70:557–61.

Bhutada MK, Phanachet I, Whittle T, Peck CC, Murray GM. Regional properties of the superior head of human lateral pterygoid muscle. Eur J Oral sci. 2008;116:518–24.

Bhutada MK, Phanachet I, Whittle T, Wanigaratne K, Peck CC, Murray GM. Threshold properties of single motor units in superior head of human lateral pterygoid muscle. Arch Oral Biol. 2007;52:552–61.

Blanksma NG, Van Eijden TM. Electromyographic heterogeneity in the human temporalis muscle. J Dent Res. 1990;69:1686–90.

Blanksma NG, Van Eijden TM. Electromyographic heterogeneity in the human temporalis and masseter muscles during static biting, open/close excursions, and chewing. J Dent Res. 1995;74:1318–27.

Blanksma NG, Van Eijden TM, Weijs WA. Electromyographic heterogeneity in the human masseter muscle. J Dent Res. 1992;71:47–52.

Bordoni B, Zanier E. Clinical and symptomatological reflections: the fascial system. J Multidiscip Healthc. 2014;7:401–11.

Bottinelli R, Betto R, Schiaffino S, Reggiani C. Unloaded shortening velocity and myosin heavy chain and alkali Light chain isoform composition in rat skeletal muscle fibres. J Physiol. 1994;478(Pt 2):341–9.

Browne PA, Clark GT, Yang Q, Nakano M. Sternocleidomastoid muscle inhibition induced by trigeminal stimulation. J Dent Res. 1993;72:1503–8.

Brunel G, El-Haddioui A, Bravetti P, Zouaoui A, Gaudy JF. General organization of the human intra-masseteric aponeuroses: changes with ageing. Surg Radiol Anat. 2003;25:270–83.

Cao R, Huang F, Wang P, Chen C, Zhu G, Chen L, Wu G. Chronic sleep deprivation alters the myosin heavy chain isoforms in the masseter muscle in rats. Br J Oral Maxillofac Surg. 2015;53(5):430.

Cioffi I, Gallo LM, Palla S, Erni S, Farella M. Macroscopic Analysis of human masseter compartments assessed by magnetic resonance imaging. Cells Tissues Organs. 2012;195:465–72.

Ciuffolo F, Manzoli L, Ferritto AL, Tecco S, D'attilio M, Festa F. Surface electromyographic response of the neck muscles to maximal voluntary clenching of the teeth. J Oral Rehabil. 2005;32:79–84.

Clark GT, Browne PA, Nakano M, Yang Q. Co-activation of sternocleidomastoid muscles during maximum clenching. J Dent Res. 1993;72:1499–502.

Commisso MS, Martinez-Reina J, Ojeda J, Mayo J. Finite element Analysis of the human mastication cycle. J Mech Behav Biomed Mater. 2015;41:23–35.

Cvetko E, Karen P, Erzen I. Myosin heavy chain composition of the human sternocleidomastoid muscle. Ann Anat. 2012;194:467–72.

Davies JC, Charles M, Cantelmi D, Liebgott B, Ravichandiran M, Ravichandiran K, Agur AM. Lateral pterygoid muscle: a three-dimensional Analysis of neuromuscular partitioning. Clin Anat. 2012;25:576–83.

Ehrlich R, Garlick D, Ninio M. The effect of jaw clenching on the Electromyographic activities of 2 neck and 2 trunk muscles. J Orofac Pain. 1999;13:115–20.

El Haddioui A, Bravetti P, Gaudy JF. Anatomical study of the arrangement and attachments of the human medial pterygoid muscle. Surg Radiol Anat. 2007;29:115–24.

El Haddioui A, Laison F, Zouaoui A, Bravetti P, Gaudy JF. Functional anatomy of the human lateral pterygoid muscle. Surg Radiol Anat. 2005;27:271–86.

Eriksson PO, Haggman-Henrikson B, Nordh E, Zafar H. Co-ordinated mandibular and head-neck movements during rhythmic jaw activities in man. J Dent Res. 2000;79:1378–84.

Farella M, De Oliveira ME, Gallo LM, Laubli T, Tomatis L, Muller C, Obrenovic R, Palla S. Firing duration of masseter motor units during prolonged low-level contractions. Clin Neurophysiol. 2011;122:2433–40.

Farella M, Palumbo A, Milani S, Avecone S, Gallo LM, Michelotti A. Synergist coactivation and substitution pattern of the human masseter and temporalis muscles during sustained static contractions. Clin Neurophysiol. 2009;120:190–7.

Forsberg CM, Hellsing E, Linder-Aronson S, Sheikholeslam A. Emg activity in neck and masticatory muscles in relation to extension and flexion of the head. Eur J Orthod. 1985;7:177–84.

Foucart JM, Girin JP, Carpentier P. Innervation of the human lateral pterygoid muscle. Surg Radiol Anat. 1998;20:185–9.

Gaudy JF, Zouaoui A, Bravetti P, Charrier JL, Guettaf A. Functional organization of the human masseter muscle. Surg Radiol Anat. 2000;22:181–90.

Giannakopoulos NN, Hellmann D, Schmitter M, Kruger B, Hauser T, Schindler HJ. Neuromuscular interaction of jaw and neck muscles during jaw clenching. J Orofac Pain. 2013a;27:61–71.

Giannakopoulos NN, Schindler HJ, Rammelsberg P, Eberhard L, Schmitter M, Hellmann D. Co-activation of jaw and neck muscles during submaximum clenching in the supine position. Arch Oral Biol. 2013b;58:1751–60.

Grunheid T, Langenbach GE, Korfage JA, Zentner A, Van Eijden TM. The adaptive response of jaw muscles to varying functional demands. Eur J Orthod. 2009;31:596–612.

Guzman-Venegas RA, Biotti Picand JL, De La Rosa FJ. Functional compartmentalization of the human superficial masseter muscle. PLoS One. 2015;10:E0116923.

Hannam AG, Mcmillan AS. Internal organization in the human jaw muscles. Crit Rev Oral Biol Med. 1994;5:55–89.

Hannam AG, Stavness I, Lloyd JE, Fels S. A dynamic model of jaw and hyoid biomechanics during chewing. J Biomech. 2008;41:1069–76.

Haralur S, Al-Gadhaan S, Al-Qahtani A, Mossa A, Al-Shehri W, Addas M. Influence of functional head postures on the dynamic functional occlusal parameters. Ann Med Health Sci Res. 2014;4:562–6.

He ZH, Bottinelli R, Pellegrino MA, Ferenczi MA, Reggiani C. Atp consumption and efficiency of human single muscle fibers with different myosin isoform composition. Biophys J. 2000;79:945–61.

Herring SW, Grimm AF, Grimm BR. Functional heterogeneity in a multipinnate muscle. Am J Anat. 1979;154:563–76.

Hsu CW, Shiau YY, Chen CM, Chen KC, Liu HM. Measurement of the size and orientation of human masseter and medial pterygoid muscles. Proc Natl sci Counc Repub China B. 2001;25:45–9.

Hu JW, Yu XM, Vernon H, Sessle BJ. Excitatory effects on neck and jaw muscle activity of inflammatory irritant applied to cervical paraspinal tissues. Pain. 1993;55:243–50.

Iida T, Komiyama O, Obara R, Baad-Hansen L, Kawara M, Svensson P. Repeated clenching causes plasticity in corticomotor control of jaw muscles. Eur J Oral sci. 2014;122:42–8.

Johansson AS, Westberg KG, Edin BB. Task-dependent control of the jaw during food splitting in humans. J Neurophysiol. 2014;111:2614–23.

Kent RD. The uniqueness of speech among motor systems. Clin Linguist Phon. 2004;18:495–505.

Klingler W, Velders M, Hoppe K, Pedro M, Schleip R. Clinical relevance of fascial tissue and dysfunctions. Curr Pain Headache Rep. 2014;18:439.

Komoda Y, Iida T, Kothari M, Komiyama O, Baad-Hansen L, Kawara M, Sessle B, Svensson P. Repeated tongue lift movement induces neuroplasticity in corticomotor control of tongue and jaw muscles in humans. Brain Res. 2015;1627:70–9.

Koolstra JH, Naeije M, Van Eijden TM. The three-dimensional active envelope of jaw border movement and its determinants. J Dent Res. 2001;80:1908–12.

Koolstra JH, Van Eijden TM. Dynamics of the human masticatory muscles during a jaw open-close movement. J Biomech. 1997;30(9):883.

Korfage JA, Koolstra JH, Langenbach GE, Van Eijden TM. Fiber-type composition of the human jaw muscles--(part 1) origin and functional significance of fiber-type diversity. J Dent res. 2005a;84:774–83.

Korfage JA, Koolstra JH, Langenbach GE, Van Eijden TM. Fiber-type composition of the human jaw muscles--(part 2) role of hybrid fibers and factors responsible for inter-individual variation. J Dent Res. 2005b;84:784–93.

Lear CS, Flanagan JB Jr, Moorrees CF. The frequency of deglutition in man. Arch Oral Biol. 1965;10:83–100.

Lee JY, Kim JN, Kim SH, Choi HG, Hu KS, Kim HJ, Song WC, Koh KS. Anatomical verification and designation of the superficial layer of the temporalis muscle. Clin Anat. 2012;25:176–81.

Lindman R, Eriksson A, Thornell LE. Fiber type composition of the human male trapezius muscle: enzyme-histochemical characteristics. Am J Anat. 1990;189:236–44.

Miles TS. Postural control of the human mandible. Arch Oral Biol. 2007;52:347–52.

Minami I, Akhter R, Albersen I, Burger C, Whittle T, Lobbezoo F, Peck CC, Murray GM. Masseter motor unit recruitment is altered in experimental jaw muscle pain. J Dent Res. 2013;92:143–8.

Minowa K, Inoue N, Ashikaga Y, Yoshida S, Totsuka Y, Nakamura M. Comparison of magnetic resonance imaging and gross findings regarding masseter muscle aponeuroses in cadavers. Oral Surg Oral med Oral Pathol Oral Radiol Endod. 1998;86:275–9.

Morquette P, Kolta A. How do we walk and chew gum at the same time? Elife. 2014;3:E03235.
Murray GM, Bhutada M, Peck CC, Phanachet I, Sae-Lee D, Whittle T. The human lateral pterygoid muscle. Arch Oral Biol. 2007;52:377–80.
Murray GM, Phanachet I, Uchida S, Whittle T. The role of the human lateral pterygoid muscle in the control of horizontal jaw movements. J Orofac Pain. 2001;15:279–92. Discussion 292–305.
Murray GM, Phanachet I, Uchida S, Whittle T. The human lateral pterygoid muscle: a review of some experimental aspects and possible clinical relevance. Aust Dent J. 2004;49:2–8.
Naidoo LC, Juniper RP. Morphometric Analysis of the insertion of the upper head of the lateral pterygoid muscle. Oral Surg Oral Med Oral Pathol Oral Radiol Endod. 1997;83:441–6.
Neunhauserer D, Zebedin M, Obermoser M, Moser G, Tauber M, Niebauer J, Resch H, Galler S. Human skeletal muscle: transition between fast and slow fibre types. Pflugers Arch. 2011;461:537–43.
Ogawa T, Kawata T, Tsuboi A, Hattori Y, Watanabe M, Sasaki K. Functional properties and regional differences of human masseter motor units related to three-dimensional bite force. J Oral Rehabil. 2006;33:729–40.
Phanachet I, Whittle T, Wanigaratne K, Murray GM. Functional properties of single motor units in the inferior head of human lateral pterygoid muscle: task firing rates. J Neurophysiol. 2002;88:751–60.
Pollak KA, Swenson JD, Vanhaitsma TA, Hughen RW, Jo D, White AT, Light KC, Schweinhardt P, Amann M, Light AR. Exogenously applied muscle metabolites synergistically evoke sensations of muscle fatigue and pain in human subjects. Exp Physiol. 2014;99:368–80.
Salame TH, Peck CC, Murray GM. A new method for lateral pterygoid Electromyographic electrode placement. J Prosthet Dent. 2007;98:224–31.
Saverino D, De Santanna A, Simone R, Cervioni S, Cattrysse E, Testa M. Observational study on the occurrence of muscle spindles in human digastric and mylohyoideus muscles. Biomed Res Int. 2014;2014:294263.
Schindler HJ, Hellmann D, Giannakopoulos NN, Eiglsperger U, Van Dijk JP, Lapatki BG. Localised task-dependent motor-unit recruitment in the masseter. J Oral Rehabil. 2014;41:477–85.
Schindler HJ, Rues S, Turp JC, Lenz J. Heterogeneous activation of the medial pterygoid muscle during simulated clenching. Arch Oral Biol. 2006;51:498–504.
Schindler HJ, Rues S, Turp JC, Schweizerhof K, Lenz J. Jaw clenching: muscle and joint forces, optimization strategies. J Dent Res. 2007;86:843–7.
Schmidt JE, Carlson CR, Usery AR, Quevedo AS. Effects of tongue position on mandibular muscle activity and heart rate function. Oral Surg Oral Med Oral Pathol Oral Radiol Endod. 2009;108:881–8.
Sedlmayr JC, Kirsch CF, Wisco JJ. The human temporalis muscle: superficial, deep, and zygomatic parts comprise one structural unit. Clin Anat. 2009;22:655–64.
Shaw SM, Martino R. The normal swallow: muscular and neurophysiological control. Otolaryngol Clin North Am. 2013;46:937–56.
Stienen GJ, Kiers JL, Bottinelli R, Reggiani C. Myofibrillar atpase activity in skinned human skeletal muscle fibres: fibre type and temperature dependence. J Physiol. 1996;493(Pt 2):299–307.
Tingey EM, Buschang PH, Throckmorton GS. Mandibular rest position: a reliable position influenced by head support and body posture. Am J Orthod Dentofac Orthop. 2001;120:614–22.
Torisu T, Tanaka M, Murata H, Wang K, Arendt-Nielsen L, De Laat A, Svensson P. Modulation of neck muscle activity induced by intra-oral stimulation in humans. Clin Neurophysiol. 2014;125:1006–11.
Turker KS. Reflex control of human jaw muscles. Crit Rev Oral Biol Med. 2002;13:85–104.
Valdes C, Astaburuaga F, Falace D, Ramirez V, Manns A. Effect of tongue position on masseter and temporalis Electromyographic activity during swallowing and maximal voluntary clenching: a cross-sectional study. J Oral Rehabil. 2014;41:881–9.
Van Eijden TM, Koolstra JH, Brugman P. Architecture of the human pterygoid muscles. J Dent Res. 1995;74:1489–95.
Van Eijden TM, Korfage JA, Brugman P. Architecture of the human jaw-closing and jaw-opening muscles. Anat Rec. 1997;248:464–74.
Van Eijden TM, Turkawski SJ. Morphology and physiology of masticatory muscle motor units. Crit Rev Oral Biol Med. 2001;12:76–91.
Widmer CG, English AW, Morris-Wiman J. Developmental and functional considerations of masseter muscle partitioning. Arch Oral Biol. 2007;52:305–8.
Yilmaz G, Ugincius P, Sebik O, Turker KS. Tonic activity of the human temporalis muscle at mandibular rest position. Arch Oral Biol. 2015;60:1645–9.
Zhang J, Luo P, Ro JY, Xiong H. Jaw muscle spindle afferents coordinate multiple orofacial motoneurons via common premotor neurons in rats: an electrophysiological and anatomical study. Brain Res. 2012;1489:37–47.

The Temporomandibular Joint

5

Istvan A. Hargitai, James M. Hawkins,
and A. Dale Ehrlich

Abstract

A joint is a site or junction between two bones with the function of providing movement or flexibility to the structures of the body. The joint which receives the greatest attention within the field of dentistry is the temporomandibular joint. It represents the union between the maxilla and mandible which house the dentition. Its function may be impacted by restorative, reconstructive, and orthodontic procedures. Understanding the anatomy, histology, and physiology of this joint in health and disease is important so treatments that target joint pain and function can have the greatest degree of success.

5.1 Introduction

The temporomandibular joint (TMJ) is a synovial joint involved in mastication, speaking, and swallowing. The TMJ has many unique features differentiating it from other synovial joints in the body. It is classified as a ginglymoarthrodial joint. It has the features of a hinging movement characteristic of a ginglymus joint, as well as a sliding movement characteristic of an arthrodial joint. It is also a biaxial joint, meaning there are two principal axes of movement corresponding to the right and left TMJ. Furthermore, the TMJ is also a diarthrodial joint. A diarthrodial joint is one that allows maximum movement such as a shoulder or knee. This type of joint is characterized by the presence of fibrocartilage or hyaline cartilage, which forms a lining on the articular surfaces. Diarthrodial joints also feature synovial fluid within the joint, which acts as a lubricant and as a source of nutrient and metabolic transport.

5.2 Articulating Surfaces

The TMJ is formed by an articulation between the maxilla and the mandible. The mandible is the only movable bone in the human skull. The

I.A. Hargitai (✉)
Naval Postgraduate Dental School,
Bethesda, MD, USA
e-mail: Istvan.a.hargitai.mil@mail.mil

J.M. Hawkins
Naval Medical Center San Diego,
San Diego, CA, USA
e-mail: James.m.hawkins77.mil@mail.mil

A. Dale Ehrlich
Louisiana State University School of Dentistry,
New Orleans, LA, USA
e-mail: aehrli@lsuhsc.edu

© Springer International Publishing AG 2018
H.A. Gremillion, G.D. Klasser (eds.), *Temporomandibular Disorders*,
https://doi.org/10.1007/978-3-319-57247-5_5

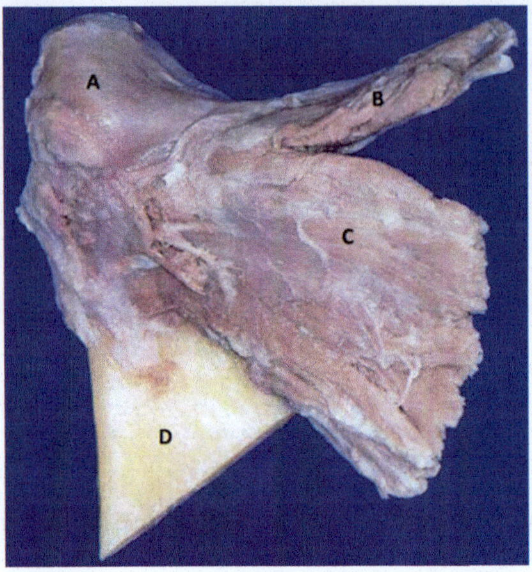

Fig 5.1 Sagittal, gross anatomical view of the temporomandibular joint complex. For orientation purposes, the anterior is to the right and superior is to the top of the picture. (**a**) TMJ disc which overlies the mandibular condyle. (**b**) Superior head of the lateral pterygoid muscle. (**c**) Inferior head of the lateral pterygoid muscle. (**d**) Ramus of the mandible

mandible at its distal ends forms a condylar process. The condylar process is composed of a thinner neck as the ascending ramus tapers superiorly with a bulbous condyle at its most superior aspect. The condyle interfaces with the glenoid fossa which is part of the squamous portion of the temporal bone (Fig 5.1). The glenoid fossa is rather thin at its most superior aspect being just several millimeters in thickness. Superior to the glenoid fossa is the middle cranial fossa and the temporal lobe of the brain. Owing to the thinness of the bone separating the two fossae, there are clinical implications. Traumatic blows to the mandible in a superior direction may implode the condyle into the brain, while surgical procedures such as osteoplasty in the vicinity of the glenoid fossa and the articular eminence may result in cerebrospinal fluid leaks if the bone is perforated.

The glenoid fossa is wider mediolaterally (ML) than anteroposteriorly (AP) which corresponds well with the dimensions of the condyle, which is also wider ML than AP. The condyle is convex in form being approximately 10 mm wide in an AP direction while being approximately 20 mm wide in a ML direction (Piette 1993).

The anatomical areas to be discussed in this chapter will include the articular cartilage, the articular disc, the synovial fluid, the retrodiscal tissues, and the associated ligaments of the TMJ. While there are similarities, for instance, between the composition of the fibrocartilage of the condyle and glenoid fossa with that of the dense fibrous connective tissue of the TMJ disc, there are several differences that will be discussed separately.

5.2.1 Articular Cartilage

Both the glenoid fossa and the superior aspect of the condyle are lined with fibrocartilage, unlike most synovial joints of the body which contain hyaline cartilage. The only other anatomic parts in the human body to consist of fibrocartilage are the sternoclavicular joint, the pubic symphysis, and the intervertebral discs (Ross and Romrell 1989). This distinction gives the TMJ some unique properties but also some inherent vulnerability.

Architecture The bony surfaces below the cartilage are made up of a cortical plate with cancellous bone beneath. The fibrocartilage of the condyle consists of four histologic zones overlying the subchondral bone. Moving from the exterior surface inward, they are the fibrous zone, proliferative zone, mature zone, and hypertrophic zone (Fig 5.2). The fibrocartilage consists of type I collagen, various proteoglycans, and water (Haskin et al. 1995). The collagen fibers are oriented in an AP fashion and with a correspondingly greater stiffness in the AP direction compared to other directions (Singh and Detamore 2009). However, there are numerous zones that exhibit structural heterogeneity that facilitate adaptations in those regions in terms of morphology and functionality. The articular cartilage is avascular and aneural. The extracellular matrix (ECM) consists of interstitial fluid and other components. Condylar cartilage may vary

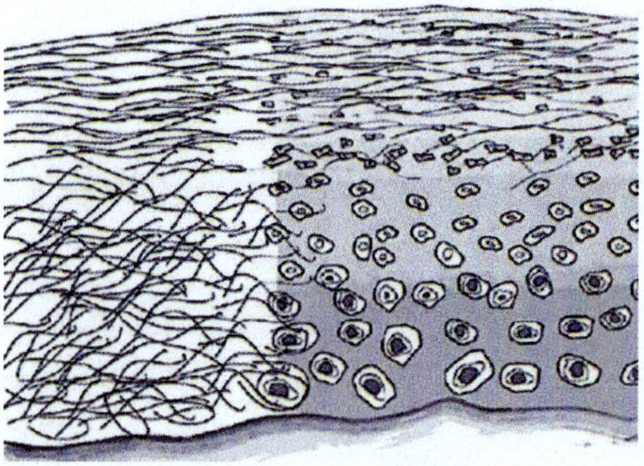

Fig. 5.2 A schematic depicting the histologic zonal organization of the TMJ fibrocartilage. The fibrous zone is the outermost layer adjacent to the articular surface. The figure highlights fiber organization and cellular composition of these zones (Reproduced from Singh and Detamore 2009 with permission)

in thickness from region to region, ranging from approximately 0.15 to 0.5 mm in thickness (Singh and Detamore 2009).

Cellular Content The cellular component of fibrocartilage consists of fibroblasts, fibrocytes, and fibrochondrocytes (Haskin et al. 1995). Fibrochondrocytes can synthesize and degrade the cartilage matrix, while fibroblasts are found in the articular zone of the cartilage and synthesize collagen (Dijkgraaf et al. 1995).

Water Content The extracellular matrix is the acellular component of TMJ articular cartilage, the main component of which consists of water. The other components of the ECM include collagen, proteoglycans, and elastin. The contents of the ECM are produced by fibroblasts and fibrochondrocytes. For comparative purposes, it is noteworthy that water content in hyaline cartilage is 60–80%, while it is somewhat less in the fibrocartilage of the TMJ (Dijkgraaf et al. 1995).

Collagen The articular cartilage of the TMJ is composed mainly of type I collagen. The articular cartilage can be found lining the load-bearing aspect of the condyle and the glenoid fossa with at least 60% of the dry weight of the TMJ cartilage being attributed to collagen (Dijkgraaf et al. 1995). The AP orientation of collagen provides increased resistance to shear forces associated with the AP motion of the condyle-disc complex (Singh and Detamore 2009). The orientation of collagen becomes more concentric at the periphery of the disc compared to articular collagen. Due to the collagen orientation, both the disc and articular cartilage withstand intermittent compressive forces better than sustained compression. Furthermore, from a functional perspective, TMJ articular cartilage resists tensile forces better than compressive ones.

Proteoglycans Another substance present in the ECM of TMJ articular cartilage is proteoglycans. Proteoglycans are glycoproteins that have a long, protein filament core with shorter glycosaminoglycan (GAG) side chain moieties that attach to the protein core (Fig 5.3). Together, the proteoglycans have a test-tube brush appearance. The GAG side chain molecules are composed of various types. The most important ones include chondroitin sulfate (CS), dermatan sulfate (DS), and hyaluronic acid (HA), also called hyaluronan. Unlike other GAG, HA is non-sulfated and can form very large complexes. Other GAG found in articular cartilage are keratin sulfate (KS) and heparan sulfate (HS). The combination of the protein core with either uniform or assorted GAG side chains gives rise to a variety of proteoglycans. A generic proteoglycan is shown here:

$$\text{Proteoglycan} = \text{protein core} + \text{GAG}$$

Large proteoglycans are demonstrated below:

$$\text{Aggrecan} = \text{protein core} + \text{CS GAG} + \text{KS GAG}$$

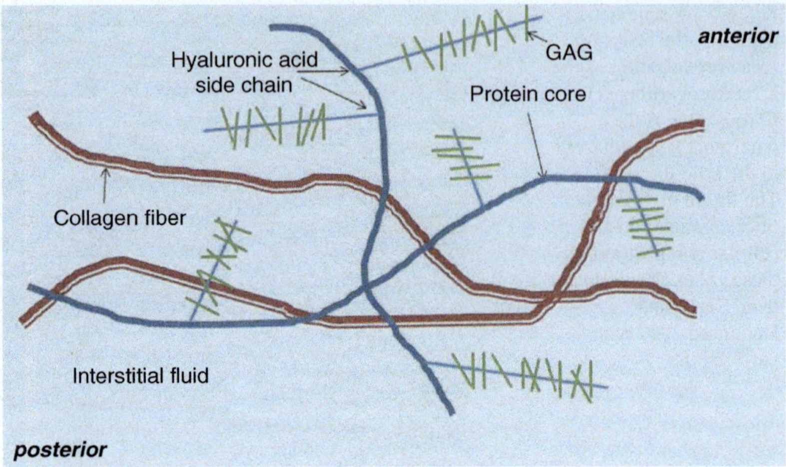

Fig 5.3 Cartilaginous matrix of TMJ fibrocartilage depicting the type I collagen network (*red*) intertwining with proteoglycans. Note the thistle-shaped appearance of the glycosaminoglycan side chains (*green*) branching off of a protein core (*blue*) and the relative AP orientation of the collagen fibers with periodic sharp turns (Courtesy of Dr. Istvan Hargitai)

$$\text{Perlecan} = \text{protein core} + \text{CS GAG} + \text{HS GAG}$$

$$\text{Versican} = \text{protein core} + \text{CS GAG} + \text{DS GAG}$$

Small proteoglycans have very few side chains. Biglycan, for example, exhibits just two GAG side chain, either a CS or a DS (Schaefer and Iozzo 2008). Examples include:

$$\text{Biglycan} = \text{protein core} + \text{two GAG} \left(\text{either CS or DS}\right)$$

$$\text{Decorin} = \text{protein core} + \text{one GAG} \left(\text{either CS or DS}\right)$$

$$\text{Lumican} = \text{protein core} + \text{KS GAG only}$$

Proteoglycans link up with one another via HA chains. Proteoglycans enhance the tensile properties of collagen. When proteoglycans intertwine and run parallel with collagen, it effectively increases the collagen's diameter. The proteoglycan aggregates are hydrophilic and intertwine through the collagen, giving the cartilage mass. The collagen is slightly hydrophobic counteracting proteoglycan's hydrophilic swelling. Proteoglycans account for 20–40% of cartilage weight (Dijkgraaf et al. 1995).

Other Contents There exists an entire class of enzymes that are capable of degrading cartilage, and they are called proteases. Proteases are secreted by chondrocytes, synovial cells, and inflammatory cells. The four proteases are (1) aspartic proteases, (2) cysteine proteases, (3) serine proteases, and (4) matrix metalloproteinases. Aspartic and cysteine proteases operate mostly under acidic pH, while serine and matrix metalloproteinases (i.e., MMP-1, MMP-2, MMP-3) operate best under neutral pH. These proteases are also inducible by other molecules. In general, cytokines such as the interleukins, tumor necrosis factor, and interferon are capable of activating proteases that then go on to degrade the ECM. Alternatively, growth factors such as insulin-like growth factor, fibroblast growth factor, and platelet-derived growth factor build cartilage (Dijkgraaf et al. 1995).

Mechanical Properties Understanding the mechanical properties of the articular cartilage lining the condyle and glenoid fossa within each TMJ enables us to appreciate the joint's function and the importance of each property to clinical practice**.** Compressive strength is the ability of a substance to resist compression forces that attempt to shrink the mass of the substance. Tensile strength is the ability of a substance to withstand elongating forces. Shear strength is the ability of a substance to withstand failure to a sliding force parallel to the substance's surface. Stiffness is the ability of a substance to withstand deformation when a force is applied to it which is quantified by the modulus of elasticity.

Condylar cartilage is stiffer in the AP direction than in the ML direction (Singh and Detamore 2009). Articular cartilage will deform in the presence of sustained compression. With greater loads, cartilage will respond with increased stiffness particularly in the anteromedial regions of the condyle and other areas that exhibit regional thickness (Singh and Detamore 2009). The presence of aggrecan in the deeper layers of the cartilage, proximal to the subchondral bone, confers an ability to resist compressive forces (Singh and Detamore 2009).

Loading of the TMJ has been an area of much study and controversy. Clinical decision making must be based on an understanding of normal responses to joint loading. Some findings that are variants of normal are due to adaptation in the presence of excess loading or as a normal part of the aging process. Some of the excess loading conditions in the patient population may include clenching (while awake and/or during sleep), coarse diets, medication-induced bruxism, and other parafunctional behaviors to include, but not limited to, chewing gum, biting on pencils and fingernails, etc. (Fujisawa et al. 2013; Chen et al. 2007; Bostwick and Jaffee 1999). Loading is beneficial for joint development and homeostasis. Remodeling is a normal, adaptive response to normal functional demands (Tanaka and Koolstra 2008). Joint hyperfunction may be detrimental to cartilage integrity and thickness but so may be the case in hypofunctional joints (Ikeda et al. 2014). In regard to the aging process, systemic disease and hormonal influences can be cofactors (Tanaka and Koolstra 2008; Westesson and Rohlin 1984). At this point, there are no agreed-upon normal values for loading forces.

Fibrocartilage is more resistant to shear forces than compressive forces, whereas in hyaline cartilage, it is the reverse (Milam 2005). Fibrocartilage is found in areas where resilience to physical impact is required. Hence, the TMJ is well-suited to be a load-bearing joint. The predominant collagen type in fibrocartilage is type I, while in hyaline cartilage, it is type II. Type I collagen produces thicker bundles and a denser cartilage framework (Ross and Romrell 1989). Therefore, if one is to contemplate the total joint reconstruction of the TMJ with synthetic implants, it should be fabricated with materials able to withstand heavy loading forces.

5.2.2 Articular (TMJ) Disc

The condyle and glenoid fossa are separated by an articular disc. The disc of the TMJ has formerly been incorrectly referred to as a meniscus. In the TMJ, the disc divides the joint cavity into superior and inferior joint spaces with attachments circumferentially around the disc. The disc functions as an actual articulating surface, thus actively factoring into TMJ movements. On the other hand, a meniscus is defined as a crescent-shaped piece of cartilage attached on only one side of the capsule, and it does not divide the joint space (Okeson 2008). As an example, a meniscus may be found in the knee joint. Like the condyle, the disc is wider in the ML direction than the AP, with dimensions of approximately 19 × 13 mm (Rees 1954). While the articular disc may have vascularization and innervation at its peripheral aspects, the vast majority of the disc in load-bearing areas are avascular and aneural (Rees 1954; Piette 1993). The disc prevents bone-on-bone attrition and facilitates joint function to include serving as a "shock absorber" or "load disperser" to distribute forces that may occur during mastication, trauma, or parafunctional behaviors such as clenching or grinding of the teeth.

The disc is roughly shaped like a bow tie: thinner in the middle and thicker at the periphery. The thinner portion is referred to as the intermediate zone (IZ). In a sagittal view, gross anatomically, there can be seen a thick anterior band (AB) and an even thicker posterior band (PB), relative to the thinner IZ. Disc collagen is wider in diameter on the lateral aspects of the disc than the center and may account for its shape. The TMJ disc is interposed between the articulating surfaces of the condyle and the glenoid fossa. The thicker PB of the disc will be positioned at the most superior point of the condyle. If the head of the condyle is likened to the face of a clock when viewed sagitally, the IZ of the TMJ disc will be situated on the right-side condyle at the 1 o'clock position, and for the left condyle, the IZ will be situated at the 11 o'clock position. It should be noted that the above-described position is considered the "normal" position. However, variations from this normal position are frequently found. Numerous anatomic and imaging studies within the non-painful, general population have consistently and repeatedly found the disc to be anteriorly displaced in approximately 30–33% of this population. This same finding is present in a temporomandibular disorder (TMD) pain population where it may be observed in approximately 37–40% of this group (Emshoff et al. 2003; Katzberg et al. 1996). Consequently, the clinician will need to make finer distinctions during history intake and clinical exam as to whether or not disc position is relevant in a patient who complains of TMJ pain with or without dysfunction.

As the disc is mostly avascular, nutrient and metabolic exchange to and from the disc occurs via passive diffusion along concentration gradients. The exchange occurs via synovial fluid and the capillaries in the retrodiscal tissues and those near the basement membrane of the synovial lining of the capsule. The consumption of nutrients and elaboration of by-products by metabolism within disc cells, however few they are, create a concentration gradient along which diffusion can take place. Solutes exchanged include oxygen, ions, and glucose. Disruptions in metabolic exchange are thought to have negative consequences. It has been found that increasing mechanical strain on the disc will impede ionic diffusion resulting, at times, in joint dysfunction (Wright et al. 2013).

The thickness of the TMJ disc varies from 0.5 mm at its thinnest aspect to 3 mm at its thickest (Nickel et al. 2001). Thinner discs produce friction faster, and this may be due to diminished weeping lubrication (Nickel et al. 2001). Detailed information regarding synovial fluid and lubrication will be discussed later in the chapter (see Sect. 5.4).

Architecture The disc of the TMJ may be categorized into a cellular component and an acellular component (Table 5.1). The vast acellular component is essentially the ECM. The interstitial fluid is comprised mainly of water which accounts for the majority of the ECM. The major acellular, non-water, molecular components of the disc primarily consist of type I collagen with interspersed proteoglycans and some elastin fibers (Detamore and Athanasiou 2003). This network of collagen and proteoglycans within the ECM assists in dispersing loading forces during jaw function and distributes these forces over a wider surface area. In this way, no singular point in the disc or articular cartilage becomes overwhelmed or compromised by bearing the entire load.

Cellular Content The disc is composed of dense fibrous connective tissue instead of fibrocartilage since there are no mature chondrocytes. The cellular component consists of fibroblasts, fibrocytes, and cells resembling fibrochondrocytes or chondrocyte-like cells (Stankovic et al. 2013; Detamore and Athanasiou 2003). This cellular component exhibits clusters of these chondrocyte-like cells throughout the disc with greater density in the center portions of the AB, IZ, and PB. The chondrocyte-like cells are fewer and are found paralleling the AP collagen bundle orientation (Mills et al. 1994). The presence of certain intermediate filament proteins associated

Table 5.1 Cellular content of fibrocartilage and the fibrous connective tissue of the disc

Component		Function
Cells	Fibrochondrocytes[a]	Secrete a cartilage matrix consisting of collagen and proteoglycans
	Fibroblasts	Synthesize extracellular matrix and collagen
	Fibrocytes	Mesenchymal cell, when activated, gives rise to fibroblasts
Intermediate filament proteins	Nestin	Indicates cells' ability to differentiate into other cells
	Glial fibrillary acidic protein	Present in maturing cells of the TMJ disc

[a]Absent within disc fibrous connective tissue network

with these cells gives hints to the behavior of that cell. Nestin is one such intermediate filament protein, and its presence suggests that the cell may differentiate to another cell as part of an adaptive response to disc damage (Stankovic et al. 2013). Glial fibrillary acidic protein (GFAP), when present within disc cells, suggests that the disc is maturing in response to an occlusal load resulting in a TMJ load, during dental development (Miyako et al. 2011).

Water Content The water content accounts for 66–80% of the weight of the TMJ disc (Detamore and Athanasiou 2003). In a porcine TMJ disc model, water content did not vary much from specimen to specimen ranging from 69–72% (Willard et al. 2012). Water content appears to decrease with the aging process (Nakano and Scott 1989). The water content is important as it plays a role not only in giving the disc its mass but also liberating water into the joint spaces. The ability of the disc to contribute to lubrication relative to condylar and articular fibrocartilage has been questioned (Zimmerman et al. 2015).

Collagen The major component of the ECM of the disc is type I collagen. Collagen type II is present in only trace amounts (Detamore et al. 2005). While type II collagen is found near the chondrocyte-like cells, type I collagen is found throughout the disc. Type I collagen is thicker and packs quite densely, clinically making the TMJ able to withstand heavy forces intermittently. Collagen generally runs in an undulating AP direction in the IZ but will take sudden turns into other directions as the fiber approaches the periphery (Detamore and Athanasiou 2003). These turns occur primarily from an AP direction to either a medial or a lateral one and little if any with superior or inferior turns (Mills et al. 1994). The collagen also displays crimps at a periodicity of every 10–30 microns (Berkovitz 2000). The crimping may impart an ability for the collagen network to withstand and rebound like a spring when loaded. In the periphery, collagen orientation may take on a ringlike formation (Shi et al. 2013; Detamore et al. 2005). Additionally, the diameter of the collagen fibers seems to be thinner in the IZ and wider in the periphery, possibly due to the primary load applied to the IZ. The diameter of collagen fibers is 18 ± 9 microns (Detamore et al. 2005). As measured in dry weight percentage, collagen accounted for 74–87% of disc weight, with central portions of the disc being at the lower end of the range (Willard et al. 2012). Other researchers have reported the dry weight of collagen to be lower at 60–62% (Dijkgraaf et al. 1995; Stankovic et al. 2013).

Proteoglycans As stated earlier in the section on articular cartilage, proteoglycans are glycoproteins that have a protein filament core with short GAG side chains. Proteoglycans are also abundant in the disc and are secreted by chondrocyte-like cells (Mills et al. 1994). GAG content within the disc assumes approximately 1% of the dry weight of the ECM in some studies (Fazaeli et al. 2016) but is reported to be higher in other studies, in the range of 5.3 ± 2% (Detamore et al. 2005). There are a variety of GAG types based on the particular chemical composition of the side chains. The most abundant GAG is chondroitin sulfate, accounting for 74% of the total GAG content (Detamore et al. 2005). The next most abundant GAG is dermatan sulfate. Collectively chondroitin sulfate and dermatan sulfate account for 84–90% of the total population of GAG within the disc ECM. These sulfated GAG proteoglycans are preferentially concentrated in the band areas of the disc, with a slight predilection toward the PB more than the AB (Mills et al. 1994). Hyaluronic acid is found in smaller amounts, reported to be 5–20% of the total GAG population. Keratan sulfate and heparin sulfate are present in trace amounts (Detamore and Athanasiou 2003).

Chondroitin sulfate proteoglycans (CSPG) are larger, are $>10^6$ Da, are predominantly of the chondroitin-6-sulfate variety, and are more numerous in the periphery. Dermatan sulfate proteoglycans (DSPG) are smaller and include biglycan (DS-PG1) and decorin (DS-PGII). Biglycan is weakly and evenly stained throughout the disc. Decorin is more intense at the anterior and posterior junctions of the disc and the periphery. Other proteoglycan types found in the disc ECM include aggrecan, fibromodulin, and lumican (Stankovic et al. 2013). Lumican is expressed more during inflammatory processes, particularly in the presence of interleukin-1 beta (Kiga et al. 2011).

Elastin Elastin fibers run parallel to collagen and are found predominantly in the posterior attachment of the TMJ but are also found throughout the disc (Mills et al. 1994). They are found in greater numbers in the periphery of the disc compared to the central portions and greater amounts in the superior layers of the disc than the inferior (Gross et al. 1999). Elastin infers upon the disc a resistance to elongation, or increased tensile strength. Along with the ECM proteoglycan content, elastin contributes to the osmotic swelling of the disc and thereby increasing its ability to withstand loading forces (Mills et al. 1994).

Mechanical Properties When a substance possesses different properties when analyzed in different directions, it is said to have anisotropy. The TMJ disc is one such anisotropic substance. Tested values in one location on the disc can differ from another location. For instance, when measuring diffusion gradients in the posterior aspect of the disc, the diffusion gradients in the ML direction are significantly faster than in the AP or supero-inferior direction (Shi et al. 2013).

The proteoglycan content of the disc enhances its stiffness. Proteoglycans also increase the disc's permeability to water. The disc modulus is reported to be 1.5–3.5 MPa, greater in the center and greater medially versus laterally. The modulus is 2–3 times greater in the center of the disc compared to more peripheral areas. According to studies of the disc in fresh cadaver specimens, faster loading speeds yielded an increase in disc stiffness (Chin et al. 1996). However, faster plowing speeds to assess friction over the surfaces of porcine discs in AP and mediolateral directions did not alter friction, but friction did decrease as plowing loads increased (Zimmerman et al. 2015).

With regard to internal friction within the disc, shear modulus increases with *compressive* strain and loading frequency but decreases somewhat with *shear* strain (Tanaka et al. 2004). The clinical correlate to the above information implies that the TMJ is well adapted to reduce friction within its articulating surfaces when greater loading forces are required during an initial bite into food or when chewing a bolus of food with a tougher consistency. In addition to the underlying bony structures, the collagenous component of the disc has great importance in resisting compressive forces. Experimentally disrupting the collagen network of the TMJ disc by the application of collagenase reduces its compressive strength by 50–90% (Fazaeli et al. 2016). This underscores the importance of collagen in resisting compressive forces.

As a unit, the AP orientation of collagen provides increased shear resistance to the AP motion of the condyle-disc complex. Overall, the disc and articular cartilage are best suited to undergo intermittent compression rather than sustained compression. Joint nutrition is maintained by diffusion of the synovial fluid as it is released during function and is dependent upon the positive and negative pressures within the superior and inferior joint spaces associated with condylar translation and seating. Logic dictates that clinical strategies used which interrupt persistent joint loading may have beneficial effects when the pain and dysfunction is intracapsular in nature.

Other areas of variability occur more at a macro level in terms of patient response variability. We know that normal loading forces help maintain joint architecture in the TMJ. We know that the TMJ is quite adaptable to normal, functional demands. The joint can adapt by remodeling its shape and architecture to maintain its integrity, most often without pain and dysfunction. A continuum between function, hyperfunction, and hypofunction along with minimal loading, physiologic loading, and excessive loading or parafunction all must be considered when analyzing TMJ joint dynamics (Ikeda et al. 2014). Over the course of the aging process, it is natural for joint remodeling and other changes to occur (Tanaka and Koolstra 2008; Westesson and Rohlin 1984).

Animal studies involving rabbit or porcine TMJ components are often used as models for the human TMJ. One such porcine study demonstrated that the friction coefficient of the disc is greater than that of the condyle. Other differences were found in that condylar friction decreased when the speed of a dynamic load increased, whereas friction was independent of load magnitude. While speed had no impact on disc friction, friction did decrease when heavier loads were applied. In both tissues, friction was less in an AP direction than a ML one. In disc displacements, the condyle may not align with the disc. Therefore, during mouth opening and subsequent disc reduction (in patients where the disc is reducible), this would result in the condyle contacting the disc in directions other than AP. Yet, condylar position was not related to the presence or absence of osseous changes in a radiographic study (Ren et al. 1995). Hence, while animal findings may show preferred mechanical directionality, it may not necessarily correlate to clinical implications.

Interestingly, TMD patients tend to be young-to middle-aged adults, while the elderly seem not to suffer from TMD pain. TMD once was considered a progressive condition, but a 30-year longitudinal study did not agree with this supposition (De Leeuw et al. 1995a, b, c). Compared to matched controls, patients with internal derangement of the disc and osteoarthrosis showed progression of radiographic degenerative joint disease (DJD). However, pain did not progress; instead, it diminished greatly and the majority reported undisturbed chewing function. The majority of the subgroup with a reducing disc remained so over this time course and displayed minimal DJD progression. The subgroup with a nonreducing disc showed more extensive radiographic changes, but this stabilized over time. The radiographic changes were mainly the development of condylar flattening and sclerosis which is thought to represent either a healing process or simply an adaptive response to joint loading versus an erosive appearance which indicates DJD progression.

5.2.3 Movement

The mandible articulates with the glenoid fossa and articular eminence of the temporal bone. As stated earlier, the articular disc is interposed between the load-bearing surfaces of the condyle and the glenoid fossa.

Movement is accomplished by the activity of the muscles of mastication. These traditionally include the masseter, temporalis, lateral pterygoid, and medial pterygoid bilaterally. Other muscles may assist as well, to include the anterior digastrics and activity of the cervical muscles to stabilize the head. The muscles of mastication receive their motor innervation from the third division of the trigeminal nerve. In turn, within the central nervous system, the nucleus responsible for the outflow of motor function is the trigeminal motor nucleus found within the trigeminal brain stem complex, situated adjacent to the trigeminal main sensory nucleus.

Initial opening comes with simultaneous contraction of the inferior lateral pterygoids along with the anterior digastric muscles, which depress the mandible inferiorly. Within the early process of opening, the condyle rotates along the inferior aspect of the disc (hinge axis). At roughly the 15–20 mm level of opening, the condyles continue to rotate, but now a translational movement of the mandible ensues. In other words, due to the contraction of the inferior lateral pterygoids, the condyle-disc complex moves in an anteroinferior direction downward and forward along the articular eminence. As a point of reference, maximum opening among the normal population is quite variable and ranges between 35 and 55 mm (Scrivani et al. 2008). As a general principle, rotation takes place in the inferior joint space between the articulating surfaces of the condyles and inferior portion of the disc. Translational movement takes place in the superior joint space between the slopes of the articular eminentiae and the superior aspect of the disc.

Near maximum opening, the mandible will continue to translate and rotate as the disc reaches the terminal movement position. It should be noted that during opening, the disc moves posteriorly relative to its starting location with the condyle-disc assembly seated in the fossa. During opening, as the condyle leaves its seated position, the retrodiscal tissues engorge with blood and come to fill the space created as a result of the condyle moving forward during mandibular translation. In the closed position, the condyle-disc assembly will initially articulate on its anterosuperior-medial location. At maximum opening, the condyle will articulate with the disc at its supero-posterior-lateral aspect (Helms et al. 1983).

When closing without resistance, the depressor muscles relax, blood leaves the retrodiscal tissues, and the condyle and disc return to their starting positions. When closing against resistance, the elevator muscles contract and include the masseter, temporalis, and medial pterygoid. In the presence of a bolus of food between the teeth, the superior head of the lateral pterygoid contracts and provides the so-called power stroke of mastication. Clenching and chewing activities additionally co-activate cervical muscles such as the sternocleidomastoid (Giannakopoulos et al. 2013; Clark et al. 1993). Other activities that invoke muscle activity include speaking, swallowing, and a variety of parafunctional habits such as clenching, chewing on fingernails and pencils, etc. In pathological conditions such as oromandibular dystonia, the movement is involuntary.

It is commonly found that the majority of individuals are able to open past the crest of the eminence (70–80%) (Obwegeser et al. 1987). As a variation of the normal, some individuals may open extremely wide as to bring the condyle well beyond the anterior aspect of the eminence. Clinically, this may be visually apparent as the lateral aspect of the condyle may create an elevation of the superficial tissues as it goes beyond the eminence, a visible bulge on maximum opening in the preauricular area of the face that may be accompanied by a late TMJ "thud-like" sound. If this is a momentary event and the condyle freely returns to the glenoid fossa, moving beneath the eminence, then this is termed a subluxation. For many individuals who can subluxate, this is an asymptomatic event. However, should the condyle be positioned anterior to the eminence without the ability of reducing on its own, this is termed a dislocation (open lock). In order to appreciate normal range of motion of the TMJ, anatomic studies have revealed that when viewed laterally during opening, the condyle travels 15 mm anteriorly whereas the disc travels 7 mm anteriorly relative to the closed mouth starting point (Rees 1954).

5.3 Posterior Attachment

The posterior attachment (PA), also known as the retrodiscal tissues, lays posterior to articular disc as its name implies. Previously, it was often referred to as the bilaminar zone. In contrast to the disc and articular cartilage, the PA is richly vascular and richly innervated and consists of copious fibroelastic tissue (Wilkinson and Crowley 1994). The presence of capillary fenestrations in the PA provides the means for metabolic exchange to occur between the cells and ECM of the disc and the articular cartilage. Its modulus of elasticity as a measure of stiffness is 1.54 MPa during normal condylar seating compared to 0.21 MPa at rest (Tanaka et al. 2002). The capacity of the PA to resist tensile forces has been shown as well (Tanaka et al. 2003). However, direct loading of a well-innervated, heavily vascularized structure such as the PA is not recommended as it may produce pain and inflammation.

The PA at its superior and inferior boundaries are bordered by the aptly named superior and inferior retrodiscal lamina. The superior retrodiscal lamina is coiled and loose in the closed mouth position. The superior and inferior retrodiscal laminae act as guidewires and limit the anterior movement of the disc during opening. Opening may continue as the condyle glides along the undersurface of the disc, but the disc itself will no longer move forward. These laminae do not stretch per se, but in cases of TMJ disc displacement, they elongate. Once elongated, they will not return to their original length. In the closed mouth position, the laminae are coiled. During wide jaw openings that invoke translation of the condyle, the coiled lamina straightens out. With opening movement of the jaw, the condyle translates anteriorly. The void left behind is occupied by the expansion of the PA as their capillaries engorge with blood, taking in 4–5 times the volume of blood relative to the closed mouth resting state (Wilkinson and Crowley 1994). This has been termed volumetric compensation. The function of the retrodiscal tissues may be to provide volumetric compensatory changes within the joint capsule to backfill the space voided by the condyle as it translates anteriorly within the glenoid fossa (Wilkinson and Crowley 1994).

Both the PA and the disc are soft tissues that can be visualized by magnetic resonance imaging (MRI). Comparing the PA volume in the closed mouth position and the open mouth position, it is quite obvious that the PA volume increases during opening. The PA, when traumatized, is often the location for TM joint edema, or joint effusions caused by an inflammatory response seen in some TMD patients, and is visible on MRI (Lee and Yoon 2009).

A study in 1996 by Pereira and colleagues compared histologic differences in the retrodiscal tissues and capsule of asymptomatic human TMJs with disc displacement to those with a complaint of TMJ pain with disc displacement. Asymptomatic joints showed loose and dense connective tissue with elastic fibers. Joints from the pain case group exhibited hyalinization of the connective tissues, narrowing of arterial lumens, and a tightly packed collagen network. There was no statistically significant difference between the two groups in terms of the presence of inflammatory cells and chondrocytes (Pereira et al. 1996). The study highlights that disc position is not always associated with pain. But it also shows histologic differences between the two groups of patients. Understanding the perpetuating factors that lead to adaptive remodeling in the displaced disc while leading to pain in another may yield better therapeutics targets for pain management.

5.4 Synovial Fluid

The synovial membrane (SM) which produces synovial fluid lines the TMJ except in the load-bearing areas of the condyle and fossa eminence. The SM is an extension of the lymphatic system and is thus responsible for drainage of the TMJ and its vicinity. The SM consists of two layers. The layer lining the inner aspect of the joint is termed the synovial intima, beneath which lies a layer called the subsynovial tissue (Dijkgraaf et al. 1996). The SM produces the synovial fluid (SF) which provides the joint with oxygen and provides the means for metabolic exchange between the avascular disc, the articular cartilage, and the vasculature at the periphery of the joint via fenestrations in the SM. The microcirculation of the SM is within the synovial intima and is near the joint cavity. Estimates put the depth of this microcirculatory system at 35 μm from the SM surface and may account for the high incidence of hemarthrosis associated with trauma (Levick 1995).

The SM consists of macrophage-like type A cells, near the articular space, and fibroblast-like type B cells. Type A cells can engulf and break down cellular debris and antigens. They are known to be involved in TMJ immune responses. Type B cells are noted for numerous amounts of rough endoplasmic reticulum in their cytoplasm. They secrete fibronectin, GAG, collagen, and HA (Nozawa-Inoue et al. 2003). Hyaluronic acid is important in maintaining viscosity of the synovial fluid to enhance condylar movement. There has been controversy as to whether the SM exhibits a true basement membrane. An immunohistochemical study of the rat TMJ showed that the type B cells demonstrated immunoreactivity to a laminin marker whereas type A cells did not (Nozawa-Inoue et al. 1999). This suggested that the type B cells may act as a basement membrane. This also underscores the function of type A cells. Due to their macrocytic activity, they need to have the ability to migrate. Thus, a cell-to-cell anchoring with laminin would not be expected.

Synovial fluid has two major functions: (1) metabolic exchange and (2) lubrication. The metabolic exchange, to include nutrient exchange, occurs along concentration gradients. A metabolic by-product would diffuse toward a slit, or fenestration, in the SM and travel to the synovial lymphatics or vasculature. With respect to lubrication, the SF allows for easy gliding within the TMJ and also serves as a means of protection to maintain the integrity of the articular surfaces during function.

Friction within synovial joints such as the knee or TMJ is reduced by the presence of the SF. There are two forms of lubrication: boundary lubrication and weeping lubrication. Boundary lubrication refers to the fluid that is elaborated from synovial tissues surrounding the TMJ and tends to adhere to the surfaces of the articulating surfaces. Boundary lubrication takes place with innocuous movements such as swallowing or speaking. Mucinous glycoproteins found in the SF include lubricin, albumin, and HA. Lubricin enhances boundary lubrication, reducing friction and ultimately optimizing joint mobility. Other lubricin functions include inhibition of synovial cell hyperplasia while preventing the adherence of various substances to articular surfaces. In a cohort of TMD patients compared to healthy controls, the TMD osteoarthritis subgroup had diminished lubricin concentrations in SF samples taken from the TMJ superior joint space (Wei et al. 2010). The coefficient of friction (COF) was increased in all three TMD patient groups studied (disc displacement with reduction, disc displacement without reduction, osteoarthritis), meaning that lubricin alone cannot explain the increased COF in TMD patients.

Weeping lubrication is fluid compressed out of the hydrated articular cartilage during loading events, such as biting into a bolus of food or in response to a jaw clench. As joint load increases, tissue fluid flows outward from the fibrocartilage of the condyle and the articular eminence until equilibrium is achieved (Zimmerman et al. 2015). When the load decreases, it is reabsorbed into the ECM of the fibrocartilage and fibrous connective tissue mentioned above. Increasing TMJ intracapsular pressure (ICP) above capillary perfusion pressure during clenching can impair venous return and have deleterious effects on the joint so that metabolic exchange does not properly occur. ICP in the TMJ at rest is near 0 mmHg. At maximum mouth opening, ICP is -53.8 ± 34.4 mmHg, while at maximum clench, it increases to 63.9 ± 52.2 mmHg (Nitzan 1994). These ICP recordings were measured in the anterolateral portion of the mandibular fossa in the superior joint space. Females in this study were able to generate a higher ICP than males. This was presumably due to the distance from dentition to the condylar axis representing a shorter lever arm in females, though this detail was not specifically studied. The delivery of an oral appliance in this study had the effect of decreasing ICP by 81% (Nitzan 1994).

Hyaluronic acid within the synovial fluid is a key mediator of joint lubrication. It attaches to the surface-active phospholipid layer (SAPL) of articular cartilage, itself creating a thin layer. The HA protects the SAPL from the degradative enzyme phospholipase A2 (PLA2) and also acts as an antioxidant. Reactive oxidative species and associated free radicals are produced during excessive joint loading, and this may lead to breakdown of the HA layer, thereby exposing the SAPL to PLA2. The downstream effect would be increased friction in the condyle-disc-fossa complex, perhaps acting as a precursor to TMJ internal derangements (Nitzan 2001; Milam 2005; Milam et al. 1998; Milam and Schmitz 1995; Zardeneta et al. 2000).

Much research has been conducted looking to synovial aspirates of TMD patients and comparing them to control aspirates in the hopes of finding molecular compounds that may precipitate or potentiate a degenerative process within a joint, either in the bone or its overlying layer of cartilage. Using bone as an example, as with other tissues, the bony matrix is replaced periodically through the degradative action of osteoclasts and then rebuilt via the action of osteoblasts. In a state of homeostasis, the degradation and synthesis of new bone balances each other. Should there be too much osteoclast activity or too little osteoblast activity, bone would eventually degenerate and lead to bony pathosis. Within SF, matrix metalloproteinases (MMP) are catabolic enzymes that function to break down the ECM of the cartilage. The MMP are controlled by the presence of tissue inhibitors of metalloproteinases (TIMP). Like the balance of osteoclasts with osteoblasts; the MMP/TIMP ratio must be kept in balance for optimal joint health and function. The SF aspirates of TMJ osteoarthritis (OA) patients, when compared to controls, showed elevated levels of MMP-1, MMP-2, MMP-3, and MMP-9 as well as a decrease in the MMP/TIMP ratio suggesting at least a correlation to OA, if not causation (Kanyama et al. 2000).

Other research has demonstrated that TMJ SF of OA patients show increases in interleukins (IL) and cytokines, particularly IL-12, IL-1B, IL-6, TNF-α (tumor necrosis factor), MCP-1 (monocyte chemoattractant protein), and PGE-2 (prostaglandin E2). Excess mechanical stress can activate the plasminogen activator system, leading to ECM proteolysis. TGF-1B (transforming growth factor) can induce chondrocyte apoptosis and induce MMP-9, MMP-13, and VEGF (vascular endothelial growth factor) resulting in abnormal subchondral bone remodeling (Wang et al. 2015; Kamelchuk and Major 1995; Haskin et al. 1995).

As stated previously, proteases are enzymes capable of degrading the ECM, and they are of four classes: (1) aspartic proteases, (2) cysteine proteases that operate mostly under acidic pH, (3) serine proteases, and (4) matrix metalloproteinases (MMP-1, MMP-2, MMP-3) operating best under neutral pH. Proteases are synthesized by chondrocytes, synovial cells, and inflammatory cells. In general, cytokines (IL I-XII, TNF, interferon) induce proteases which degrade the ECM, whereas growth factors such as insulin-like growth factor (IGF), fibroblast growth factor (FGF), and platelet-derived growth factor (PDGF) help build the ECM. Arachidonic acid and its metabolite classes of leukotrienes and thromboxanes can be derived from synovial cells by cytokines, especially by PGE-2, which is induced by IL-1 (Dijkgraaf et al. 1995).

Research (Milam and Schmitz 1995) investigating synovial aspirate has been performed, and this has led to the proposal for three mechanisms that can lead to articular injury. (1) Direct mechanical injury: Excess loading causes disruption of molecules and free radical formation. Arachidonic acid may be liberated at greater levels in the presence of free radicals. Hydrostatic pressure can activate heat-shock protein, which disrupts cellular cytoskeletons. (2) Hypoxia-reperfusion injury: Diminished blood flow and the accompanied decrease in oxygen in a compressed joint lead to hypoxia-nutrient deficits. When pressure is released, again free radicals, like superoxide anion, can be formed which can use the metal in hemoglobin to convert into a more reactive species, the hydroxyl anion. (3) Neurogenic inflammation: Substance P and CGRP (calcitonin gene related peptide) have been recovered from C-fiber nerve endings in the TMJ. Both these compounds are well-known mediators of pain and act on nociceptors.

Since TMD patients present with a strong female predilection, it has been proposed that hormonal influences either peripherally or centrally have an effect in nociceptive processing as estrogen receptors have been located in the TMJ (Bartley and Fillingim 2013; LeResche et al. 2003). Sex hormones may alter opioid, noradrenergic, and serotonergic modulatory activity within the central nervous system (Manson 2010). In low estrogen states, endogenous opioids are also at low levels in the thalamus, the nucleus accumbens, and the amygdala which, as a part of the limbic system, governs pain unpleasantness and the affective-motivational dimension of pain (Smith et al. 2006). This state was associated with hyperalgesia in females. The influence of hormones on the TMJ has been widely studied. Estrogen and prolactin have been shown in some models to have the net effect of bone degradation (Milam and Schmitz 1995). Estrogen is proposed to inhibit condyle chondrocyte proliferation with a net degradative effect on cartilage ECM. In contrast, estrogen is inhibitory to the harmful effects on chondrocytes exerted by nitric oxide (NO) (Wang et al. 2015).

In summary, the synovial membrane and the synovial fluid it produces are integral to the normal function and homeostasis within the TMJ. Disease states and parafunctional loads that are detrimental to the elaboration or consistency of the synovium may lead to detrimental, structural/mechanical effects.

5.5 Ligaments

A ligament is a band of dense, fibrous connective tissue that aids in mechanical reinforcement of joints. Ligaments originate from either bone or cartilage and then insert on other bones further afield. Furthermore, ligaments act as guidewires to a given joint, providing directionality and preventing extreme movements that may be harmful to the integrity of a joint. Ligaments have a very limited modulus of elasticity and in essence do not stretch. Under conditions of strain, they may elongate but will never return to their original length. In the case of TMJ anterior disc displacement, ligaments posterior to the disc elongate. TMJ surgical procedures that attempt to reposition the disc often relapse because once a ligament is elongated, it will no longer act to restrict movement in the way it had prior to the procedure.

5.5.1 Articular Capsule and Temporomandibular Joint Ligament

The fibrous articular capsule provides for the primary enclosure of the bony parts of the TMJ. The medial one half of the anterior TMJ has no capsule. The superior head of the lateral pterygoid muscle sends a small percentage of its fibers into the foot of the disc at the anteromedial aspect. Most of the lateral pterygoid superior belly fibers continue under the foot of the disc to attach into the condylar neck (pterygoid fovea). Lateral to the attachment of the muscle to the disc, the connective tissue forms a capsule-like structure with the appearance of loose areolar connective tissue.

The capsule on the medial and lateral walls of the joint is comprised of well-organized collagen fibers, but in the closed mouth position, they are not under tension. This laxity of the fibers does not firmly support the joint but allows the medial and lateral poles of the condyles to translate forward without straining or tearing the capsule. Ligaments have the primary functions of stabilization, guidance of movement, and limitations of movement. Most likely, ligaments associated with the masticatory system primarily function to limit the degree of condylar movement (Osborn 1985). The medial and lateral walls are reinforced by the medial and lateral temporomandibular joint ligaments (Hylander, 2006). The lateral TMJ ligament originates at the articular tubercle and inserts into the condylar neck. It is made up of superficial and deep components. The superficial fibers are oriented horizontally and are suggested to limit condylar retrusion thus protecting the retrodiscal tissues (Hylander 2006). The deep fibers are vertically oriented and have been suggested to be associated with limiting jaw opening (Osborn 1989; Hesse and Hansson 1988). The medial TMJ ligament is a functional thickening in the medial capsule oriented horizontally (Loughner et al. 1997). The posterior wall of the joint lacks a well-organized capsule. The loose vascular tissue (capillary bed) in this zone constitutes a meshwork of connective tissue made up of collagen, reticulin, and elastin which facilitates physiologic function during opening and closing.

5.5.1.1 Collateral Ligaments

The disc is reinforced both laterally and medially by the lateral discal ligament (LDL) and the medial discal ligament (MDL). These two ligaments are called collateral ligaments. The LDL runs from the lateral aspect of the disc to that lateral pole of the condyle, while MDL runs from the medial aspect of the disc to the medial pole. The LDL and MDL prevent lateral and medial movement of the mandible. Thus, they enable an AP movement of the mandible. Since they are reinforcing the boundaries of the inferior joint space, the movement they assist with is rotation.

5.5.2 Accessory Ligaments

There are other ligaments remote to the TMJ that are notable. The stylomandibular ligament prevents excessive protrusive mandibular movements. This ligament extends from the styloid process, runs anteriorly and inferiorly, and attaches on the medial aspect of the angle of the mandible. The sphenomandibular ligament does not appear to have a major role in jaw function, but it is of prominent size easily identified in gross anatomic sections. This ligament originates from the spine of the sphenoid bone, runs anteriorly and inferiorly, and inserts onto the spine of the lingula, which is found on the medial surface of the mandibular ramus.

5.6 Summary

There is a wide range of outcomes in any disease or condition studied in medicine. In the study of TMD, it may be helpful to think of patient factors and loading factors as determinants of clinical outcome. Symptoms such as pain and findings such as joint noises and the appearance of the TMJ on imaging must be assessed to determine if their presence is a significant contributor to the outcome. Understanding the form and function of this complex synovial joint in health will certainly enhance our ability to understand pathosis. This will result in optimal case-specific treatment outcomes.

Disclaimer The views expressed in this presentation are those of the authors and do not necessarily reflect the official policy or position of the Department of the Navy, the Department of Defense, or the US Government.

References

Bartley EJ, Fillingim RB. Sex differences in pain: a brief review of clinical and experimental findings. Br J Anaesth. 2013;111:52–8.

Berkovitz BK. Crimping of collagen in the intra-articular disc of the temporomandibular joint: a comparative study. J Oral Rehabil. 2000;27:608–13.

Bostwick JM, Jaffee MS. Buspirone as an antidote to SSRI-induced bruxism in 4 cases. J Clin Psychiatry. 1999;60:857–60.

Chen CY, Palla S, Erni S, Sieber M, Gallo LM. Nonfunctional tooth contact in healthy controls and patients with myogenous facial pain. J Orofac Pain. 2007;21:185–93.

Chin LP, Aker FD, Zarrinnia K. The viscoelastic properties of the human temporomandibular joint disc. J Oral Maxillofac Surg. 1996;54:315–8; discussion 318-9.

Clark GT, Browne PA, Nakano M, Yang Q. Co-activation of sternocleidomastoid muscles during maximum clenching. *J Dent Res*. 1993;72:1499–502.

De Leeuw R, Boering G, Stegenga B, De Bont LG. TMJ articular disc position and configuration 30 years after initial diagnosis of internal derangement. J Oral Maxillofac Surg. 1995a;53:234–41; discussion 241-2

De Leeuw R, Boering G, Stegenga B, De Bont LG. Symptoms of temporomandibular joint osteoarthrosis and internal derangement 30 years after nonsurgical treatment. Cranio. 1995b;13:81–8.

De Leeuw R, Boering G, Stegenga B, De Bont LG. Radiographic signs of temporomandibular joint osteoarthrosis and internal derangement 30 years after nonsurgical treatment. Oral Surg Oral Med Oral Pathol Oral Radiol Endod. 1995c;79:382–92.

Detamore MS, Athanasiou KA. Structure and function of the temporomandibular joint disc: implications for tissue engineering. J Oral Maxillofac Surg. 2003;61:494–506.

Detamore MS, Orfanos JG, Almarza AJ, French MM, Wong ME, Athanasiou KA. Quantitative analysis and comparative regional investigation of the extracellular matrix of the porcine temporomandibular joint disc. Matrix Biol. 2005;24:45–57.

Dijkgraaf LC, DE Bont LG, Boering G, Liem RS. The structure, biochemistry, and metabolism of osteoarthritic cartilage: a review of the literature. J Oral Maxillofac Surg. 1995;53:1182–92.

Dijkgraaf LC, De Bont LG, Boering G, Liem RS. Structure of the normal synovial membrane of the temporomandibular joint: a review of the literature. J Oral Maxillofac Surg. 1996;54:332–8.

Emshoff R, Brandlmaier I, Gerhard S, Strobl H, Bertram S, Rudisch A. Magnetic resonance imaging predictors of temporomandibular joint pain. J Am Dent Assoc. 2003;134:705–14.

Fazaeli S, Ghazanfari S, Everts V, Smit TH, Koolstra JH. The contribution of collagen fibers to the mechanical compressive properties of the temporomandibular joint disc. Osteoarthritis Cartilage. 2016;24:1292–301.

Fujisawa M, Kanemura K, Tanabe N, Gohdo Y, Watanabe A, Iizuka T, Sato M, Ishibashi K. Determination of daytime clenching events in subjects with and without self-reported clenching. J Oral Rehabil. 2013;40:731–6.

Giannakopoulos NN, Schindler HJ, Rammelsberg P, Eberhard L, Schmitter M, Hellmann D. Co-activation of jaw and neck muscles during submaximum clenching in the supine position. Arch Oral Biol. 2013;58:1751–60.

Gross A, Bumann A, Hoffmeister B. Elastic fibers in the human temporo-mandibular joint disc. Int J Oral Maxillofac Surg. 1999;28:464–8.

Haskin CL, Milam SB, Cameron IL. Pathogenesis of degenerative joint disease in the human temporomandibular joint. Crit Rev Oral Biol Med. 1995;6:248–77.

Helms CA, Katzberg RW, Morrish R, Dolwick MF. Computed tomography of the temporomandibular joint meniscus. J Oral Maxillofac Surg. 1983;41:512–7.

Hesse JR, Hansson TL. Factors influencing joint mobility in general and in particular respect of the craniomandibular articulation: a literature review. J Craniomandib Disord. 1988;2:19–28.

Hylander WL. TMDs – an evidence-based approach to diagnosis and treatment. Chicago, IL: Quintessence Publishing; 2006.

Ikeda Y, Yonemitsu I, Takei M, Shibata S, Ono T. Mechanical loading leads to osteoarthritis-like changes in the hypofunctional temporomandibular joint in rats. Arch Oral Biol. 2014;59:1368–76.

Kamelchuk LS, Major PW. Degenerative disease of the temporomandibular joint. J Orofac Pain. 1995;9:168–80.

Kanyama M, Kuboki T, Kojima S, Fujisawa T, Hattori T, Takigawa M, Yamashita A. Matrix metalloproteinases and tissue inhibitors of metalloproteinases in synovial fluids of patients with temporomandibular joint osteoarthritis. J Orofac Pain. 2000;14:20–30.

Katzberg RW, Westesson PL, Tallents RH, Drake CM. Anatomic disorders of the temporomandibular joint disc in asymptomatic subjects. J Oral Maxillofac Surg. 1996;54:147–53; discussion 153-5.

Kiga N, Tojyo I, Matsumoto T, Hiraishi Y, Shinohara Y, Makino S, Fujita S. Expression of lumican and fibromodulin following interleukin-1 beta stimulation of disc cells of the human temporomandibular joint. Eur J Histochem. 2011;55:e11.

Lee SH, Yoon HJ. The relationship between MRI findings and the relative signal intensity of retrodiscal tissue in patients with temporomandibular joint disorders. Oral Surg Oral Med Oral Pathol Oral Radiol Endod. 2009;107:113–5.

Leresche L, Mancl L, Sherman JJ, Gandara B, Dworkin SF. Changes in temporomandibular pain and other symptoms across the menstrual cycle. Pain. 2003;106:253–61.

Levick JR. Microvascular architecture and exchange in synovial joints. Microcirculation. 1995;2:217–33.

Loughner BA, Gremillion HA, Mahan PE, Watson RE. The medial capsule of the human temporomandibular joint. J Oral Maxillofac Surg. 1997;55:363–9; discussion 369-70

Manson JE. Pain: sex differences and implications for treatment. Metabolism. 2010;59(Suppl 1):S16–20.

Milam SB. Pathogenesis of degenerative temporomandibular joint arthritides. Odontology. 2005;93:7–15.

Milam SB, Schmitz JP. Molecular biology of temporomandibular joint disorders: proposed mechanisms of disease. J Oral Maxillofac Surg. 1995;53:1448–54.

Milam SB, Zardeneta G, Schmitz JP. Oxidative stress and degenerative temporomandibular joint disease: a proposed hypothesis. J Oral Maxillofac Surg. 1998;56:214–23.

Mills DK, Fiandaca DJ, Scapino RP. Morphologic, microscopic, and immunohistochemical investigations into the function of the primate TMJ disc. J Orofac Pain. 1994;8:136–54.

Miyako H, Suzuki A, Nozawa-Inoue K, Magara J, Kawano Y, Ono K, Maeda T. Phenotypes of articular disc cells in the rat temporomandibular joint as demonstrated by immunohistochemistry for nestin and GFAP. J Anat. 2011;219:472–80.

Nakano T, Scott PG. Proteoglycans of the articular disc of the bovine temporomandibular joint. I. High molecular weight chondroitin sulphate proteoglycan. Matrix. 1989;9:277–83.

Nickel JC, Iwasaki LR, Feely DE, Stormberg KD, Beatty MW. The effect of disc thickness and trauma on disc surface friction in the porcine temporomandibular joint. Arch Oral Biol. 2001;46:155–62.

Nitzan DW. Intraarticular pressure in the functioning human temporomandibular joint and its alteration by uniform elevation of the occlusal plane. J Oral Maxillofac Surg. 1994;52:671–9; discussion 679-80

Nitzan DW. The process of lubrication impairment and its involvement in temporomandibular joint disc displacement: a theoretical concept. J Oral Maxillofac Surg. 2001;59:36–45.

Nozawa-Inoue K, Ajima H, Takagi R, Maeda T. Immunocytochemical demonstration of laminin in the synovial lining layer of the rat temporomandibular joint. Arch Oral Biol. 1999;44:531–4.

Nozawa-Inoue K, Amizuka N, Ikeda N, Suzuki A, Kawano Y, Maeda T. Synovial membrane in the temporomandibular joint--its morphology, function and development. Arch Histol Cytol. 2003;66:289–306.

Obwegeser HL, Farmand M, Al-Majali F, Engelke W. Findings of mandibular movement and the position of the mandibular condyles during maximal mouth opening. Oral Surg Oral Med Oral Pathol. 1987;63:517–25.

Okeson J. Management of temporomandibular disorders and occlusion. Mosby Elsevier: St Louis, MO; 2008.

Osborn JW. The disc of the human temporomandibular joint: design, function and failure. J Oral Rehabil. 1985;12:279–93.

Osborn JW. The temporomandibular ligament and the articular eminence as constraints during jaw opening. J Oral Rehabil. 1989;16:323–33.

Pereira FJ, Lundh H, Eriksson L, Westesson PL. Microscopic changes in the retrodiscal tissues of painful temporomandibular joints. J Oral Maxillofac Surg. 1996;54:461–8; discussion 469

Piette E. Anatomy of the human temporomandibular joint. An updated comprehensive review. Acta Stomatol Belg. 1993;90:103–27.

Rees L. The structure and function of the mandibular joint. Br Dent J. 1954;96:125–33.

Ren YF, Isberg A, Westesson PL. Condyle position in the temporomandibular joint. Comparison between asymptomatic volunteers with normal disk position and patients with disk displacement. Oral Surg Oral Med Oral Pathol Oral Radiol Endod. 1995;80:101–7.

Ross M, Romrell L. Histology. Baltimore, MD: Williams & Wilkins; 1989.

Schaefer L, Iozzo RV. Biological functions of the small leucine-rich proteoglycans: from genetics to signal transduction. J Biol Chem. 2008;283:21305–9.

Scrivani SJ, Keith DA, Kaban LB. Temporomandibular disorders. N Engl J Med. 2008;359:2693–705.

Shi C, Wright GJ, Ex-Lubeskie CL, Bradshaw AD, Yao H. Relationship between anisotropic diffusion properties and tissue morphology in porcine TMJ disc. Osteoarthritis Cartilage. 2013;21:625–33.

Singh M, Detamore MS. Biomechanical properties of the mandibular condylar cartilage and their relevance to the TMJ disc. J Biomech. 2009;42:405–17.

Smith YR, Stohler CS, Nichols TE, Bueller JA, Koeppe RA, Zubieta JK. Pronociceptive and antinociceptive effects of estradiol through endogenous opioid neurotransmission in women. J Neurosci. 2006;26:5777–85.

Stankovic S, Vlajkovic S, Boskovic M, Radenkovic G, Antic V, Jevremovic D. Morphological and biomechanical features of the temporomandibular joint disc: an overview of recent findings. Arch Oral Biol. 2013;58:1475–82.

Tanaka E, Del Pozo R, Sugiyama M, Tanne K. Biomechanical response of retrodiscal tissue in the temporomandibular joint under compression. J Oral Maxillofac Surg. 2002;60:546–51.

Tanaka E, Hanaoka K, Tanaka M, Van Eijden T, Iwabe T, Ishino Y, Sasaki A, Tanne K. Viscoelastic properties of bovine retrodiscal tissue under tensile stress-relaxation. Eur J Oral Sci. 2003;111:518–22.

Tanaka E, Kawai N, Hanaoka K, Van Eijden T, Sasaki A, Aoyama J, Tanaka M, Tanne K. Shear properties of the temporomandibular joint disc in relation to compressive and shear strain. J Dent Res. 2004;83:476–9.

Tanaka E, Koolstra JH. Biomechanics of the temporomandibular joint. J Dent Res. 2008;87:989–91.

Wang XD, Zhang JN, Gan YH, Zhou YH. Current understanding of pathogenesis and treatment of TMJ osteoarthritis. J Dent Res. 2015;94:666–73.

Wei L, Xiong H, Li B, Cheng Y, Long X. Boundary-lubricating ability and lubricin in synovial fluid of patients with temporomandibular joint disorders. J Oral Maxillofac Surg. 2010;68:2478–83.

Westesson PL, Rohlin M. Internal derangement related to osteoarthrosis in temporomandibular joint autopsy specimens. Oral Surg Oral Med Oral Pathol. 1984;57:17–22.

Wilkinson TM, Crowley CM. A histologic study of retrodiscal tissues of the human temporomandibular joint in the open and closed position. J Orofac Pain. 1994;8:7–17.

Willard V, Arzi B, Athanasiou K. The attachements of the temporomandibular joint disc: a biochemical and histological investigation. Arch Oral Biol. 2012;57:599–606.

Wright GJ, Kuo J, Shi C, Bacro TR, Slate EH, Yao H. Effect of mechanical strain on solute diffusion in human TMJ discs: an electrical conductivity study. Ann Biomed Eng. 2013;41:2349–57.

Zardeneta G, Milam SB, Schmitz JP. Iron-dependent generation of free radicals: plausible mechanisms in the progressive deterioration of the temporomandibular joint. J Oral Maxillofac Surg. 2000;58:302–8; discussion 309

Zimmerman BK, Bonnevie ED, Park M, Zhou Y, Wang L, Burris DL, Lu XL. Role of interstitial fluid pressurization in TMJ lubrication. J Dent Res. 2015;94:85–92.

Part III

Dysfunction of the Masticatory System

Myogenous Disorders

6

Heidi Crow, Yoly Gonzalez,
and Shehryar N. Khawaja

Abstract

Temporomandibular disorders (TMD) involving the muscles are the most common form of TMD. Various theories have been proposed as to why masticatory muscles may become painful and lead to TMD or even influence the shift from an acute to a chronic form. No single etiologic factor has been identified, and so myalgia has been classified as "multifactorial," which ultimately makes it more challenging to identify risk factors and their unique contributions to the disease process. Even more, this multi-domain characterization of these conditions equally challenges the transfer of these concepts to clinical care including potential prevention or early intervention. New validated diagnostic criteria, however, have the potential to clearly identify what disorders are being investigated and may lead to targeted therapeutic solutions with clearly defined outcome measures.

6.1 Introduction

In the area of orofacial pain (OFP), particularly temporomandibular disorders (TMD), muscle disorders are the most common presentation, representing greater than 50% of diagnoses within representative samples. This fact is not trivial; particularly taking into account that OFP affects approximately 39 million adults in the USA (Renton et al. 2012). Population-based studies suggest the prevalence of TMD has been estimated to range from 2.8 to 10.5%. These estimates are modified by gender, age, race, and socioeconomic status (Isong et al. 2008; Janal et al. 2008).

H. Crow (✉)
Oral Diagnostic Sciences, University at Buffalo, Buffalo, New York, NY, USA
e-mail: hccrow@buffalo.edu

Y. Gonzalez, DDS, MS, MPH
Oral Diagnostic Sciences, TMD and Orofacial Pain, University at Buffalo, Buffalo, New York, NY, USA
e-mail: ymg@buffalo.edu

S.N. Khawaja, BDS, MS
Graduate, Oral and Maxillofacial Pain, Department of Oral and Maxillofacial Surgery, Massachusetts General Hospital, Boston, MA, USA
e-mail: Khawaja_Nasir@hsdm.harvard.edu

© Springer International Publishing AG 2018
H.A. Gremillion, G.D. Klasser (eds.), *Temporomandibular Disorders*,
https://doi.org/10.1007/978-3-319-57247-5_6

More so, within the spectrum of signs and symptoms among most masticatory muscle diagnoses, pain is widely accepted as the most common feature or chief complaint, and it is probably the most frequent and disabling symptom in medicine. In addition, signs and symptoms may include limited range of motion and compromised function, which may be patient reported and/or clinically evident.

In the clinical arena, the goal is to provide the most efficacious care, which is based on proper diagnosis and the best understanding of the phenomenology or explanatory models involved in the conditions under study. Therefore, diagnosis should be based upon criteria in which validated methodological principles are followed by an evidence-based approach.

This chapter will first discuss the postulated models of etiologies of muscle pain. Secondly, it will explore the various etiologies of muscle conditions, such as direct and indirect trauma, parafunction, and psychosocial and genetic factors. Lastly, the current diagnostic classification of masticatory muscle conditions will be presented. From diagnostic and management perspectives, it is important to understand the nature of the relationship between masticatory muscle pain and motor function. Over the years, multiple theories have been postulated in an attempt to explain this association. Different explanatory models have been discussed in the literature. Among them, as outlined above, are the Vicious Cycle of Pain Model, the Pain Adaptation Model, the Integrated Pain Adaptation Model, and the Motor Adaptation to Pain Model.

6.2 Vicious Cycle of Pain Model

The Vicious Cycle of Pain Model (VCPM), presented by Travell et al. (1942), asserts that cycles of muscle hyperactivity and pain are self-perpetuating. It suggests that an initiating factor, such as an abnormal posture, excessive or aberrant movement, or stress, results in muscle pain. Moreover, it proposes that muscle pain, in turn, leads to hyperactivity of the muscle itself or fatigue, which leads to further muscle pain and dysfunction, thus perpetuating the cycle (Murray and Peck 2007; Peck et al. 2008).

The suggested mechanism of the VCPM is that activation of muscle nociceptors results in the increased firing of muscle spindle-afferent neurons through the direct excitation of gamma-motor neurons (Johansson and Sojka 1991). This neuronal excitation clinically translates as an increase in muscle activity. However, this results in the deterioration in the functional capability of muscle spindle-afferent transmission, a loss of proprioceptive acuity, poor muscular coordination, and the increased accumulation of inflammatory substances, which results in muscle pain or fatigue (Peck et al. 2008; Johansson and Sojka 1991).

The literature in support of this association between muscle pain and muscle hyperactivity is confounding and limited. Furthermore, the findings have been inconsistent, possibly due to methodological problems associated with the characterization of muscle activity. Most of these past studies have used oral parafunctional behaviors as a surrogate to muscle activity. Moreover, they have relied on non-validated and non-standardized questionnaires and/or clinical oral examinations for the assessment of oral parafunctional behaviors, and the focus has been restricted to clenching and bruxism only (Manfredini and Lobbezoo 2009; Manfredini and Lobbezoo 2010). Investigations using the exogenous model of pain, such as an injection of hypertonic saline into the muscle, reported no changes in muscle activity (Svensson et al. 1998; Matre et al. 1998).

Clinical studies using surface electromyographic (EMG) activity recordings demonstrated some success in determining an association between muscle hyperactivity and pain (Glaros and Burton 2004; Raphael et al. 2013). It has been suggested that a possible explanation for such findings may be attributed to the contamination of surface jaw muscle EMG activity recordings from activity in the muscles of facial expression (Cecere et al. 1996). However, surface electrodes may have advantages over fine-wire electrodes when characterizing "whole-muscle" behavior rather than single motor units.

Nevertheless, recent investigations using surface EMG or standardized validated questionnaires in a multivariate statistical model have suggested an association between psychological characteristics and muscle activity, whereas no association has been found between muscle pain and muscle activity (Khawaja et al. 2015a, b).

The VCPM oversimplifies the intricate association between muscle pain and activity. It does not take into consideration the multidimensional nature of pain, neuroplasticity associated with the chronicity of pain, or the effect of supraspinal pathways on pain.

6.3 Pain Adaptation Model

The Pain Adaptation Model (PAM) described by Lund et al. (1991) proposes that alterations in muscle activity are a consequence of the presence of pain. This model is based on the review of literature on chronic musculoskeletal pain conditions, such as temporomandibular disorders, chronic lower back pain, fibromyalgia, and post-exercise muscle soreness (Murray and Peck 2007; Peck et al. 2008; Johansson and Sojka 1991).

The proponents of this model hypothesize that the presence of pain results in the inhibition of alpha-motor neurons during the agonist phase of muscle activity, whereas the effects of pain are proposed to be reversed during the antagonist phase of muscle movement. These changes are expressed as a reduction in maximum muscle contraction, range of movement, and velocity of motion. These authors speculate that these changes are "adaptive" and thereby protect the muscle from potential damage (Lund et al. 1991). If the PAM is valid, then some of the parafunctional behaviors, such as clenching and grinding, may not be considered as perpetuating factors in the continuity of masticatory muscle pain.

Multiple clinical and animal investigations on alterations in masticatory muscle function, secondary to experimentally introduced pain in the musculoskeletal region, support this model. These studies have found a reduction in masseter muscle activity during mandibular-closing movements and an increase in masseter muscle activity during mandibular-opening movements (Lund et al. 1991; Svensson et al. 1996; Falla et al. 2007; Farina et al. 2005).

However, there are several studies that do not support the PAM. Some investigations have reported no effect of pain on the alteration of muscle activity or the force of contraction (Khawaja et al. 2015c; Kumar et al. 2015; Ro et al. 2002). Similar effects have also been observed in investigations on the effects of pain on paraspinal muscles (van Dieen et al. 2003) and forelimb muscle activity (Ervilha et al. 2004).

The PAM parallels the principles of physiological homeostasis and neurophysiology. However, it does not take into account the psychosocial aspect of pain, neuroplasticity, genetics, and inter- or intraindividual variations in pain behavior. Similarly, no information is available regarding the onset or perpetuation of the nociception or the pain in the orofacial region. Alternatively, a broader model called the Integrated Pain Adaptation Model (IPAM) has been posited, which includes the existing PAM as a subset (Murray and Peck 2007; Peck et al. 2008).

6.4 Integrated Pain Adaptation Model

The IPAM proposed that the effect of pain on motor activity relies on the complex interaction of distinctive biopsychosocial characteristics, as well as the anatomical and functional complexity of the individual sensory-motor system (Murray and Peck 2007; Peck et al. 2008). The model is based on the premise that the masticatory system is adaptable and can perform a required task using multiple muscle recruitment pathways.

The model states that under non-painful circumstances, the brain will activate the appropriate motor units required to produce a specific movement. However, in the presence of pain, it suggests that pain interacts with the sensorimotor system to result in a unique characteristic pattern of muscle activation. The type of characteristic pattern is dependent on the anatomic and functional complexity of the jaw sensorimotor system, as well as the sensory-discriminative, motivational-affective, and cognitive-evaluative aspects of pain.

Alteration in the excitability of the primary motor cerebral cortex has been suggested as a possible proposed mechanism for the modification in recruitment pathways of masticatory muscles in this model (Murray and Peck 2007; Peck et al. 2008). This assumption is based on multiple experimental pain model investigations that have shown an inhibition of the excitability of primary motor cerebral cortex (Farina et al. 2001; Falla 2004). However, the inhibitory effect of nociceptive activity on facial motor cortical function has yet to be demonstrated in humans (Murray and Peck 2007; Peck et al. 2008).

The IPAM is, in part, a unification of components from the VCPM and the PAM. The Integrated Pain Adaptation Model theorizes that a unique motor response will be generated with the intention of minimizing pain and its associated distresses, similar to the PAM. However, it also postulates that in some individuals it may result in the aggravation of pain and associated disabilities, analogous to the VCPM. The factors influencing the type of individualistic response have not yet been determined. This may not be an easy task since the IPAM consists of various factors, which are postulated to interact in a complex manner with each other.

6.5 Motor Adaptation to Pain Model

The Motor Adaptation to Pain Model (MAPM), an enhancement of the IPAM, promotes the concept that noxious stimulation at a site results in a redistribution of activity within and between muscles. Furthermore, it incorporates the concept that changes in higher centers of the brain (e.g., psychosocial aspects) are an important feature in determining the final nature of the redistributed motor activity (Hodges and Tucker 2011).

The MAPM is based upon existing data at the micro (motor neuron discharge) and macro (whole-muscle behavior) levels. This theory incorporates five key elements that expand on the premise that the purpose for adaptation to pain is to reduce pain and protect the painful part but with a more flexible solution than what has been proposed by either the VCPM or the PAM and to a lesser extent than the IPAM. The key elements consist of the following principles:

1. Pain/injury or threat thereof involves the redistribution of activity within and between muscles.
2. This results in changes to the mechanical behavior of the musculature such as modified movement (direction/load distribution) and stiffness.
3. This leads to protection from further pain or injury or from threatened pain or injury.
4. This adaptation cannot be explained by simple changes in excitability but involves changes at multiple levels of the motor system, and these changes may be complementary, additive, or competitive.
5. Adaptation to pain results in short-term benefit but with the potential to develop long-term consequences due to factors such as increased load, decreased movement, and decreased variability.

Although this new theory for the motor adaptation to pain is consistent with clinical and experimental observations and provides a range of testable hypotheses, it requires additional validation and longitudinal studies to confirm whether non-resolution of adaptation is associated with long-term consequences.

In summary, the core mechanisms causing pain in most muscle conditions are not completely elucidated. Although there has been a focus on the role of the peripheral and central hyperexcitability as structural mechanisms, the influence of the biopsychosocial domains cannot be denied, and an integrative model will better explain not only the causation but also the perpetuation and prognostic outcomes (Table 6.1).

Table 6.1 Explanatory models of muscle pain

Theory	Author, year	Main idea
Vicious Cycle of Pain Model (VCPM)	Travell et al. (1942)	"Limitation of motion is primarily a reaction to pain, rather than the result to structural lesion. Muscle spasm causes pain and pain reflexly produce muscle spasm as a self-perpetuating pain vicious cycle"
Pain Adaptation Model (PAM)	Lund et al. (1991)	"In order to prevent further damage and promote healing, dysfunction that is characteristic of several types of chronic musculoskeletal pain is a normal protective adaptation and is not a cause of pain"
Integrated Pain Adaptation Model (IPAM)	Murray and Peck (2007)	"Pain results in a new, optimized recruitment strategy of motor units that represents the individual's integrated motor response to the sensory-discriminative, motivational-affective, and cognitive-evaluative components of pain. This recruitment strategy aims to minimize pain and maintain homeostasis"
Motor Adaptation to Pain Model (MAPM)	Hodges and Tucker (2011)	"Movement is changed in pain due to: redistribution of activity between muscles rather than stereotypical inhibition or excitation of muscles; modification of mechanical behavior in a variable manner with the objective to "protect" the tissues from further pain or injury, or threatened pain or injury; involvement of changes at multiple levels of the motor system that may be complementary, additive or competitive; and results in short-term benefit, but with potential long-term consequences"

6.6 Etiologies

The idea that we can find a single cause for the development of myalgia in TMD has long been discarded. The "multifactorial" nature of TMD has led to numerous theories and attempts at the identification of potential risk factors, none of which clearly explain why a given individual develops masticatory and/or cervical myalgia. Much of the literature is based on retrospective reviews, which often lack adequate data or exhibit deficiencies in standardization, which are fundamental methodological limitations (Scott et al. 1997). An additional limitation of the existing literature is that it has often utilized questionnaires which do not allow for a diagnosis of a muscle disorder as opposed to utilizing standardized validated clinical examinations such as the DC/TMD (Diagnostic Criteria for Temporomandibular Disorders) (Schiffman et al. 2014). However, a recent addition to the literature attempts to overcome these limitations by providing a prospective, longitudinal cohort study on the incidence of first-onset TMD—the OPPERA (Orofacial Pain: Prospective Evaluation and Risk Assessment) study (Bair et al. 2013). Given that the prevalence of TMD has been estimated in approximately 10% in the adult population (Janal et al. 2008) and the incidence of TMD in 3.7% (Slade et al. 2013), the risk of becoming an onset case increases with the presence of other comorbid painful conditions (Sanders et al. 2013).

Various risk factors have been proposed as etiologic factors; however, this chapter will focus on the characteristics that have been identified through case-control methods, predominantly through the OPPERA baseline case-control study (Maixner et al. 2011). The risk factors identified include direct trauma, indirect trauma, parafunction or microtrauma, psychological, and genetic factors (Table 6.2).

Direct trauma would seem to be a reasonable risk factor for developing myogenous TMD, and in an acute situation, it can be associated with the development of myositis or transient myalgia. However, chronic TMD does not have as clear of an association with direct trauma. In a study of martial arts professional fighters, there was an increased prevalence of myogenous TMD in high-performance mixed martial arts participants compared to non-athletes (Bonotto et al. 2016). However, when retrospectively looking at individuals who had mandibular

Table 6.2 Etiology of muscle pain

	Main idea	Supports	Does not support	Study design
Direct trauma	External jaw trauma will lead to the development of TMD	Certain types of hard and/or soft tissue injuries including fractures may be associated with increased TMD signs and symptoms (Tabrizi et al. 2014)	History of external jaw trauma was not associated with first-onset TMD (Ohrbach et al. 2013)	Ohrbach et al. (2013) prospective cohort study Tabrizi et al. (2014) retrospective cohort study
Indirect trauma	Is flexion-extension injury (whiplash), as a form of indirect trauma, related to developing TMD	A recent systematic review showed that the prevalence of flexion-extension injury trauma in TMD patients is higher than in non-TMD controls (Häggman-Henrikson et al. 2014). A case-control study reported a higher frequency of disc displacement and myofascial pain in patients also diagnosed with late (symptoms persisting 6 months or longer after injury) flexion-extension (Marini et al. 2013). A recent systematic review also indicated that incidence rates of TMD may also be higher in flexion-extension trauma (Häggman-Henrikson et al. 2013)	A controlled prospective study utilizing a standardized exam did not demonstrate increased incidence of TMD (Kasch et al. 2002)	Kasch et al. (2002) prospective cohort study Häggman-Henrikson et al. (2014) systematic review Marini et al. (2013) case-control series Häggman-Henrikson et al. (2013) systematic review
Parafunction and microtrauma	Repetitive oral behaviors lead to muscle overuse and/or joint overload	Self-report of frequent and/or multiple parafunctional behaviors are associated with first-onset TMD (Ohrbach et al. 2013)		Ohrbach et al. (2013) prospective cohort study
Psychological factors	Certain psychological factors may contribute to the first onset of TMD	Somatic symptoms have the strongest association with first-onset TMD (Kasch et al. 2002)		Kasch et al. (2002) prospective cohort study
Genetics	Certain genetic domains may predispose an individual to the development of TMD	Increased risk of myofascial pain in COMT polymorphism (Fillingim et al. 2013)	OPPERA did not find significant differences in the panel of genes they tested between those that developed or did not develop TMD (Mladenovic et al. 2016)	Mladenovic et al. (2016) prospective cohort study Fillingim et al. (2013) cross-sectional case control

TMD temporomandibular disorders, *COMT* catechol-O-methyltransferase, *OPPERA* Orofacial Pain: Prospective Evaluation and Risk Assessment

fractures (Tabrizi et al. 2014), only certain types of fractures resulted in an increased prevalence of TMD. When evaluating the incidence of first-time TMD, direct trauma did not have an association with developing TMD (Ohrbach et al. 2013).

Indirect trauma to the orofacial region has been associated with extension-flexion injuries (Smith et al. 2011). There are extensive reports in the literature, both associated and non-associated with extension-flexion injuries. One issue with many of these reports is that they are based on a history of extension-flexion or cervical injury without a reasonable time sequence associated with the onset of myogenous TMD (Häggman-Henrikson et al. 2016). Two prospective studies of acute extension-flexion injuries have differing outcomes, one demonstrating no increased incidence in developing myogenous TMD (Kasch et al. 2002) and the other with an increased incidence of developing TMD symptoms as determined by questionnaire (Häggman-Henrikson et al. 2016).

Additional evidence is needed utilizing standardized exams and recording the timeframe from the indirect injury to the development of myogenous TMD symptoms.

Parafunction or microtrauma has been suspected in contributing to myogenous TMD without much direct evidence that it is related to causing myogenous TMD. However, recent evaluations resulting from the OPPERA study show that frequent self-reports of multiple types of parafunctional activities are increased in individuals reporting first-onset myogenous TMD (Ohrbach et al. 2013).

Case-control studies have highlighted an association of psychological factors with chronic pain, including chronic myogenous TMD. These studies have limited value in terms of identifying risk factors for TMD, since the question remains whether the psychologic factor developed due to the chronic myogenous TMD pain or acted as an increased risk factor for developing painful myogenous TMD. By evaluating a number of psychological factors based on a large cohort of individuals without myogenous TMD, and then following them for an average of approximately 3 years, the OPPERA study was able to ascertain various factors that were associated with the development of first-onset myogenous TMD (Fillingim et al. 2013). Increased somatic symptoms remained a robust risk factor, potentially highlighting an increased general symptomatology (a widespread collection of body symptoms) or an increased body awareness and potential preoccupation with symptoms. Additional factors highlighted in univariate analysis included negative mood, stress, and other general psychological symptoms (Fillingim et al. 2013).

Genetic variations using DNA sampling methods were analyzed in the OPPERA baseline case-control study and determined various associations between certain genes and TMD (Smith et al. 2011). Furthermore, in another cross-sectional study (Mladenovic et al. 2016), a relationship between catechol-O-methyltransferase (COMT) polymorphism and myofascial pain using the RDC/TMD (Research Diagnostic Criteria for Temporomandibular Disorders) criteria was reported. The findings in the prospective OPPERA study, evaluating whether any of the selected genetic panels were associated with the onset of myogenous TMD, were less positive (Smith et al. 2013). None of the panels were directly associated; however, there were associations with intermittent predictors of myogenous TMD, as listed previously. There is speculation that the initial onset of myogenous TMD, as evaluated by the OPPERA study, may not have direct genetic risk factors; however, transitioning from acute to chronic myogenous TMD may have some genetic influences.

6.7 Diagnostic Classification

Historically, multiple classification systems have been presented in the literature; among them is that by the American Academy of Orofacial Pain (2013), which has been strongly endorsed by clinicians, as well as the RDC/TMD criteria (Dworkin and LeResche 1992), which has not only been recently validated but has also evolved into the DC/TMD (Schiffman et al. 2014). One of the great improvements associated with this new classification system is that it does not target a particular audience, as it is presented for both clinical and research practices. It also provides the strongest internal and external validity, allowing for a transition from content validity to data-driven criterion. It is important to emphasize that this diagnostic criteria has maintained, similarly to its predecessor, a dual Axis system: Axis I, also known as physical diagnoses, and Axis II, or an assessment of psychosocial and behavioral factors.

Table 6.3 Validated muscle diagnoses

Muscle diagnosis	Criteria		
Criterion validity: based on sensitivity and specificity estimates using appropriate reference standard diagnosis			
	History	Clinical	Sensitivity/specificity
Myalgia (Schiffman et al. 2014)	Pain localized in the muscles of mastication, modified by either function or parafunction	Confirmed localization of the pain in the areas of interest. Familiar pain[a] upon vertical range of motion or muscle palpation	90% and 99%
Myofascial pain with referral (Schiffman et al. 2014)	Same as above	Confirmed localization of the pain in the areas of interest. Familiar pain upon muscle palpation is beyond the boundary of the muscle palpated	86% and 98%
Headaches attributed to TMD (Schiffman et al. 2014)	Headache localized exclusively in the temporal region, which is modified by function and parafunction. Conditioned to the pre- or coexistence of painful TMD diagnoses	Confirmed localization of the headache on the temporal region. Familiar headache upon vertical and horizontal range of motion and/or palpation of the temporal muscles	89% and 87%

TMD temporomandibular disorder
[a]Familiar pain: defined as similar or like the pain the individual has experienced in the last 30 days

Specifically for the pain-related classifications presented in Table 6.3, the DC/TMD provides acceptable validity, supported by both sensitivity and specificity values; this group of conditions represents the most common conditions among the umbrella of TMDs as well. These definitive diagnoses are based on self-reported items, which address the pain history in conjunction with the structure of a standardized clinical examination, which address the patient's clinical characterization. During the structured clinical examinations, the clinician not only has to verbalize clear commands in order to establish an efficient level of understanding and communication with the patient but also to gather information in a consistent and reliable manner. In regard to the examination technique, it is equally important that the clinician adopts the concept of calibration in order to maintain the clinical skills, for example, reaching and maintaining a target pressure of 1 kg for the palpation of the masseter and temporalis muscles for a period of 5 s in several areas of the muscles. It is important to recognize that the Axis II assessment does not influence the diagnostic classification; however, it may contribute to the onset and perpetuation of the TMD (Schiffman and Ohrbach 2016).

Myalgia and myofascial pain with referral are defined as pain of the muscle origin that is modified by function and/or parafunction. The information, in regard to the chief complaint of pain localized in the masticatory structures, is obtained from the history questionnaire. Specifically in the DC/TMD, the time frame utilized is within the last 30 days. Additional relevant questions in this instrument cover the concepts of modification by function or parafunction, which are assessed within the same time frame of 30 days (Schiffman et al. 2014).

A common question in clinical practice concerns the presence of pain upon awakening. Even though data suggests that pain-related awakening occurs in about 30% of patients with persistent pain conditions and is associated with pain intensity (Benoliel et al. 2009), this particular item is sometimes taken as a surrogate of sleep-related parafunctional activity and does not stand out in the validated criterion. However, it is a question included in the TMD pain screener instrument (Gonzalez et al. 2011). This screening instrument is considered a component of the DC/TMD

(Schiffman et al. 2014) and provides sensitivity and specificity values of 99% and 97%, respectively (Gonzalez et al. 2011).

The concept of familiar pain which has been previously presented (Gonzalez and Mohl 2006) is present in the DC/TMD as a diagnostic criterion, being a surrogate of replication of the chief complaint of pain. This familiar or similar pain, which is provoked upon palpation, represents the conceptualized mechanical pain model, which involves the application of pressure stimulation to induce pain from deep structures as a response from receptors in deep somatic tissues, such as muscle, fascia, and aponeuroses (Graven-Nielsen and Arendt-Nielsen 2010).

It is important to realize that even though the DC/TMD for the muscle disorders localized the replication of familiar pain either during mandibular movement or palpation at the masseter and/or temporalis muscles, the intention was not to omit other muscles that could be involved. Although other muscles can be examined to assess the construct of familiar pain during mandibular movement and palpation, the clinician must be aware that such locations including the lateral pterygoid, temporalis tendon, and posterior and submandibular regions had low reliability (Schiffman et al. 2010). The last condition within the validated group of diagnoses is headache attributed to TMD. The criterion for this diagnosis is parallel to myalgia. Therefore, the history component includes presence of headache in the temporal region during the last 30 days and the modification of such headaches by function and parafunction. The clinical component consists of confirmed localization of the headaches in the temporal region and replication of headaches during mandibular movement or during palpation of the temporalis muscle. The International Headache Society (IHS) in their most current classification of headache disorders (Headache Classification Committee of the International Headache Society (IHS) 2013) attempted to include this validated criteria and recommended the use of the DC/TMD (Schiffman et al. 2014). Nevertheless, the IHS failed by maintaining the need for clinical or imaging evidence of temporomandibular joint pathology while there is evidence supporting that joint structural changes may not be associated with pain. In addition the inclusion of replication or familiar pain during provocation construct that is pivotal to the diagnostic criterion was ignored.

The groups of diagnoses presented in Table 6.4 represent a group of conditions that do not have estimates of sensitivity and specificity but have construct and content validity; these are not as common but still have clinical relevance for the profession. These conditions were presented by Peck and colleagues in the expanded taxonomy of the DC/TMD (Peck et al. 2014). They are tendonitis, neoplasms, movement disorders, and masticatory muscle pain attributed to systemic/central pain disorders. Their criteria were consensus-based derived from expert opinion and review of the literature using as a context the AAOP taxonomy (The American Academy of Orofacial Pain 2013).

These postulated pain diagnoses provide a framework to assess progression from a localized muscle pain condition such as localized myalgia to myofascial pain or myofascial pain with referral, representing different levels of severity, which may require unique treatment approaches and prognostic characteristics and mechanisms ranging from a local phenomenon to a centrally mediated condition (Peck et al. 2014).

In summary, various theories have been postulated to describe the mechanism behind the development and etiology of muscle pain. The IPAM and further enhanced MAPM are the most adequate models to explain the mechanism by which chronic muscle pain occurs, integrating the sensory-motor system and the multidimensional nature of pain.

Temporomandibular disorders are still considered to be multifactorial, due to the fact that no unique or singular exposure can explain causation. With the development of the DC/TMD, however, the ability to adequately characterize patients and the disease process allows the clinician to target personalized treatment modalities for the management of muscle TMDs subgroups.

Table 6.4 Non-validated muscle diagnoses

Muscle diagnosis	Criteria		
Construct and content validity: based on expert opinion and review of the literature			These diagnoses do not have sensitivity and specificity values
	History	Clinical	Sensitivity/specificity
Local myalgia (Schiffman et al. 2014)	As myalgia	Confirmation of localization of pain in the temporalis and masseter muscle Familiar pain with palpation Pain with palpation localized to the immediate site of the palpating finger	N.A.[a]
Myofascial pain (Schiffman et al. 2014)	As myalgia	Familiar pain upon palpation of masseter or temporalis with **spreading** beyond the site of palpation but within the boundary of the muscle	N.A.
Myositis (Peck et al. 2014)	Pain of muscle origin with inflammatory characteristics. Secondary to acute trauma or chronic autoimmune conditions (Calcification of the muscle can occur)	Local pain, presence of edema, erythema, and increase in temperature Limited range of motion Non-specific serologic test, such as creatine kinase and inflammatory markers	N.A.
Spasm (Peck et al. 2014)	Sudden onset of myalgia Immediate report of limited range of motion	Myalgia as above in any masticatory muscle Limited range of motion in the direction that elongates the affected muscle Laboratory testing: elevated intramuscular EMG activity when compared to the contralateral unaffected side	N.A.
Contracture (Peck et al. 2014)	Muscle shortening due to fibrosis Progressive loss of range of motion	Unassisted and assisted opening are limited <40 mm Firm, resistance to assisted movements	N.A.
Hypertrophy (Peck et al. 2014)	Muscle enlargement usually a non-painful condition associated with overuse, familial, or genetic origin Evidence of enlargement confirmed by photographs or previous records	Evidence of the enlargement through photographs and confirmed by examination	N.A.

[a]N.A.: sensitivity/specificity not assessed

References

American Academy of Orofacial Pain. Diagnosis and management of TMDs. In: de Leeuw R, Klasser GD, editors. Orofacial pain guidelines for assessment, diagnosis, and management. Illinois: Quintessence; 2013. p. 127–86.

Bair E, Brownstein NC, Ohrbach R et al. Study protocol, sample characteristics, and loss to follow-up: the OPPERA prospective cohort study. J Pain. 2013;14(12 Suppl):T2–19.

Benoliel R, Eliav E, Sharav Y. Self-reports of pain-related awakenings in persistent orofacial pain patients. J Orofac Pain. 2009;23(4):330–8.

Bonotto D, Namba EL, Veiga DM, et al. Professional karate-do and mixed martial arts fighters present with a high prevalence of temporomandibular disorders. Dent Traumatol. 2016;32(4):281–5.

Cecere F, Ruf S, Pancherz H. Is quantitative electromyograpphy reliable? J Orofac Pain. 1996;10:38–47.

Dworkin SF, LeResche L. Research diagnostic criteria for temporomandibular disorders: review, criteria, examinations and specifications critique. J Craniomandib Disord. 1992;6(4):301–55.

Ervilha UF, Arendt-Nielsen L, Duarte M, et al. The effect of muscle pain on elbow flexion and coactivation tasks. Exp Brain res. 2004;156:174–82.

Falla D. Unravelling the complexity of muscle impairment in chronic neck pain. Man Ther. 2004;9:125–33.

Falla D, Farina D, Dahl MK, et al. Muscle pain induces task-dependent changes in cervical agonist/antagonist activity. J Appl Physiol. 2007;102(2):601–9.

Farina S, Valeriani M, Rosso T, et al. Transient inhibition of the human motor cortex by capsaicin-induced pain. A study with transcranial magnetic stimulation. Neurosci Lett. 2001;314:97–101.

Farina D, Arendt-Nielsen L, Graven-Nielsen T. Experimental muscle pain reduces initial motor unit discharge rates during sustained submaximal contractions. J Appl Physiol. 2005;98:999–1005.

Fillingim RB, Ohrbach R, Greenspan JD, et al. Psychological factors associated with development of TMD: the OPPERA prospective cohort study. J Pain. 2013;14(12 Suppl):T75–90.

Glaros AG, Burton E. Parafunctional clenching, pain, and effort in temporomandibular disorders. J Behav med. 2004;27:91–100.

Gonzalez YM, Mohl ND. Masticatory muscle pain and dysfunction. In: Laskin DM, Greene CS, Hylander WL, editors. TMDs: an evidence-based approach to diagnosis and treatment. 1st ed. Illinois: Quintessence; 2006. p. 255–69.

Gonzalez YM, Schiffman E, Gordon S, et al. Development of a brief and effective temporomandibular disorder pain screener questionnaire: reliability and validity. J Am Dent Assoc. 2011;142(10):1183–91.

Graven-Nielsen T, Arendt-Nielsen L. Assessment of mechanisms in localized and widespread musculoskeletal pain. Nat Rev Rheumatol. 2010;6:599–606.

Häggman-Henrikson B, List T, Westergren HT, et al. Temporomandibular disorder pain after whiplash trauma: a systematic review. J Orofac Pain. 2013;27(3):217–26.

Häggman-Henrikson B, Rezvani M, List T. Prevalence of whiplash trauma in TMD patients: a systematic review. J Oral Rehabil. 2014;41(1):59–68.

Häggman-Henrikson B, Lampa E, Marklund S, et al. Pain and disability in the jaw and neck region following whiplash trauma. J Dent Res. 2016;95(10):1155–60.

Headache Classification Committee of the International Headache Society (IHS). The international classification of headache disorders, 3rd edition (beta version). Cephalalgia. 2013;33(9):629–808.

Hodges PW, Tucker KJ. Moving differently in pain: a new theory to explain the adaptation to pain. Pain. 2011;152:S90–8.

Isong U, Gansky SA, Plesh O. Temporomandibular joint and muscle disorder-type pain in the U.S. adults: the National Health Interview Survey. J Orofac Pain. 2008;22(4):317–22.

Janal MN, Raphael KG, Nayak S, Klausner J. Prevalence of myofascial temporomandibular disorder in US community women. J Oral Rehabil. 2008;35(11):801–9.

Johansson H, Sojka P. Pathophysiological mechanisms involved in genesis and spread of muscular tension in occupational muscle pain and in chronic musculoskeletal pain syndromes: a hypothesis. Med Hypotheses. 1991;35:196–203.

Kasch H, Hjorth T, Svensson P, et al. Temporomandibular disorders after whiplash injury: a controlled, prospective study. J Orofac Pain. 2002;16(2):118–28.

Khawaja SN, Nickel JC, Iwasaki LR, et al. Association between waking-state oral parafunctional behaviours and bio-psychosocial characteristics. J Oral Rehabil. 2015a;42(9):651–6.

Khawaja SN, Iwasaki LR, Dunford R, et al. Association of masseter muscle activities during awake and sleep periods with self-reported anxiety, depression, and somatic symptoms. J Dent Health Oral Disord Ther. 2015b;2(1)

Khawaja SN, McCall W Jr, Dunford R, et al. Infield masticatory muscle activity in subjects with pain-related temporomandibular disorders diagnoses. Orthod Craniofac Res. 2015c;18(Suppl 1):137–45.

Kumar A, Castrillon E, Svensson KG, et al. Effects of experimental craniofacial pain on fine jaw motor control: a placebo-controlled double-blinded study. Exp Brain Res. 2015;233:1745–59.

Lund JP, Donga R, Widmer CG, et al. The pain-adaptation model: a discussion of the relationship between chronic musculoskeletal pain and motor activity. Can J Physiol Pharmacol. 1991;69:683–94.

Manfredini D, Lobbezoo F. Role of psychosocial factors in the etiology of bruxism. J Orofac Pain. 2009;23:153–66.

Manfredini D, Lobbezoo F. Relationship between bruxism and temporomandibular disorders: a systematic review of literature from 1998 to 2008. Oral Surg Oral Med Oral Pathol Oral Radiol Endod. 2010;109:e26–50.

Marini I, Paduano S, Bartolucci ML, et al. The prevalence of temporomandibular disorders in patients with late whiplash syndrome who experience orofacial pain: a case-control series study. J Am Dent Assoc. 2013;144(5):486–90.

Matre DA, Sinkjaer T, Svensson P, Arendt-Nielsen L. Experimental muscle pain increases the human stretch reflex. Pain. 1998;75:331–9.

Maixner W, Diatchenko L, Dubner R, et al. Orofacial pain prospective evaluation and risk assessment study – the OPPERA study. J Pain. 2011;12(11 Suppl):T4–11.

Mladenovic I, Supic G, Kozomara R, et al. Genetic polymorphisms of catechol-O- methyltransferase: association with temporomandibular disorders and postoperative pain. J Oral Facial Pain Headache. 2016;30(4):30210.

Murray GM, Peck CC. Orofacial pain and jaw muscle activity: a new model. J Orofac Pain. 2007;21:263–78.

Ohrbach R, Bair E, Fillingim RB, et al. Clinical orofacial characteristics associated with risk of first-onset TMD: the OPPERA prospective cohort study. J Pain. 2013;14(12 Suppl):T33–50.

Peck CC, Murray GM, Gerzina TM. How does pain affect jaw muscle activity? The integrated pain adaptation model. Aust Dent J. 2008;53:201–7.

Peck CC, Goulet JP, Lobbezoo F, et al. Expanding the taxonomy of the diagnostic criteria for temporomandibular disorders (DC/TMD). J Oral Rehabil. 2014;41(1):2–23.

Raphael KG, Janal MN, Sirois DA, et al. Masticatory muscle sleep background electromyographic activity is elevated in myofascial temporomandibular disorder patients. J Oral Rehabil. 2013;40:883–91.

Renton T, Durham J, Aggarwal VR. The classification and differential diagnosis of orofacial pain. Exp Rev Neurother. 2012;12(5):569–76.

Ro JY, Svensson P, Capra N. Effects of experimental muscle pain on electromyographic activity of masticatory muscles in the rat. Muscle Nerve. 2002;25:576–84.

Sanders AE, Slade GD, Bair E, et al. General health status and incidence of first- onset temporomandibular disorder: the OPPERA prospective cohort study. J Pain. 2013;14(12 Suppl):T51–62.

Scott BA, Clark GM, Al HJP e. Comparing prospective and retrospective evaluations of temporomandibular disorders after orthognathic surgery. J Am Dent Assoc. 1997;128(7):999–1003.

Schiffman EL, Ohrbach R, Trulove EL, et al. The research diagnostic criteria for temporomandibular disorders V: methods used to establish and validate revised Axis I diagnostic algorithms. J Orofac Pain. 2010;24(1):63–78.

Schiffman E, Ohrbach R, Trulove E, et al. Diagnostic criteria for temporomandibular disorder (DC/TMD) for clinical and research applications: recommendations of the international RDC/TMD consortium network and orofacial pain special interest group. J Oral Facial Pain Headache. 2014;28(1):6–27.

Schiffman E, Ohrbach R. Executive summary of the diagnostic criteria for temporomandibular disorders for clinical and research applications. J Am Dent Assoc. 2016;147(6):438–45.

Slade GD, Fillingim RB, Sanders AE, et al. Summary of findings from the OPPERA prospective cohort study of incidence of first-onset temporomandibular disorder: implications and future directions. J Pain. 2013;14(12 Suppl):T116–24.

Smith SB, Maixner DW, Greenspan JD, et al. Potential genetic risk factors for chronic TMD: genetic associations from the OPPERA case control study. J Pain. 2011;12(11 Suppl):T92–101.

Smith SB, Mir E, Bair E, et al. Genetic variants associated with development of TMD and its intermediate phenotypes: the genetic architecture of TMD in the OPPERA prospective cohort study. J Pain. 2013;14(12 Suppl):T91–101.

Svensson P, Arendt-Nielsen L, Houe L. Sensory-motor interactions of human experimental unilateral jaw muscle pain: a quantitative analysis. Pain. 1996;64:241–9.

Svensson P, De Laat A, Graven-Nielsen T, Arendt-Nielsen L. Experimental jaw-muscle pain does not change heteronymous H-reflexes in the human temporalis muscle. Exp Brain Res. 1998;121:311–8.

Tabrizi R, Bahramnejad E, Mohaghegh M, et al. Is the frequency of temporomandibular dysfunction different in various mandibular fractures? J Oral Maxillofac Surg. 2014;72(4):755–61.

Travell J, Rinzler S, Herman M. Pain and disability of the shoulder and arm treatment by intramuscular infiltration with procaine hydrochloride. J Am Med Assoc. 1942;120(6):417–22.

van Dieen JH, Selen LP, Cholewicki J. Trunk muscle activation in low-back pain patients, an analysis of the literature. J Electromyog Kinesiol. 2003;13:333–51.

Arthrogenous Disorders

7

John H. Campbell, Yoly Gonzalez, and Heidi Crow

Abstract

Disease involving the temporomandibular joint (TMJ) can be painful (arthralgia) and may involve disc disorders and/or bony destruction of the joint. Theories of progression of joint disorders, from displaced discs with reduction to displaced discs without reduction to degenerative joint disease (DJD), have been proposed but are not well supported in longitudinal studies. This chapter reviews proposed mechanical, hormonal, and inflammatory models that may lead to dysfunction and discusses current validated diagnostic schemes which may ultimately lead to more focused research protocols.

7.1 Introduction

Temporomandibular disorders (TMD) involving the temporomandibular joint (TMJ) can be placed into two general categories: pain, and functional disorders involving jaw movements. These are not mutually exclusive, and the range of dysfunction can range from a minor inconvenience to severe limitations in jaw function. This chapter will review the structural elements involved in TMJ disorders, theories behind pain development and maintenance within the joint, and clinical classifications and risk factors in development of the disorders.

7.2 Intra-articular Considerations

Temporomandibular articular disc disorders, commonly referred to as "internal derangements" (ID), have long been thought to be the primary etiological factors in functional joint disturbances and pain in patients with temporomandibular dysfunction. In the most common iteration, some precipitating event—trauma, for

J.H. Campbell, DDS, MS, FACS
Oral and Maxillofacial Surgery, University at Buffalo, Buffalo, NY, USA
e-mail: jc294@buffalo.edu

Y. Gonzalez, DDS, MS, MPH
Oral Diagnostic Sciences, TMD and Orofacial Pain, University at Buffalo, Buffalo, NY, USA
e-mail: ymg@buffalo.edu

H. Crow, DMD, MS (✉)
Oral Diagnostic Sciences, University at Buffalo, Buffalo, NY, USA
e-mail: hccrow@buffalo.edu

© Springer International Publishing AG 2018
H.A. Gremillion, G.D. Klasser (eds.), *Temporomandibular Disorders*,
https://doi.org/10.1007/978-3-319-57247-5_7

instance—would cause anterior displacement of the disc. This would initially present as a displaced disc that reduces upon opening (clicking), often without pain, and progresses to a nonreducing disc (clicking disappears). The disc would then become a mechanical block to opening, and pain would result as the condyle functioned on the heavily innervated posterior attachment (retrodiscal tissues). Degenerative joint disease (DJD) would ultimately result, with crepitus, bony erosions and osteophytes, and even perforation of disc attachments (Wilkes 1989). In late stages, pain may resolve, but functional disturbances may persist (Rasmussen 1981). While this theory seems elegant in its simplicity, it cannot account for the finding that many individuals without a history of either pain or limited opening are found to have disc displacement (Katzberg et al. 1986). Neither can it explain the many patients with debilitating pain who have no evidence of disc derangement. In addition, recent evidence suggests that while this classical scenario may occur, disc displacement without reduction is not a necessary precursor for the development of degenerative joint disease. Indeed, in long-term follow-up, disc displacement and DJD remain stable over time with the potential for disease regression (Schiffman and Ohrbach 2016).

Clearly, disc position cannot be the sole etiology of joint pain and dysfunction. Over the past 20 years, significant strides have been made in delineation of possible molecular mechanisms that initiate a cascade of events hypothesized to lead to degeneration of joint structures (Milam 2005; Haskin et al. 1995). These proposed molecular events provide plausible explanations for destructive processes that lead to both functional disturbances and pain. While these mechanisms are addressed further elsewhere in this chapter, this section will focus on their possible effects on the disc, its function, and associated degenerative changes within the joint capsule.

Unlike most synovial joints, the TMJ is surfaced with fibrocartilage rather than hyaline cartilage. This is one reason that proposed mechanisms of disease associated with other joints may not be fully applicable to the TMJ. The disc, which completely separates the joint into two compartments in the normal state, is composed neither of hyaline nor fibrocartilage but rather of dense fibrous connective tissue.

The TMJ is a synovial joint, and in the normal state, synovium produces lubricating fluid that aids in joint movement and hence joint function. It is hypothesized by some that it is the breakdown of this lubricating system that predisposes to hypomobility and ultimately disc displacement in susceptible individuals (Nitzan 2003; Nitzan et al. 2004).

It should be noted that there are two proposed mechanisms for joint hypomobility associated with disc derangements. The first, previously described, is anterior disc displacement that does not reduce on jaw opening. The second, described by Nitzan, is the "anchored disc phenomenon" (ADP), whereby a normally positioned disc becomes "stuck" to the articular fossa either through excessive intraarticular pressure as a result of hyperfunction (suction cup phenomenon) or by way of degradation of the articular surfaces as a result of oxidative stress (Nitzan and Marmary 1997; Nitzan and Etsion 2002). Anchored disc phenomenon is thought to be distinct from anterior disc displacement, as the anchored disc resolves with joint lavage (arthrocentesis), while the nonreducing displaced disc responds less favorably to such intervention (Nitzan et al. 2002).

In each of the above scenarios (disc displacement or anchored disc), altered joint lubrication is the proposed mechanism for disc dysfunction. It is theorized that direct mechanical stresses generate reactive oxygen species that degrade components of synovial fluid, in particular hyaluronic acid (HA). As HA is thought to protect surface-active phospholipids (SAPLs) lining the articular surfaces from degradation by phospholipases, its degradation would expose the SAPLs to destruction by lipases and reduce the smooth lubrication function of the joint (Nitzan 2001). This could be the cause of ADP, and there is evidence that ADP joints are less able to cope with oxidative stress (Nitzan et al. 2002). With mouth opening, it is proposed that the increased friction causes elongation of disc attachments as the condyle moves over the lagging disc, ultimately resulting in disc displacement (Nitzan 2001). Chronic inflammation in an animal model has demonstrated deterioration of mechanical properties of the disc and alteration of its surface morphology (Wang et al. 2014). Finite element analysis suggests disc displacement during clenching is associated with increased stress in the articular capsule and retrodiscal tissues of the contralateral (unaffected) joint, which could theoretically lead to weakening of the tissues which maintain the disc in its normal position and possibly contribute to disc displacement (Hattori-Hara et al. 2014).

Other proposed molecular models of joint dysfunction may also have relevance to disc dysfunction. These include direct mechanical injury, hypoxia-reperfusion injury, and neurogenic inflammation. The common pathway for each is oxidative stress, that is, generation of free radicals which damage joint structure and function through multiple mechanisms (Milam et al. 1998; Milam and Schmitz 1995). Indeed, in a rat synovium model, injection of free radical precursors resulted in tissue changes consistent with free radical damage that included adhesion formation similar to that seen in human TMJ disease (Sheets et al. 2006). A mounting body of evidence supports the concept that free radicals may, in fact, play a role in TMJ degenerative disease. For example, lavage fluid obtained from superior joint space arthrocentesis has demonstrated the presence of denatured hemoglobin that could contribute ferrous iron in quantities sufficient to catalyze reactions that lead to free radical formation (Zardeneta et al. 1997, 2000). The presence of modified and cleaved proteins in lavage fluid from symptomatic patients provides at least some suggestion that they have been subjected to oxidative stress. Furthermore, high oxidative stress levels can contribute to the formation of cross-linked proteins that could serve as scaffolds for joint adhesions (Dijkgraaf et al. 2003).

The direct mechanical trauma model of degenerative temporomandibular disease hypothesizes that mechanical forces in the joint are, in susceptible individuals, sufficient to generate free radicals that could act in progressive joint deterioration (Haskin et al. 1995; Milam 2005). Shearing forces within the joint (i.e., mechanical stress) can generate radicals in both the organic and inorganic components of the bone (Symons 1988). Altered joint loading appears to be associated with condylar fibrocartilage degeneration prior to any detectable changes in the histological, biochemical, or mechanical properties of the disc, suggesting that molecular events affecting the bony components of the joint precede disc degeneration (Henderson et al. 2015).

The hypoxia-reperfusion model proposes that excessive joint loading exceeds the end capillary perfusion pressures of blood vessels in joint tissues. If persistent—as in chronic clenching—tissue hypoxia may result. As blood flow is restored during mandibular opening or relaxation, excessive amounts of reactive oxygen species are generated. These can damage not only disc tissue as indicated above but also may have damaging effects on cells and other extracellular components. In fact, intra-articular pressures have been demonstrated to be greater than capillary perfusion pressure during clenching, and significantly higher compressive forces in the superior compartment of the joint have been demonstrated in females compared to males, although there is conflicting data regarding such gender differences (Nitzan 1994; Casares et al. 2014). This could, if true, help to partially explain the higher prevalence of internal derangement in females. In addition, opening the bite with an oral appliance significantly reduces intra-articular pressure, a possible explanation for the palliative effect of appliances for some patients (Nitzan 1994).

The neurogenic inflammation hypothesis suggests that proinflammatory neuropeptides contained in retrodiscal tissues and other parts of the TMJ may be released by mechanical stimulation and indirectly prompt an inflammatory response. The final common pathway is, again, production of free radicals that promote degenerative changes in susceptible individuals. Neuropeptides, including calcitonin gene-related peptide, substance P, vasoactive intestinal polypeptide, and neuropeptide Y, have been observed in human disc autopsy specimens that showed no evidence of arthritic change (Haeuchi et al. 1999). While the significance is unclear, these substances could be involved in both regulation of blood flow and nociception. Interestingly, neuropeptides have also been isolated from human TMJs in patients with rheumatoid arthritis and other arthropathy signs and symptoms, although there did not appear to be any correlation between the concentration of neuropeptides and clinical signs and symptoms or arthroscopic findings (Appelgren et al. 1991; Holmlund et al. 1991).

Reported sexual dimorphism in the presence of estrogen receptors suggests that response to estrogen is an additional factor in development of joint damage leading to disc and joint dysfunction. Estrogen may be indirectly implicated in joint laxity and fibrocartilage degeneration through its effects on enhancing cellular responses to relaxin, known to stimulate matrix metalloproteases (Milam 2005). It has also been hypothesized that inflammatory pain in temporomandibular disorders may be enhanced by the effect of estrogen on specific sodium channels, contributing to the gender difference in TMD prevalence (Bi et al. 2015).

Another possible contributing factor to TMJ osteoarthritis (OA) may include alteration in the vascular supply to the bone. Since the fibrocartilage surfacing the joint relies, at least in part, on nutrients supplied by the underlying bone, obstruction of the bone's vascularity could be anticipated to alter the structural and functional integrity of the overlying cartilage. In support of this concept, a rat model of chemically induced hemolysis and disseminated thrombosis has demonstrated histological and radiographic features consistent with OA. Further study will better elucidate what effect vascular obstruction might have in the pathogenesis of temporomandibular OA (Amir et al. 2011).

While these proposed mechanisms, especially taken together, provide plausible possibilities for temporomandibular arthritides including disc derangements, they have not been definitively proven. Much of the data comes from non-primate animal studies, and much of the human data has been gleaned from analysis of fluids and tissues derived from symptomatic patients. Even "control" patients in some publications had either some joint abnormality or were thought to be suffering from "hysteric dysfunction" (i.e., a conversion disorder in which psychological stress is manifested by physical complaints) and therefore had "normal" joints (Nitzan et al. 2002; Nitzan 1994). Until better analysis of the normal situation can be achieved, our understanding of disease will continue to remain incomplete. Nonetheless, the preponderance of evidence at present suggests that molecular events that adversely affect the cartilage, bone, synovium, and lubrication system of the joint precede disc displacement. Thus, disc displacement is probably not the sole, or even primary, dysfunctional process in TMJ disease.

7.3 Inflammatory Models of Pain Development

Pain in the joint, commonly referred to as arthralgia, has been frequently associated with inflammation in the synovial lining (Gynther et al. 1998). However, arthralgia is not necessarily an inflammatory process. Free nerve endings as well as sensory nerve end organs have been identified in the disc itself (Asaki et al. 2006), but the underlying mechanism of their activation is not known. Most animal models of TMJ pain involve rodents, with inflammatory products inducing a nociceptive response, which then can be further evaluated (Table 7.1). The OA models also start with a traumatic event, which triggers a cascade of various neuromodulated events resulting in pain and inflammatory breakdown in the joint complex. Moving from animal models to human subjects, however, does not provide such a clear picture, and the inflammatory progression models demonstrated in animals do not mimic what is seen in longitudinal studies in humans. In the TMJ Impact study, 14% of the magnetic resonance imaging (MRI) images

Table 7.1 Rodent models of osteoarthrosis and cytokine release

Authors	Animal model	Methods	Outcome
Wang et al. (2012)	72 female rats	Injection of monosodium iodoacetate (MIA) into the upper compartment TMJ	Progression of OA, nociceptive response corresponds to inflammatory changes
Oliveira-Fusaro et al. (2012)	124 male rats	5-Hydroxytryptamine (5-HT) injected into TMJ	Nociceptive response directly to 5-HT, as well as 5-HT induced release of prostaglandins and norepinepherine
Hawkins and Durham (2016)	50 male rats	Prolonged jaw opening	Increased nocifensive responses until day 14
			Increased cytokines in the trigeminal ganglion and upper cervical spinal cord after nocifensive behavior ceased

Table 7.2 Cytokine studies, knee versus TMJ

Authors	Demographics	Methods	Joint	Inflammatory markers
Bigoni et al. (2013)	48 male subjects with acute ACL tears	Analysis of synovial fluid	Knee	Increased IL-1β, IL-6, IL-8; decreased IL-1ra; no difference TNF-α
Bigoni et al. (2017)	46 males; 23 females; 30–72 years of age with chronic meniscal tears	Analysis of synovial fluid	Knee	Increased IL-6, IL-8, IL-10, TNF-α; decreased IL-1ra
Kellesarian et al. (2016)		Systematic review, 15 studies included	TMJ	80% (12/15 studies) showed a positive correlation between cytokine levels (see Table 7.3) and TMJD

Proinflammatory interleukins (IL): IL-1β, IL-6, IL-8; tumor necrosis factor (TNF)-α; anti-inflammatory interleukins IL-1ra and IL-10; temporomandibular joint dysfunction (TMJD)

of the TMJ showed progression of disease as compared to 86% that were unchanged or improved over an approximate 8-year period. The hard tissue evaluation for DJD of the TMJ demonstrated similar findings, with progression in 15% of the joints and unchanged or improved findings in 85% of the joints (Schiffman and Ohrbach 2016).

Analysis of joint aspirations for various inflammatory cytokine levels has yielded plenty of information, but how to interpret the information has proved difficult. A recent systematic review (Kellesarian et al. 2016) yielded fifteen papers where control groups were used to compare amounts of various cytokine levels (Tables 7.2 and 7.3). These articles compared OA subjects with internal disc derangement (ID) and control subjects. However, some of the studies separated ID subjects from OA subjects, and some grouped them together. In addition, the variability of inclusion criteria used to determine the groups of patients made it difficult to ensure that the studies were consistent with uniformity of patient populations.

One further area of concern in the cytokine measurement studies is that while various amounts may be considered statistically different, it is unknown if there is clinical significance. Only one study in the systematic review grouped patients according to pain (Lee et al. 2010), which would presumably correlate with inflammation. While this group recorded higher values of IL-6 and TNF-α, the values were not statistically significant. In addition, relative values have not yielded diagnostic categories that can be used to assess joint health or progression of disease, limiting clinical value in aspirate analysis. At this time, biochemical markers in TMJ aspirations remain an area of interest but have unknown implications in disease progression.

Table 7.3 Studies which used control groups to compare various joint aspirates with patient groups (*Adapted from Kellesarian et al. 2016)

Cytokine	Articles that report different levels in patients vs. controls	Articles that report no difference in levels between patients vs. controls	Comments
IL-1β	↑ in patients Takahashi et al. (1998) Kubota et al. (1998) Kaneyama et al. (2002) Kaneyama et al. (2005) Vernal et al. (2008)	Shinoda and Takaku (2000) Kaneyama et al. (2003)	Takahashi et al. (1998) and Kaneyama et al. (2002) had four groups: ID with clicking, ID with locking, OA, and controls. Kubota combined ID and OA in one group. Kaneyama et al. (2003, 2005) had three groups: ID, OA, and controls. Shinoda had four groups: control, TMJD without osseous change, with osseous change, and with osseous change and disc damage
IL-2	↑ in patients (OA) Vernal et al. (2008)	Wake et al. (2013)	Wake: compared controls to TMJ chondromatosis patients
IL-6	↑ in patients Fu et al. (1995) Takahashi et al. (1998) Kubota et al. (1998) Shinoda and Takaku (2000) Kaneyama et al. (2002) Kaneyama et al. (2004) Kaneyama et al. (2005) Wake et al. (2013)	Vernal et al. (2008) Lee et al. (2010)	Fu: DJD higher levels than muscle disorder patients but no difference in levels DJD compared to ID
IL-8	↑ in patients Takahashi et al. (1998) Kaneyama et al. (2002)	Wake et al. (2013)	
IL-10		Fang et al. (1999)	Fang: undetectable in either OA, ID, or controls
IL-11	↑ in patients Kaneyama et al. (2004)		Higher in joints with osseous change
IL-12	↑ expression in controls Vernal et al. (2008)		
IL-17	↑ in patients Vernal et al. (2008)	Kaneyama et al. (2004)	
TNF-α	↑ in patients Takahashi et al. (1998) Fu et al. (1995) Kaneyama et al. (2002) Kaneyama et al. (2005) Lee et al. (2010) Vernal et al. (2008)	Kaneyama et al. (2003) Wake et al. (2013) Lee et al. (2010)	Fu: higher DJD than ID Lee: grouped as control, those in pain, those with limited opening, and those with clicking
TNF-β	↑ in patients Vernal et al. (2008)	Fang et al. (1999) Wake et al. (2013) (both found no detectable levels in either group)	
IFN-γ	↑ in patients Takahashi et al. (1998) Vernal et al. (2008)	Wake et al. (2013) (no detectable levels in either group)	
TGF-β1	↑ in patients Fang et al. (1999)		Higher levels in OA than internal derangement
EG-VEGF	↑ in controls Herr et al. (2011)		Higher level in controls
OCIF/OPG	↑ in patients Kaneyama et al. (2003)		

IL interleukin, *TNF* tumor necrosis factor, *IFN* interferon, *TGF* tumor growth factor, *OCIF/OPG* osteoclastogenesis inhibitory factor/osteoprotegerin, *EG-VEGF* endocrine gland-derived vascular endothelial growth factor, *ID* internal derangement, *OA* osteoarthritis, *TMJD* temporomandibular joint dysfunction, *DJD* degenerative joint disease

7.4 Diagnostic Classification

The study of temporomandibular disorders (TMD) is complex because of the variety of conditions that are under this umbrella. Among these conditions, we can identify some that are pain related, while others are mechanical in nature. In addition, developmental and congenital conditions have been described as well. Therefore, to evaluate the etiology, natural history, and diagnostic procedures of these conditions becomes a challenge not only for researchers but also for clinicians.

Furthermore, the validity of the diagnostic criteria, explanatory models, theories, and belief systems used in everyday practice comes into question. It is universally accepted that in order to advance understanding in the field, we need to have reliable and valid classification systems and diagnostic criteria.

Among the variety of conditions affecting the TMJ, the most prevalent has been described as noninflammatory, although there is a change or deterioration of the articular cartilage and subsequently the hard tissue, followed by secondary inflammatory changes (Tanaka et al. 2008). It has been postulated that such degenerative changes could be the result of dysfunctional remodeling due to a failure of the host adaptive capacity (Tanaka et al. 2008).

One of the most common conditions affecting the TMJ is DJD, currently defined as a degenerative disorder involving the TMJ and characterized by deterioration of the articular tissue, including osseous changes in the condyle and/or articular eminence (Schiffman et al. 2014). This condition has been previously described as osteoarthrosis and osteoarthritis in the literature, and in a recent study, using a convenience sample, the prevalence of osteoarthrosis and osteoarthritis was 14% and 32%, respectively. Specifically, disc displacement with reduction was 31%. Meanwhile disc displacement without reduction without limited opening was 33% and 10% with limited opening (Schiffman et al. 2010).

Several classifications have been presented, describing a continuum from disc displacement with reduction to OA, based on a combination of signs and symptoms. Among these signs and symptoms are joint sounds, pain, limited range of motion, and imaging findings. This is linked to an important milestone in the field of TMD, which includes the establishment of a standardized criterion for the assessment of imaging, such as MRI and computed tomography (CT). The presentation of this comprehensive image criteria and establishment of radiologist reliability (Ahmad et al. 2009) allowed for the testing of the validity of the diagnostic criteria for pain-related and intra-articular conditions (Schiffman et al. 2014). In particular, for soft tissue assessment, MRI has excellent reliability for determining disc position, while CT has similar characteristics for the assessment of hard tissues (Ahmad et al. 2009).

It is important to realize that these are clinical diagnoses, which include examination and self-report components. The validity of these clinical diagnoses was assessed using the imaging characterization as "reference standards" for the intra-articular conditions and consensus diagnosis for the pain-related condition (Ahmad et al. 2009; Schiffman et al. 2014).

7.5 Arthralgia

Among the TMD pain-related conditions, the Diagnostic Criteria for Temporomandibular Disorders (DC/TMD) describes arthralgia as pain of TMJ origin, which is modified by function or parafunction. It is relevant to clarify that arthralgia as presented by the DC/TMD is a diagnostic category with clear criteria and not simply joint pain. In addition to the self-reported history items, during the clinical examination, confirmation of pain localization in the TMJs and replication of such pain is needed. Pain replication can be provoked during mandibular movements, including opening, closing, lateral, and protrusive, or during palpation of the lateral pole and/or around the pole. It is important to note that palpation, both static on the lateral pole and dynamic around the pole, is done with 1 and 2 kg of pressure, respectively. The sensitivity and specificity of arthralgia are 89% and 98%, respectively;

Table 7.4 Criteria for arthralgia

Arthralgia		
Pain of joint origin affected by jaw movement, function, or parafunction, and replication of this pain occurs with provocation testing of the TMJ		
Criteria	History	Patient reports pain in the jaw, temple, ear, or in front of the ear Patient reports pain modified with jaw movement, function, or parafunction
	Exam	Localization of pain confirmed in the area of the TMJ Report of familiar pain in the TMJ with at least one of the following provocation test: palpation of the lateral or around the pole **or** during maximum unassisted and assisted opening, lateral, and protrusive movements
	Validity	Sensitivity 0.89; specificity 0.98
Note		The pain is not accounted for by another pain diagnosis

these values endorse diagnostic validity, providing clinicians the certainty to identify subjects who in fact have arthralgia. A summary of the criteria is presented in Table 7.4.

7.6 Disc Displacements

Among the intra-articular conditions are disc displacements and DJD. As a group, disc displacement is described as an intracapsular biomechanical disorder involving the condyle-disc complex. The four categories presented are in the sagittal plane, although medial and lateral displacement may be present. These clinical diagnoses are presented with clear diagnostic criteria, and their validity was tested using MRI interpretation as a reference standard (Schiffman et al. 2014). Illustration of the anatomical landmarks and reference position are described in Figs. 7.1 and 7.2 for open and closed mouth position, respectively.

Disc displacement with reduction integrates a history of joint sound by self-report or reported by the patient during the examination with joint sounds, specifically clicks identified by the examiner. The presence of clicks during two mandibular movements in at least one out of three repetitions is required, as presented in Table 7.5. Disc displacement with reduction with intermitting locking has an additional parameter, which is a history of momentary inability to open the mouth, which may present during the clinical examination (Table 7.6). MRI technique was used as a reference standard to evaluate the position of the disc in both open and closed mouth. In a closed mouth, the anatomical reference is the posterior band of the disc, which is positioned anterior to the 11:30 position and the intermediate zone of the disc being anterior to the condyle and articular eminence. These characteristics are presented in Fig. 7.3. In open mouth position, the intermediate zone is back in its normal position, located between the condyle and the articular eminence as presented in Fig. 7.4 (Schiffman et al. 2014).

Disc displacement without reduction, as represented in Fig. 7.5, is displayed in the closed and open mouth position. Furthermore, this group is classified as being with and without limited opening. These conditions share common characteristics including history of inability to achieve previous maximum opening, which implies locking and functional severe interference. The distinction between with and without limited opening depends upon the ability to achieve a minimum opening of 40 mm (information summarized in Tables 7.7 and 7.8). The sensitivity and specificity of disc displacement with reduction are 34 and 92%, for disc displacement with intermitting locking 38 and 98%, for disc displacement without reduction with limited opening 80 and 97%, and for disc displacement without reduction without limited opening 54 and 79%. Except for disc displacement without reduction with limited opening, which has sufficient validity, caution in interpretation is still recommended, as all other disc displacement clinical diagnoses have poor diagnostic validity. Therefore, if significant mechanical and functional problems are present or if treatment has been unsuccessful in management of presenting symptomatology, imaging is indicated (Schiffman and Ohrbach 2016).

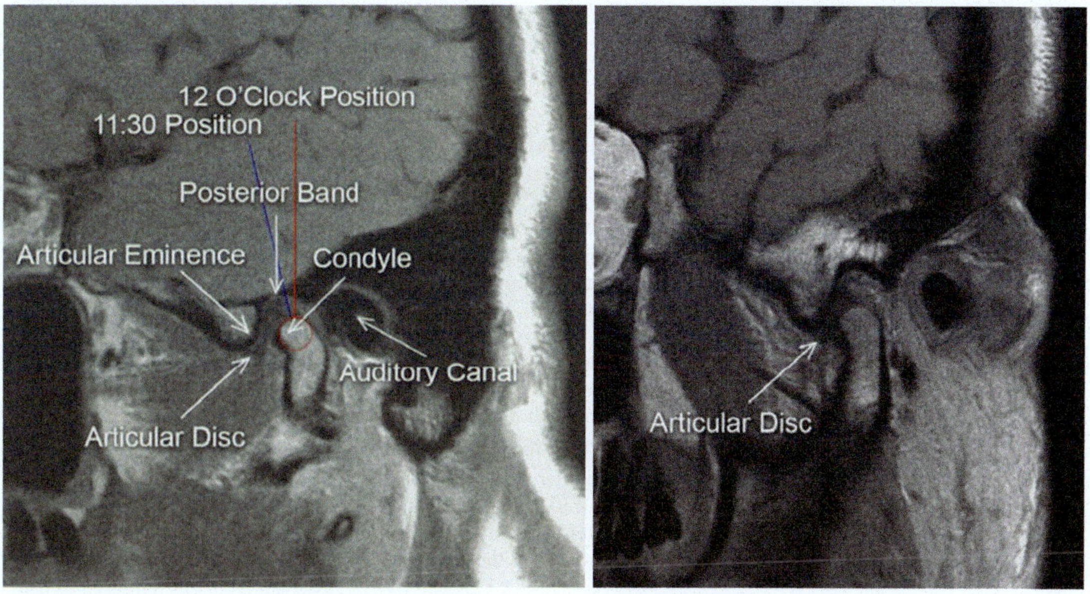

Fig. 7.1 Sagittal views in closed mouth showing normal anatomical position of the articular disc

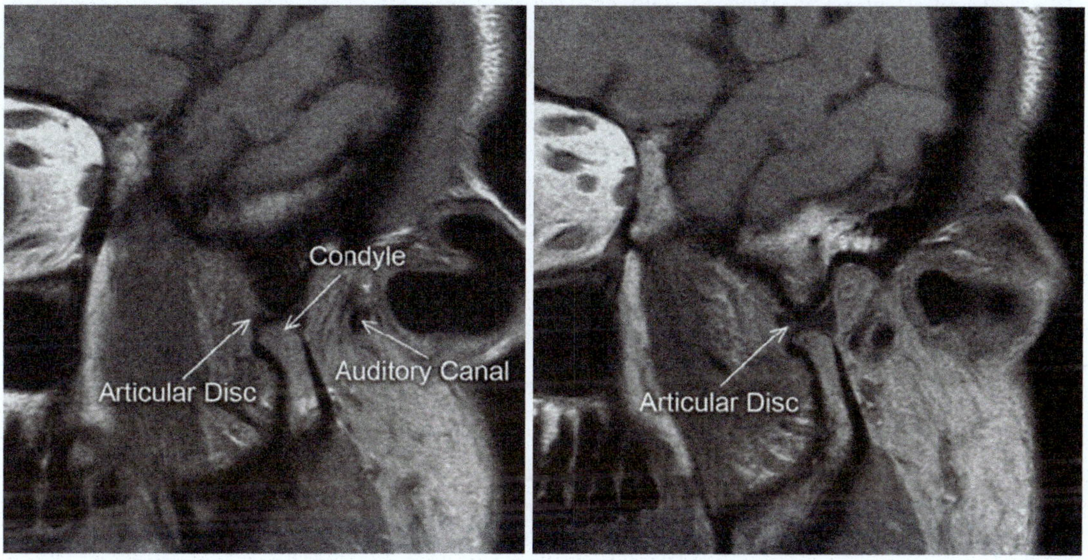

Fig. 7.2 Sagittal views in open mouth showing normal anatomical position of the articular disc

7.7 Degenerative Joint Disease

Based on the DC/TMD, DJD is described as deterioration of the articular tissue with concurrent osseous changes in the condyle and/or articular eminence. Patient-reported history of joint sounds or sounds noted during the examination composes the history component, while identification of crepitus by the examiner is the clinical element of this criterion (Table 7.9). In addition, the reference standard for the assessment of DJD is the CT. The use of panoramic imaging and MRI for the evaluation of DJD is inferior and not recommended based on poor to fair reliability and low to mar-

Table 7.5 Disc displacement with reduction

Disc displacement with reduction		
In the closed mouth position, the disc is in an anterior position relative to the condyle and reduces upon mouth opening. Clicking, popping, or snapping noises may occur		
Criteria	History	Patient reports any TMJ noise(s) present with jaw movement or function in the last 30 days **or** patient reports any noises of joint sounds during the exam
	Exam	Clicking, popping, or snapping noise in at least one of the three repetitions either during both opening and closing (vertical range of motion) [two vertical clicks] **or** a combination during vertical ROM and lateral or protrusive movements (horizontal ROM) [one vertical and one horizontal clicks]
	Validity	Sensitivity 0.34; specificity 0.92
Reference standard	Imaging	In the maximum intercuspal position, the posterior band of the disc is located anterior to the 11:30 position, the intermediate zone of the disc is anterior to the condyle, **and,** on full opening, the intermediate zone of the disc is located between the condyle and the articular eminence

Table 7.6 Disc displacement with reduction with intermittent locking

Disc displacement with reduction with intermittent locking		
In the closed mouth position, the disc is in an anterior position relative to the condyle and intermittently reduces upon mouth opening. When the disc does not reduce with opening of the mouth, intermittent limited mandibular opening occurs. Clicking, popping, or snapping noises may occur		
Criteria	History	Patient reports any TMJ noise(s) present with jaw movement or function in the last 30 days **or** patient reports any noises of joint sounds during the exam **and** patient reports lockjaw with limited mouth opening, even for a moment, and then unlocks in the last 30 days
	Exam	Clicking, popping, or snapping noise in at least one of the three repetitions either during both opening and closing (vertical ROM) [two vertical clicks] **or** a combination during vertical ROM and lateral or protrusive movements (horizontal ROM) [one vertical and one horizontal click]
	Validity	Sensitivity 0.38; specificity 0.98
Reference standard	Imaging	The same as disc displacement with reduction. If locking occurs during imaging, a diagnosis of DD without reduction will be given, and clinical confirmation of reversion to intermittent locking is needed
Note		Although not required, when the disorder is clinically present, inability to open to a normal amount, even momentarily, without the clinician or the patient performing a maneuver to reduce the locking is observed

ginal sensitivity using these techniques to detect osseous parameters (Ahmad et al. 2009). More so, the sensitivity and specificity of the clinical criteria are 55% and 61%, respectively, and it has been recommended to use this diagnostic allocation as a means of screening for clinical application (Schiffman and Ohrbach 2016) since the reference standard is the radiographic diagnosis.

The radiographic parameters for the diagnosis of DJD include the presence of generalized

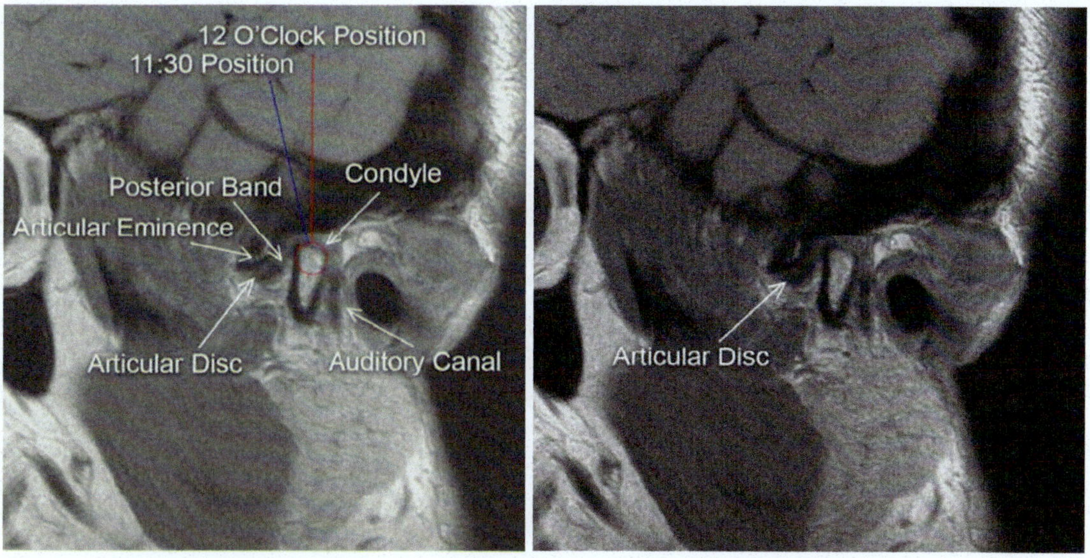

Fig. 7.3 Sagittal views in closed mouth position showing the articular disc anteriorly displaced

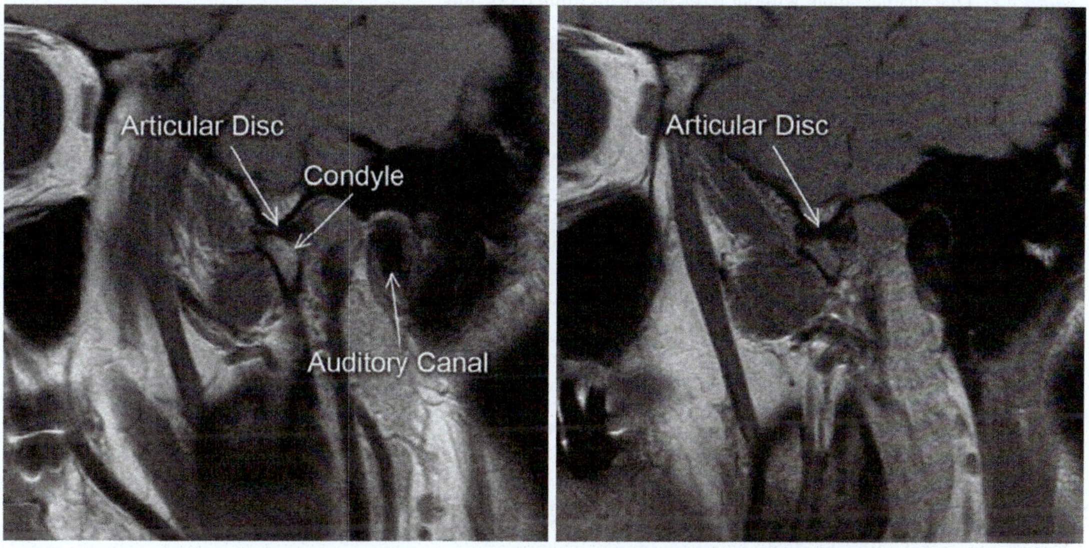

Fig. 7.4 Sagittal views in open mouth position showing reduction of the articular disc

sclerosis, erosion, subcortical cyst, and osteophyte(s) (Figs. 7.6 and 7.7) (Ahmad et al. 2009; Ahmad and Schiffman 2016). These parameters are defined as follows: Sclerosis is an increase in thickness of the cortical plate in the load-bearing areas probably as a result of increased loading in the joint or from normal loading if there is a displaced disc; marginal sclerosis may be interpreted as indeterminate and may represent aging or functional remodeling. Erosion is a loss of the continuity of the articular cortex of the condyle and/or articular fossa. Subcortical cyst is a cavity below the articular surface that deviates from normal, indicating loss of the trabeculation. Osteophyte is defined as an angular and exophytic osseous formation (Ahmad and Schiffman 2016). These parameters are further used in order to establish

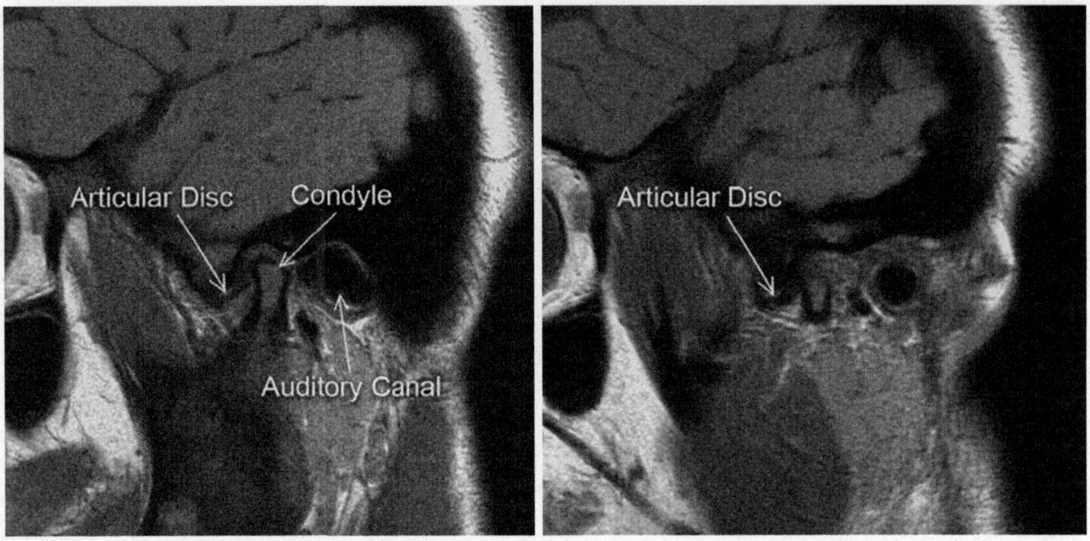

Fig. 7.5 Sagittal views in closed and open mouth position, respectively showing anteriorly displaced discs

Table 7.7 Disc displacement without reduction with limited opening

Disc displacement without reduction with limited opening		
In the closed mouth position, the disc is in an anterior position relative to the condyle, and the disc does not reduce with opening of the mouth. "Closed lock" is associated with persistent limited mandibular opening that does not improve (reduce) with the clinician or patient performing a manipulative maneuver		
Criteria	History	Jaw is locked so that the mouth would not open all the way Limitation in jaw opening severe enough to limit jaw opening and interfere with ability to eat
	Exam	Maximum assisted opening (passive stretch) movement including incisal overlap <40
	Validity	Sensitivity 0.80; specificity 0.97
Reference standard	Imaging	In the maximum intercuspal position, the posterior band of the disc is located anterior to the 11:30 position, and the intermediate zone of the disc is anterior to the condyle On full opening, the intermediate zone of the disc is located anterior to the condyle
Note		Presence of TMJ noise does not exclude this diagnosis

Table 7.8 Disc displacement without reduction without limited opening

Disc displacement without reduction without limited opening		
In the closed mouth position, the disc is in an anterior position relative to the condyle, and the disc does not reduce with opening of the mouth. This disorder is not associated with current limited opening		
Criteria	History	Jaw locked so that the mouth would not open all the way Limitation in jaw opening severe enough to limit jaw opening and interfere with ability to eat
	Exam	Maximum assisted opening (passive stretch) movement including incisal overlap ≥ 40
	Validity	Sensitivity 0.54; specificity 0.79
Reference standard	Imaging	In the maximum intercuspal position, the posterior band of the disc is located anterior to the 11:30 position, and the intermediate zone of the disc is anterior to the condyle On full opening, the intermediate zone of the disc is located anterior to the condyle
Note		Presence of TMJ noise does not exclude this diagnosis

Table 7.9 Degenerative joint disease

Degenerative joint disease		
Characterized by the deterioration of the articular tissue with concomitant osseous changes in the condyle and/or articular eminence		
Criteria	History	Patient reports any TMJ noise(s) present with jaw movement or function in the last 30 days **or** patient reports any noises during the assessment of joint sounds during the exam
	Exam	Crepitus detected during assessment of joint sounds during at least one of the mandibular movements: opening, closing, lateral, or protrusion
	Validity	Sensitivity 0.55; specificity 0.61
Reference standard	Imaging	Positive for one of the following: generalized sclerosis, subchondral cyst(s), erosion(s), or osteophyte(s)
Note		Presence of TMJ noise does not exclude this diagnosis

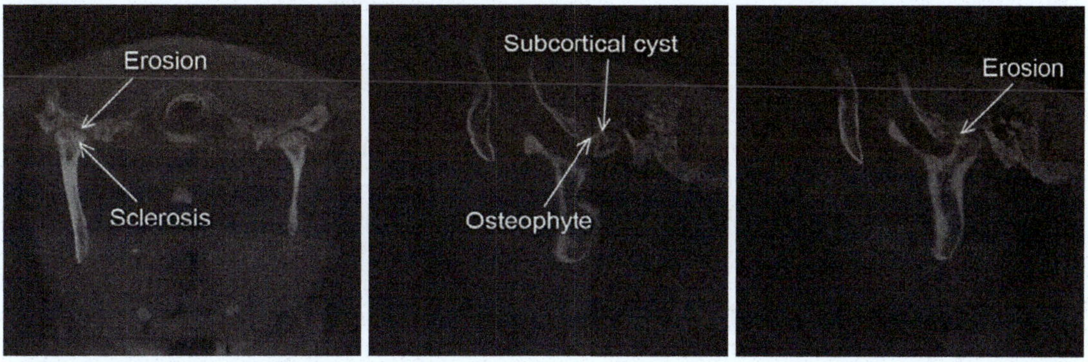

Fig. 7.6 CBCT on corrected coronal and sagittal orientations from the same individual showing structural changes consistent with erosion and generalized sclerosis as parameters of DJD

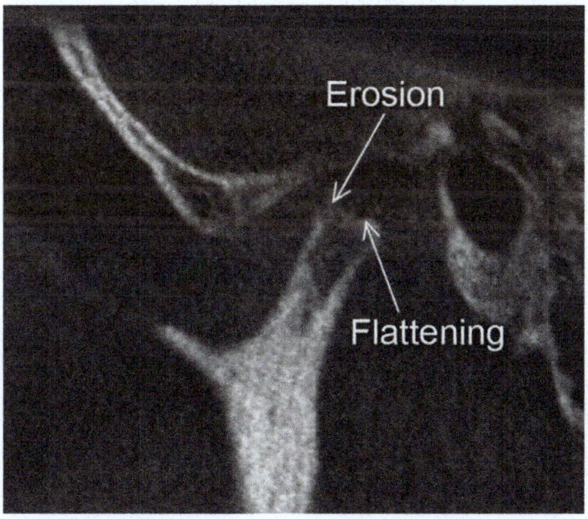

Fig. 7.7 CBCT on corrected sagittal orientation showing structural changes consistent with erosion and flattening as parameters of DJD

a level of severity for DJD, as presented in Table 7.10.

Although the DC/TMD expresses that crepitus is present during palpation, the intent was for the sound to be detected during the examination of joint sounds, during which no pressure is applied to the TMJ.

The availability of validated criteria for the diagnosis of common joint conditions represents a great source of information for clinicians and researchers. For clinicians, these current data demonstrate that the former belief that joint sounds are useful for the definitive diagnosis of joint conditions only maintains us in a state of clinical uncertainty. It is relevant to emphasize that at the validation study (Schiffman et al. 2010), the assessment of joint

Table 7.10 Postulated criteria for further classification of DJD

Degenerative joint disease (DJD)	Parameters	Grade 1	Grade 2
	Osteophyte	Measured <2 mm from the tip to the expected contour viewed in the corrected sagittal plane	Measured ≥2 mm from the tip to the expected contour as viewed in the corrected sagittal plane
			and/or
	Erosion	The greatest dimension is <2 mm in depth and width and limited to a single occurrence	The greatest dimension is ≥ 2 mm in depth and width and limited to a single occurrence or more than one erosion of any size
			and/or
	Subcortical pseudocyst	The greatest dimension is <2 mm in depth and width and limited to a single occurrence	The greatest dimension is ≥2 mm in depth and width and limited to a single occurrence or more than one pseudocyst of any size
			and/or
			Two or more imaging signs of grade 1

sounds was done exhaustively characterizing them not only by palpation but also using a stethoscope during multiple repetitions and multiple jaw movements, with a definitive outcome assessment by palpation deemed best fit for clinical characterization of disc displacements. Nonetheless, these clinical characterizations can only be interpreted at the screening level, and responsibility will rest at the provider level for best clinical practice to determine if imaging is needed not only to reduce uncertainty but also to influence the treatment pathway.

For researchers, having validated diagnostic criteria is of unique significance since most of the methodological limitations of previous studies are associated with the lack of clear operationalization of the condition or conditions. Homogeneity among research groups will allow for the evaluation of factors associated with the conditions and mechanisms involved. One of the most recent examples is data presented by Schiffman and Ohrbach (2016) clearly illustrating that in most TMJ conditions, 70% are maintained for a period of 7 years. This is in contrast to the previous biomedical model of TMJ disease progression, which, until that time, was thought to be linear.

7.8 Summary

Since the majority of TMJ conditions remain stable over time, what are the phenotypic characteristics including biomechanical, functional, and biopsychosocial properties that would permit us to identify who among those with intra-articular manifestations will progress or even regress? At this time the answer is not yet available to be integrated into clinical practice. Looking ahead, however, the ultimate goal is a constant interaction between clinical research and practice to enrich the field and most importantly provide the best possible care to our patients.

References

Ahmad M, Hollender L, Anderson Q, et al. Research diagnostic criteria for temporomandibular disorders (RDC/TMD): development of image analysis criteria and examiner reliability for image analysis. Oral Surg Oral Med Oral Pathol Oral Radiol Endod. 2009;107(6):844–60.

Ahmad M, Schiffman EL. Temporomandibular joint disorders and orofacial pain. Dent Clin North Am. 2016;60(1):105–24.

Amir G, Goldfarb AW, Nyska M, et al. 2-Butoxyethanol model of haemolysis and disseminated thrombosis in female rats: a preliminary study of the vascular mechanism of osteoarthritis in the temporomandibular joint. Br J Oral Maxillofac Surg. 2011;49:21–5.

Appelgren A, Appelgren B, Eriksson S, et al. Neuropeptides in temporomandibular joints with rheumatoid arthritis: a clinical study. Scand J Dent Res. 1991;99:519–21.

Asaki S, Sekikawa M, Kim YT. Sensory innervation of the temporomandibular joint disk. J Orthop Surg. 2006;14(1):3–8.

Bi RY, Ding Y, Gan YH. A new hypothesis of sex-differences in temporomandibular disorders: estrogen enhances hyperalgesia of inflamed TMJ through modulating voltage-gated sodium channel 1.7 in trigeminal ganglion? Med Hypotheses. 2015;84:100–3.

Bigoni M, Sacerdote P, Turati M, et al. Acute and late changes in intraarticular cytokine levels following anterior cruciate ligament injury. J Orthop Res. 2013;31(2):315–21.

Bigoni M, Turati M, Sacerdote P, et al. Characterization of synovial fluid cytokine profiles in chronic meniscal tear of the knee. J Orthop Res. 2017;35(2):340–6.

Casares G, Thomas A, Carmona J, et al. Influence of oral stabilization appliances in intra-articular pressure of the temporomandibular joint. Cranio. 2014;32:219–23.

Dijkgraaf LC, Zardeneta G, Cordewener FW, et al. Crosslinking of fibrinogen and fibronectin by free radicals: a possible initial step in adhesion formation in osteoarthritis of the temporomandibular joint. J Oral Maxillofac Surg. 2003;61:101–11.

Fang PK, Ma XC, Ma DL, KY F. Determination of interleukin-1 receptor antagonist, interleukin-10, and transforming growth factor-beta1 in synovial fluid aspirates of patients with temporomandibular disorders. J Oral Maxillofac Surg. 1999;57(8):922–8.

Fu K, Ma X, Zhang Z, Chen W. Tumor necrosis factor in synovial fluid of patients with temporomandibular disorders. J Oral Maxillofac Surg. 1995;53(4):424–6.

Gynther GW, Dijkgraaf LC, Reinholt FP, et al. Synovial inflammation in arthroscopically obtained biopsy specimens from the temporomandibular joint: a review of the literature and a proposed histologic grading system. J Oral Maxillofac Surg. 1998;56(11):1281–6.

Haeuchi Y, Matsumoto K, Ichikawa H, Maeda S. Immunohistochemical demonstration of neuropeptides in the articular disk of the human temporomandibular joint. Cells Tissues Organs. 1999;164:205–11.

Haskin CL, Milam SB, Cameron IL. Pathogenesis of degenerative joint disease in the human temporomandibular joint. Crit Rev Oral Biol Med. 1995;6:248–77.

Hattori-Hara E, Mitsui SN, Mori H, et al. The influence of unilateral disc displacement on stress in the contralateral joint with a normally positioned disc in a human temporomandibular joint: An analytic approach using the finite element method. J Craniomaxillofac Surg. 2014;42:2018–24.

Hawkins JL, Durham PL. Prolonged jaw opening promotes nociception and enhanced cytokine expression. J Oral Facial Pain Headache. 2016;30(1):34–41.

Henderson SE, Lowe JR, Tudares MA, et al. Temporomandibular joint fibrocartilage degeneration from unilateral dental splints. Arch Oral Biol. 2015;60:1–11.

Herr MM, Fries KM, Upton LG, Edsberg LE. Potential biomarkers of temporomandibular joint disorders. J Oral Maxillofac Surg. 2011;69(1):41–7.

Holmlund A, Ekblom A, Hansson P, et al. Concentrations of neuropeptides substance P, neurokinin A, calcitonin gene-related peptide, neuropeptide Y, and vasoactive intestinal polypeptide in synovial fluid of the human temporomandibular joint: a correlation with symptoms, signs, and arthroscopic findings. Int J Oral Maxillofac Surg. 1991;20:228–31.

Kaneyama K, Segami N, Nishimura M, et al. Importance of proinflammatory cytokines in synovial fluid from 121 joints with temporomandibular disorders. Br J Oral Maxillofac Surg. 2002;40(5):418–23.

Kaneyama K, Segami N, Nishimura M, et al. Osteoclastogenesis inhibitory factor/osteoprotegerin in synovial fluid from patients with temporomandibular disorders. Int J Oral Maxillofac Surg. 2003;32(4):404–7.

Kaneyama K, Segami N, Sato J, et al. Interleukin-6 family of cytokines as biochemical markers of osseous changes in the temporomandibular joint disorders. Br J Oral Maxillofac Surg. 2004;42(3):246–50.

Kaneyama K, Segami N, Sun W, et al. Analysis of tumor necrosis factor-a, interleukin-6, interleukin-1b, soluble tumor necrosis factor receptors I and II, interleukin-6 soluble receptor, interleukin-1 soluble receptor type II, interleukin-1 receptor antagonist, and protein in the synovial fluid of patients with temporomandibular joint disorders. Oral Surg Oral Med Oral Pathol Oral Radiol Endod. 2005;99(3):276–84.

Katzberg RW, Westesson P-L, Tallens RH, et al. Anatomic disorders of the temporomandibular joint disc in asymptomatic subjects. J Oral Maxillofac. 1986;54:147–53.

Kellesarian SV, Al-Kheraif AA, Vohra F, et al. Cytokine profile in the synovial fluid of patients with temporomandibular joint disorders: a systematic review. Cytokine. 2016;77:98–106.

Kubota E, Kubota T, Matsumoto J, et al. Synovial fluid cytokines and proteinases as markers of temporomandibular joint disease. J Oral Maxillofac Surg. 1998;56(2):192–8.

Lee JK, Cho YS, Song SI. Relationship of synovial tumor necrosis factor alpha and interleukin 6 to temporomandibular disorder. J Oral Maxillofac Surg. 2010;68(5):1064–8.

Milam SB, Schmitz JP. Molecular biology of temporomandibular joint disorders: proposed mechanisms of disease. J Oral Maxillofac Surg. 1995;53:1448–54.

Milam SB, Zardeneta G, Schmitz JP. Oxidative stress and degenerative temporomandibular joint disease: a proposed hypothesis. J Oral Maxillofac Surg. 1998;56:214–23.

Milam SB. Pathogenesis of degenerative temporomandibular joint arthritides. Odontology. 2005;93:7–15.
Nitzan DW. Intraarticular pressure in the functioning human temporomandibular joint and its alteration by uniform elevation of the occlusal plane. J Oral Maxillofac Surg. 1994;52:671–9.
Nitzan DW, Marmary Y. The "anchored disc phenomenon": a proposed etiology for sudden-onset, severe, and persistent closed lock of the temporomandibular joint. J Oral Maxillofac Surg. 1997;55:797–802.
Nitzan DW. The process of lubrication impairment and its involvement in temporomandibular joint disc displacement: a theoretical concept. J Oral Maxillofac Surg. 2001;59:36–45.
Nitzan DW, Etsion I. Adhesive force: the underlying cause of the disc anchorage to the fossa and/or eminence in the temporomandibular joint-a new concept. Int J Oral Maxillofac Surg. 2002;31:94–9.
Nitzan DW, Goldfarb A, Gati I, Kohen R. Changes in the reducing power of synovial fluid from temporomandibular joints with "anchored disc phenomenon". J Oral Maxillofac Surg. 2002;60:735–40.
Nitzan DW. "Friction and adhesive forces" possible underlying causes for temporomandibular joint internal derangement. Cells Tissues Organs. 2003;174:6–16.
Nitzan DW, Kreiner B, Zeltser R. TMJ lubrication system: its effect on the joint function, dysfunction, and treatment approach. Compendium. 2004;25:437–48.
Oliveira-Fusaro MC, Clemente-Napimoga JT, Teixeira JM, et al. 5-HT induces temporomandibular joint nociception in rats through the local release of inflammatory mediators and activation of local β adrenoceptors. Pharmacol Biochem Behav. 2012;102(3):458–64.
Rasmussen OC. Description of population and progress of symptoms in a longitudinal study of temporomandibular arthropathy. Scand J Dent Res. 1981;89:196–203.
Schiffman EL, Truelove EL, Ohrbach R, et al. The research diagnostic criteria for temporomandibular disorders I: overview and methodology for assessment of validity. J Orofac Pain. 2010;24(1):7–24.
Schiffman E, Ohrbach R, Trulove E, et al. Diagnostic Criteria for Temporomandibular Disorders (DC/TMD) for clinical and research applications: recommendations of the International RDC/TMD consortium network and orofacial pain special interest group. J Oral Facial Pain Headache. 2014;28(1):6–27.
Schiffman E, Ohrbach R. Executive summary of the diagnostic criteria for temporomandibular disorders for clinical and research applications. J Am Dent Assoc. 2016;147(6):438–45.
Sheets Jr DW, Okamoto T, Dijkgraaf LC, et al. Free radical damage in facsimile synovium: Correlation with adhesion formation in osteoarthritic TMJs. J Prosthodont. 2006;15:9–19.
Shinoda C, Takaku S. Interleukin-1beta, interleukin-6, and tissue inhibitor of metalloproteinase-1 in the synovial fluid of the temporomandibular joint with respect to cartilage destruction. Oral Dis. 2000;6(6):383–90.
Symons MC. Formation of radicals by mechanical processes. Free Radic Res Commun. 1988;5:131–9.
Takahashi T, Kondoh T, Fukuda M. Proinflammatory cytokines detectable in synovial fluids from patients with temporomandibular disorders. Oral Surg Oral Med Oral Pathol Oral Radiol Endod. 1998;85(2):135–41.
Tanaka E, Detamore MS, Mercuri LG. Degenerative disorders of the temporomandibular joint: etiology, diagnosis and treatment. J Dent Res. 2008;87:296–307.
Vernal R, Velásquez E, Gamonal J, et al. Expression of proinflammatory cytokines in osteoarthritis of the temporomandibular joint. Arch Oral Biol. 2008;53(10):910–5.
Wake M, Hamada Y, Kumagai K, et al. Up-regulation of interleukin-6 and vascular endothelial growth factor-A in the synovial fluid of temporomandibular joints affected by synovial chondromatosis. Br J Oral Maxillofac Surg. 2013;51(2):164–9.
Wang XD, Kou XX, He DQ. Progression of cartilage degradation, bone resorption and pain in rat temporomandibular joint osteoarthritis induced by injection of iodoacetate. PLoS One. 2012;7(9):e45036.
Wang XD, Cui SJ, Liu Y, et al. Deterioration of mechanical properties of discs in chronically inflamed TMJ. J Dent Res. 2014;93:1170–6.
Wilkes CH. Internal derangements of the temporomandibular joint: pathological variations. Arch Otolaryngol Head Neck Surg. 1989;115:469–77.
Zardeneta G, Milam SB, Schmitz JP. Presence of denatured hemoglobin deposits in diseased temporomandibular joints. J Oral Maxillofac Surg. 1997;55:1242–8.
Zardeneta G, Milam SB, Schmitz JP. Iron-dependent generation of free radicals: plausible mechanisms in the progressive deterioration of the temporomandibular joint. J Oral Maxillofac Surg. 2000;58:302–8.

Part IV

Management Principles

Muscle-Based Conditions

8

Steven L. Kraus, Steven D. Bender,
and Janey Prodoehl

Abstract

Among the most common pain-related temporomandibular disorders (TMDs) are disorders arising from muscular sources. Lacking a single etiology, treatment for TMD and myofascial pain (MP) is directed toward identifying and treating the source of the patient's pain. Successful management of chronic TMD problems often requires a multidisciplinary approach utilizing a team of professionals working in conjunction with the individual patient. Evidence-based conservative treatment options to reduce the signs and symptoms of TMD, with special attention on MP, will be discussed in this chapter. These include patient education and biobehavioral strategies, therapeutic exercises, manual procedures, trigger point dry needling and therapeutic modalities offered by physical therapists, pharmacotherapy, and evidence-based oral appliances offered by dentists. In addition, the role of occlusion and occlusal oriented treatments will be discussed.

8.1 Introduction

Among the most common pain-related temporomandibular disorders (TMDs) are disorders arising from muscular sources. Myalgia is a general term used to describe pain of muscular origin. The terms "myalgia," "muscle pain," "myofascial pain," "myofascial pain with referral," and myofascial trigger points (MTrPs) are often used interchangeably, but throughout this chapter, unless stated otherwise, these will collectively be referred to as myofascial pain (MP). Symptoms associated with masticatory MP that are modified by jaw function or parafunction may consist of headache (located in the temporalis muscle) as

S.L. Kraus, PT, OCS, MTC, CCTT, CODN
Physiotherapy Associates, Atlanta, GA, USA
e-mail: Steve@TMDstevekraus.com

S.D. Bender, DDS
Center for Facial Pain and Sleep Medicine, Texas A&M College of Dentistry, Dallas, TX, USA
e-mail: bender@tamhsc.edu

J. Prodoehl, PT, PhD (✉)
Physical Therapy Program, Midwestern University, Downers Grove, IL, USA
e-mail: JProdo@midwestern.edu

© Springer International Publishing AG 2018
H.A. Gremillion, G.D. Klasser (eds.), *Temporomandibular Disorders*,
https://doi.org/10.1007/978-3-319-57247-5_8

well as pain, tension, achiness, and tightness located in any one or combination of the masticatory muscles, and patients may or may not complain of limited mouth opening. Pertinent to TMD, MP has been found to exist in the masticatory muscles such as the masseter, temporalis, and medial and lateral pterygoids (Simons et al. 1999). Having a good understanding of variables that cause an inordinate amount of muscle contraction that can result in the development of masticatory MP is essential for both researchers and clinicians who seek to develop appropriate intervention plans for patients with MP. It is currently recommended that unless there are specific and justifiable indications to the contrary, initial treatment of TMD, regardless of whether it is an intra-articular or myalgic type of TMD, should be based on the use of nonsurgical, reversible, and evidence-based therapeutic modalities (American Academy of Orofacial Pain et al. 2013; American Association of Dental Research Adopted 1996, revised 2010). However, successful management of chronic TMD problems often requires a multidisciplinary approach utilizing a team of professionals including dentists, physicians, physical therapists, pharmacists, and psychologists working in conjunction with the individual patient. Treatment options that meet these criteria to reduce the signs and symptoms of TMD, with special attention on MP, will be discussed in this chapter.

8.2 Etiology

Understanding the etiology of MP can assist with the development and implementation of a case-specific treatment plan. However, the etiology of TMD and MP is multifactorial. Certain cases have a clear antecedent etiologic event such as trauma, biting into something hard, or even dental treatment (Carlsson 2001). Other etiologies though are less clear and not fully understood. In 1934, Costen suggested the etiology of TMD was a malocclusion, i.e., crowding, malalignment, or structural abnormality and that malocclusion was the cause of a variety of head, facial, jaw, and throat symptoms (Costen 1934). Today, researchers have failed to reach a consensus regarding the role of occlusal interferences in the development of TMD. Current clinical perspectives on occlusal factors related to TMD and MP will be addressed later in this chapter. Since Dr. Costen's declaration of malocclusion as a causal factor of TMD, etiological theories for the development of TMD have expanded to include, although are not limited to, genetics, joint morphology, mandibular asymmetry, and structural alignment problems between the cranium and cervical spine (Greene 2001; Klasser and Greene 2009). None of these factors have consistently been found to completely explain the etiology of TMD or orofacial MP.

One etiological factor that has gained attention as contributing to excessive muscle contraction, especially to account for chronic TMD and MP, is the biopsychosocial model of pain (Klasser and Greene 2009). A biopsychosocial model takes into account the physical source of a patient's pain as well as their psychosocial distress. Psychosocial distress has consistently been found to be associated with parafunctional behaviors and masticatory MP and can have a substantial impact on muscle contraction, pain persistence, and responsiveness to treatment (Restrepo et al. 2008; Kotiranta et al. 2015; Tosato Jde et al. 2015). However, only 12% of TMD patients have the highest level of symptoms of depression, somatization, sleep dysfunction, pain-related worry, and catastrophizing/ruminative thoughts, suggesting that psychosocial distress alone cannot explain the etiology of all TMD or orofacial MP (Kotiranta et al. 2015). While a patient's level of psychosocial distress cannot be underestimated, for the vast majority of patients with TMD and masticatory MP, psychosocial distress can be addressed at the clinical level discussed later in this chapter (Sect. 8.4.1).

Though all of the previous factors may have some merit and may be associated with the onset of MP, none have been definitively determined to explain the etiology of TMD. However, regardless of the etiology of MP, concentric, eccentric, and isometric contractions can produce MP with the same pathophysiologic process as that underlying ischemic pain (Newham et al. 1994).

Regardless of the type of muscle contraction, MP can occur if a contraction is sustained, repetitious, and/or too intense.

8.3 General Management Strategies

Lacking a single etiology, treatment for TMD and MP is directed toward identifying and treating the source of the patient's pain. Of all the diagnostic subsets of TMD (Schiffman et al. 2014), MP is the most common subtype followed by arthralgia (Manfredini et al. 2012; Kraus 2014). While MP is often diagnosed without arthralgia, arthralgia is, at times, diagnosed without MP, and MP and arthralgia can exist concurrently (Kraus 2014). The temporomandibular joint (TMJ) complex is ginglymoarthrodial and requires coordinated kinematic movement between both joints and withstands significant repetitive loading during normal daily function. Restricting joint movement that is excessive and reducing abnormal joint loading by treating MP can often facilitate reduction of symptoms associated with other intra-articular disorders.

8.4 Specific Management Strategies

8.4.1 Patient Education/Self-Management and Biobehavioral Strategies

The most conservative and often most effective treatment for a patient diagnosed with masticatory MP is patient education (Aggarwal et al. 2010). Patient education generally focuses on educating the patient as to their diagnosis, their role in management, treatment options, and treatment expectations. An essential component of patient education pertinent to the treatment of MP however is behavior modification related to the elimination of harmful oral behaviors. Harmful oral behaviors may predispose, precipitate, or perpetuate masticatory MP. Patient education that focuses on the elimination or reduction of harmful oral behaviors through behavior modification is the corner stone for treatment of masticatory MP.

Changing behavior relies on patient education and a patient's willingness to change their harmful behavior. Patient education goes far beyond a passive approach of simply providing the patient with a sheet of instructions of "do's and don'ts." The clinician must invest the time necessary to educate their patient on the importance of these changes in an easily understood format. The clinician can help the patient identify obstacles that may interfere with their ability to change behavior and then provide them with suggestions regarding various strategies for resolution. A primary focus of care should be on reducing or eliminating oral parafunctional activity.

Oral parafunctional activity is any oral activity that includes habitual use of the mouth unrelated to essential activities of eating, drinking, yawning, or talking. One of the more common parafunctional activities associated with MP is bruxism, defined as repetitive jaw-muscle activity characterized by clenching or grinding of the teeth and/or by bracing or thrusting of the mandible (Klasser et al. 2015). Bruxism can occur during the awake hours or during sleep in which case it is referred to as sleep bruxism. Addressing sleep bruxism presents several challenges. To date, the etiology of sleep bruxism is unknown; however, a recent hypothesis supports the roles of the central and autonomic nervous systems in the genesis of oromandibular activity during sleep (Klasser et al. 2015). Currently, there is no therapy that has been proven to be effective in eliminating sleep bruxism. Suggested management strategies for sleep bruxism include biofeedback, hypnotherapy, cognitive behavioral therapy (CBT), pharmacotherapy, and occlusal appliances (Klasser et al. 2015). These treatments can involve considerable cost to the patient, and most are not supported by the literature or have been shown to have only transitory effects. An alternative treatment for sleep bruxism is patient education. Anecdotal evidence suggests that for some patients, patient education pertaining to sleeping postures is not only cost-effective but may be helpful in reducing sleep bruxism.

In considering alternate sleep positions, patients are informed to avoid positions that prevent relaxation of head and neck muscles and positions that place excessive force on the mandible. Anecdotal evidence suggests sleep positions that include stomach sleeping and side-lying (lateral decubitus) positions with hands placed between the mandible, and pillow can apply undue pressure on the mandible. However, empirical evidence is lacking to support a causal relationship between sleeping posture and the development of sleep bruxism. Educating patients regarding modification of sleep positions using appropriate pillow type based on their body type may still be beneficial. The pillow should be soft yet supportive enough to maintain the natural contour of the neck in the supine or side-lying position. In the side-lying position, the pillow must be able to effectively support the mandible. Analyzing and addressing the ergonomics of sleeping posture can be addressed in detail by the physical therapist as part of a comprehensive plan of care.

Individuals with masticatory muscle pain have been shown to have an increased frequency of daytime clenching episodes compared to pain-free controls (Cioffi et al. 2016). Also, individuals who self-report that they have awake bruxism, sleep bruxism, and parafunctional habits have been shown to have a greater likelihood of having jaw pain than if they report only experiencing one of those factors (Fernandes et al. 2016). It is possible that the presence of awake and sleep bruxism in conjunction with parafunctional habits may extend periods of muscle activation and reduce rest periods for masticatory muscles, thus contributing to the chronicity of MP. Since sleep bruxism is not under volitional control, one treatment approach to allow increased periods of rest for masticatory muscles is to reduce or eliminate awake bruxism. However, there is no empirical evidence to support this. There is also no evidence yet that reducing awake bruxism would lead to reduced sleep bruxism. However, patients should be educated to avoid daytime triggers for bruxism such as smoking, alcohol, and caffeine (Feu et al. 2013; van Selms et al. 2013). A simple and effective way to control awake bruxism is to educate the patient that their teeth should never make contact unless they are chewing or swallowing and, even then, contact does not always need to be made. Increased or prolonged muscle activity can lead to significantly increased occlusal loads and increased loading of the temporomandibular joints (Santana-Mora et al. 2014). Patients must be aware that during the day, they should keep their tongue relaxed and teeth apart and maintain even breathing patterns (Kraus 1994). Educating the patient on the appropriate jaw resting position can promote reduced masticatory muscle activity and rest, and patients should be instructed to return to this resting position throughout the day as they feel their jaw muscles tightening or MP increasing.

Another aspect of awake bruxism that should be addressed with the patient is bracing or thrusting the jaw forward, both of which are done with the teeth out of contact. A simple yet effective awareness exercise to lessen this behavior is to instruct the patient to move their jaw from side to side, an exercise referred to as the “wiggle at will” (Kraus 1994). It is essential that the patient understands that the goal of this exercise is not to go through a large range of motion but to perform a small rhythmical movement from side to side, ensuring that movement does not cause pain or repetitive TMJ clicking. If the patient is not coordinated to isolate small side-to-side movements with their jaw, the exercise should not be continued.

Patients must be willing to put forth the effort to increase their awareness of their jaw’s resting position and to avoid bruxing during the day by keeping their jaw relaxed. Anecdotal evidence suggests that educating patients on simple concepts of tongue position and reducing jaw bracing when confronted with daily stressors can reduce awake bruxism and subsequently MP. Patients should be made aware that when confronted with any one or a combination of daily stressors, they must be cognizant of applying the strategies taught to them to minimize increases in masticatory muscle activity. These daily stressors include periods of focused activity which include working at a computer, driving, texting, reading, or writing and activities of exertion such as pushing, pulling, and lifting and periods of physical stress or psychosocial distress.

While psychosocial distress especially fear, anxiety, anger, and depression (FAAD) has consistently been found to be associated with bruxism and masticatory muscle pain, the majority of patients fall into the no pain or low pain disability groups (Kotiranta et al. 2015). The following recommendations may eliminate or reduce psychosocial distress in patients with low levels of pain disability and may reduce psychosocial distress in patients with high pain disability:

1. Treat the source of pain:

   A patient's FAAD can develop as a result of pain, or if a patient is predisposed to FAAD, such emotions can be magnified because of pain (Giesecke et al. 2005). The medical model of pain management should still be applied, i.e., find the source of pain and eliminate the source of pain, thereby reducing any unnecessary psychosocial distress that may be a contributing factor to the pain. The best prevention against the development of chronic TMD-related pain and the enhancement of psychosocial distress is to diagnose and efficiently treat the patient's source of pain while in the acute phase of pain.
2. Understand the patient's journey to find pain relief:

   A patient's FAAD may be associated with processes of worrying and searching for a meaning of their acute or chronic pain (Bonathan et al. 2014). Patients with MP often consult with multiple healthcare professionals (Fricton and Heir 2006; Kraus 2014), and it is not unusual for patients to consult with a primary care physician; a neurologist; a physical therapist; an ear, nose, and throat specialist; a family dentist; a chiropractor; and one or more dentists who claim to be a TMD "specialist." Still, patients may not receive a definitive diagnosis, or they may receive conflicting diagnoses and treatment recommendations at variable costs. Some patients may have been informed that if they do not receive treatment soon, their condition will worsen which can promote increased FAAD. Unfortunately, FAAD may result from or be enhanced by a patient's experiences with different healthcare providers. This can be particularly problematic with healthcare providers who are not knowledgeable *and who do not apply appropriate* diagnostic criteria for TMD or who utilize treatment approaches that are not supported by current best evidence (Klasser and Greene 2007). Muscle pain that is magnified by FAAD can be minimized if the patient can find and trust a well-informed healthcare professional who takes the necessary time to provide a clear and easily understood description of their diagnosis and treatment options (Bonathan et al. 2014). Interprofessional collaboration in the management of patients with chronic TMD is an important component in minimizing FAAD.
3. Take into account a patient's willingness to change and how they respond to stressors:

   Stressors can take on many forms including interpersonal relationships at work and home, financial stress, and health-related issues with self and family members. Stressors may be associated with myogenous TMD. The severity of TMD symptoms has been shown to correlate with salivary cortisol levels and electromyographic levels of masseter and anterior temporalis muscle activity, suggesting a relationship between physical manifestations of stressors and masticatory muscle activity (Tosato Jde et al. 2015). Educating patients regarding the negative physical effects of stressors such as premature aging and cardiovascular problems may help them to accept that stressors can lead to detrimental physical effects. However, given that stressors may not ever completely be eliminated in daily life, patient education on controlling stressors in a more positive way should be included.

8.4.2 Physical Therapy

Physical therapy is well recognized as a conservative method for the management of symptoms associated with TMD (Sturdivant and Fricton 1991; Kraus 2000; McNeely et al. 2006). Physical therapy is aimed at preventing, correcting, or alleviating movement dysfunction. In relation to masticatory MP, individuals commonly experience movement problems of limited opening, deviations or deflections on mandibular movements, aberrant mandibular posturing, and/or pain associated with jaw function. Additionally, maladaptive head posture and sleep disturbances may be present. Patient education and self-management as described earlier in this chapter are central to any physical therapy plan of care for MP. Additional management strategies for the treatment of MP utilized by physical therapists include therapeutic exercise and neuromuscular reeducation, manual therapy, dry needling, treatment of cervical spine and postural contributions to muscle-related dysfunction, and therapeutic modalities. Though all physical therapists receive undergraduate training in musculoskeletal evaluation and treatment, emphasis on TMD may be a shortcoming. Physical therapists who have received post-professional training in the evaluation and management of orofacial pain and headache may be better equipped to deal with the acute and chronic headache and orofacial/TMD patient population (The Physical Therapy Board of Craniofacial & Cervical Therapeutics from www.ptbcct.org).

8.4.2.1 Therapeutic Exercise and Neuromuscular Reeducation

Physical therapists utilize a variety of therapeutic exercise and neuromuscular reeducation activities to reduce muscle activity and pain in individuals with TMD. Therapeutic exercise involving stretching and strengthening has been found to decrease pain and improve function in patients with chronic pain conditions (Karlsson et al. 2015) and in patients with myofascial TMD (Nicolakis et al. 2002). Therapeutic exercise and neuromuscular reeducation are used in the management of patients with masticatory MP. Patients with TMD have been shown to have impaired orofacial motor function (De Felicio et al. 2012; Ferreira et al. 2014), and therapeutic exercise and neuromuscular reeducation have been shown to improve mandibular motion, alter muscle coordination during jaw movement, reduce muscle tension, increase muscle strength, and improve circulation within masticatory muscles (Simons et al. 1999; Wirianski et al. 2014). Indeed, several recent systematic reviews have supported the role of exercise for treating TMD (McNeely et al. 2006; Medlicott and Harris 2006; Armijo-Olivo et al. 2016).

The physiological mechanisms underlying the effects of exercise on pain and function may be through alteration of pressure pain threshold and desensitization of muscle tissue. Exercise has been shown to lead to alterations in the concentration of glutamate, substance P, beta-endorphin, and cortisol in individuals with chronic pain (Karlsson et al. 2015). Additionally, specific types of stretching can promote reciprocal inhibition leading to reduced resting muscle tone. A focus on neuromuscular control may improve proprioception and the motor control of masticatory muscles which can lead to reduced parafunction (Wong et al. 2011). Muscular awareness relaxation training can be used to reduce resting muscle activity in elevator muscles of the mandible and improve mandibular opening and to reduce TMJ loading (Treacy 1999).

8.4.2.2 Manual Therapy

Manual therapy is a general term that is used to describe intra- and extra-articular manual therapeutic techniques. Non-thrust mobilization techniques are usually directed toward the TMJ to address intra-articular disorders involving disc displacements or adhesions (Fig. 8.1). Extra-articular

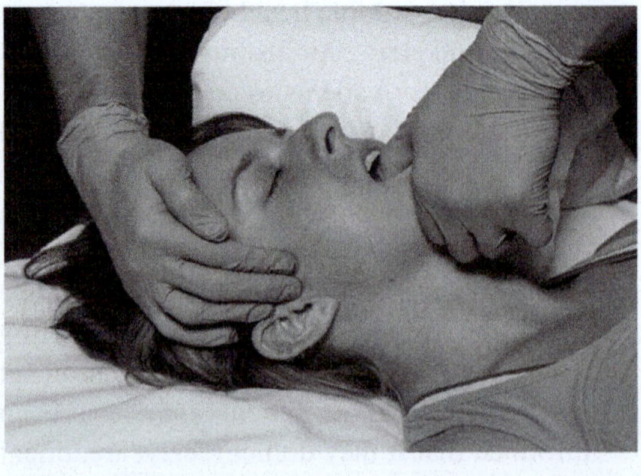

Fig. 8.1 Example of a manual therapy technique directed toward mobilizing the TMJ

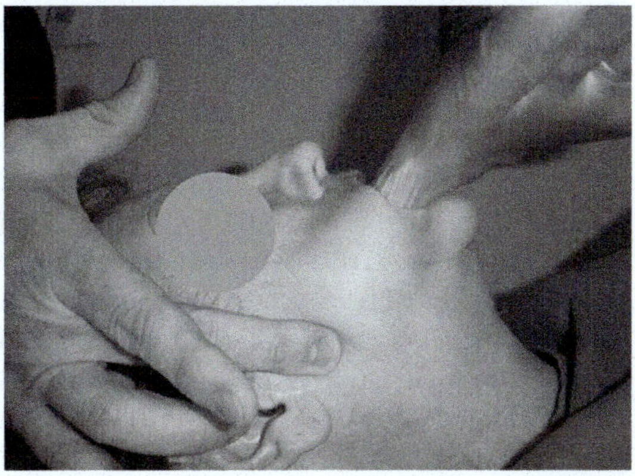

Fig. 8.2 Intraoral soft tissue mobilization of the masseter

techniques include the use of soft tissue mobilization which includes mobilization of the masticatory muscles (Fig. 8.2). The mechanism of effect of manual therapy in the treatment of musculoskeletal pain is multifaceted, but in brief, it has been suggested that introduction of a mechanical force to tissue leads to a cascade of neurophysiological responses involving the peripheral and central nervous systems that serves to reduce pain and improve clinical outcomes (Korr 1978; Bialosky et al. 2009). A number of manual techniques have been advocated for use in treating MP. Different terms have been used to describe what the clinician may be attempting such as myofascial release, neuromuscular massage, strain counter strain, soft tissue mobilization, joint mobilization and manipulation, sustained natural apophyseal glides (SNAGs), upper limb neural tension mobilization, and Graston Techniques®. No one approach has been shown to be more therapeutically beneficial than another.

Regardless of the TMD diagnostic subset, a manual approach to treatment has been shown to improve mandibular range of motion and reduce pain compared to other conservative treatments (Calixtre et al. 2015; Martins et al. 2015). For TMD of myofascial origin, patient education and behavioral modification are ongoing components of a physical therapy plan of care as previously discussed (De Laat et al. 2003). In addition, the focus of physical therapy is usually directed toward treating the source of MP. Acute muscle pain due to local ischemia results in the peripheral sensitization of local muscle nociceptors. While acute muscle pain often resolves on its own, treatment of the affected muscles may help to speed recovery (Andersen et al. 2013). However, muscle contractions that persist will lead to a cascade of molecular events that can lead to the development of myofascial trigger points (MTrPs) within the masticatory muscles. While the existence of MTrPs has not been without controversy (Dommerholt and Gerwin 2015; Quintner et al. 2015), strong evidence to support the validity of MTrPs has come through different technologies. Magnetic resonance elastography has been used to identify the presence of a taut band within the muscle (Chen et al. 2007; Chen et al. 2016), and sonoelastography and diagnostic ultrasound have been used to visualize MTrPs (Sikdar et al. 2009). Decreases in oxygen in the vicinity of an MTrP have been shown using Doppler ultrasound (Sikdar et al. 2010), and changes in chemical milieu consistent with pain and inflammation have been shown using microdialysis of an MTrP (Shah et al. 2005).

MTrPs can be an overlooked source of musculoskeletal pain in the muscles of mastication as well as in cervical muscles (International Association for the Study of Pain 1986). The development of active MTrPs may be a source of chronic MP in TMD (see Chap. 6). In brief, it has been theorized that MTrPs can become a source of chronic orofacial pain or headache when muscle contraction persists. Abnormal depolarization of the postjunctional membrane may lead to an abnormally sustained muscle fiber contraction which can promote depletion of local adenosine triphosphate (ATP). The resulting impaired calcium uptake then leads to an increased concentration of calcium, causing a local contracture of muscle fibers. Continued contraction of muscle fibers can cause blood vessel compression and local muscle ischemia, ultimately resulting in sensitization of nociceptors and a chronic pain state (Simons and Mense 1998; Simons et al. 1999; Jafri 2014). While there is some evidence to support the presence of MTrPs in muscles, the evidence to support a direct relationship between MP and MTrPs requires additional study.

Treatment of MP and MTrPs begins with an accurate diagnosis. A MTrP is palpated as a hypersensitive nodule in a taut band of the muscle (Simons et al. 1999). For patients with TMD, the masseter and temporalis are the muscles most commonly involved, and they can cause pain both locally in a predictable or unpredictable referred pattern to other areas of the face or head (Simons et al. 1999). For example, MTrP in the superficial portion of the masseter muscle can produce local pain in the muscle itself or referred pain in the lower jaw, the molar teeth and related gingiva, the maxilla, or over the eyebrow area. In contrast, MTrPs in the deep portion of the masseter muscle can produce tinnitus in the ipsilateral ear or pain in the mid cheek area, the temporomandibular joint itself, or deep in the ear (Simons et al. 1999). Myofascial trigger points can be classified as either active or latent. Active trigger points are always tender and are associated with spontaneous pain production and when palpated may produce a local "twitch" response felt by the examiner. They prevent full lengthening of the muscle and can cause muscle weakening. In contrast, while latent MTrPs can also cause muscle weakening and an inability to fully lengthen the muscle, they do not produce pain without provocation which is usually achieved via application of manual pressure to the trigger point (Simons et al. 1999). Latent MTrPs may become active by repeated muscle contraction (Celik and Mutlu 2013), and they have been associated with changes in muscle activation including increased intramuscular electromyographic activity during synergistic muscle activation and increased antagonistic muscle activity during agonist muscle contraction (Ge et al. 2014). Latent MTrPs, like active MTrPs, can also contribute to stiffness, to fatigue, and possibly to limited mouth opening (Manolopoulos et al. 2008). Sustained mechanical stimulation of latent MTrPs has been shown to induce central sensitization in healthy subjects (Xu et al. 2010). Central sensitization has been suggested as an important component in the development of many chronic musculoskeletal pain problems including TMD and headache (Sessle 2011; Coppola et al. 2013; Quartana et al. 2015). It should be noted that the 2014 Diagnostic Criteria (DC) for TMD does not consider the evaluation of latent trigger points (Schiffman et al. 2014). However, given the relationship between latent MTrPs and central sensitization, evaluation and treatment consideration should be given to both active and latent MTrPs in the orofacial region.

Treatment of MTrPs located in the muscles of mastication begins with patient education and behavioral modification as previously discussed. Sensitization of nerve fibers may be associated with excessive release of neurotransmitters in motor end plates which can lead to spontaneous electromyographic activity in parts of the muscle. Soft tissue mobilization may reduce this abnormal discharge (Fricton et al. 1985; Hong and Simons 1998). Soft tissue mobilization is used to promote muscle lengthening and relaxation, and vapocoolant spray may be used to enhance passive stretch of the muscles (Kostopoulos and Rizopoulos 2008). Soft tissue mobilization is usually performed with the patient lying in a relaxed, supported position using manual techniques such as stroking and gliding either extraorally or intraorally to increase mouth opening and reduce pain associated with MTrPs (Pierson 2011) and to improve the abnormal thickness of the masseter muscle that has been shown to be present in patients with TMD (Ariji et al. 2010).

8.4.2.3 Dry Needling

Dry needling is a skilled intervention that uses a thin filiform needle without injectate to penetrate the skin and stimulate underlying myofascial trigger points and muscular and connective tissues for the management of neuromusculoskeletal pain and movement impairments (American Physical Therapy Association 2013). The goal of MTrP dry needling is to release or inactivate trigger points and thus relieve pain (Fig. 8.3). Dry needling of muscle tissue has been shown to inactivate MTrPs (Hong 1994) and can be an effective method of relieving pain and improving the quality of life of patients with myofascial pain (Tekin et al. 2013). When comparing MTrP injection to dry needling for the reduction of cervical pain, both have been shown to be effective at reducing pain and improving range of motion,

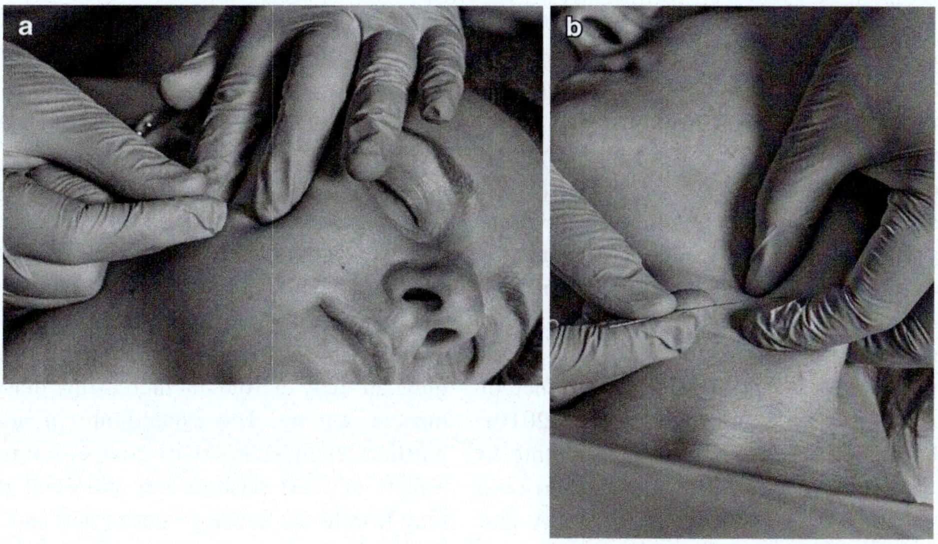

Fig. 8.3 Examples of trigger point dry needling into (**a**) masseter and (**b**) sternocleidomastoid muscles

suggesting that needling by itself constitutes the therapeutic effect and not the injected material (Ay et al. 2010).

Dry needling of MTrPs in the masseter of patients with TMD has been shown to increase pain threshold levels and maximum mouth opening distance (Fernandez-Carnero et al. 2010), and dry needling of MTrPs in the masseter, temporalis, and cervical muscles has been shown to reduce severity of symptoms in patients with myofascial pain and headache (Venancio Rde et al. 2009). Compared to trigger point injection with lidocaine or botulinum toxin, however, dry needling may be associated with increased discomfort at the insertion site during treatment and increase post-needling discomfort (Venancio Rde et al. 2009). Stretching exercises, manual therapy, and use of any modalities (Sect. 8.4.2.5) are often indicated post-needling to minimize these effects.

8.4.2.4 Cervical Spine and Postural Considerations

Symptoms of TMD and other head and orofacial pain often overlap with symptoms related to the cervical spine. Indeed, neck pain has been shown to be an associated symptom in 70% of patients diagnosed with TMD (Ciancaglini et al. 1999; Kraus 2014). The cervical spine is a primary source of headache with a prevalence of 17.8% in a general population, similar to migraine (Nilsson 1995). The pathophysiology to explain the cervical spine as a source of headache, facial, and jaw pain is based on the well-established convergence of craniofacial and cervical afferents in the trigeminocervical nucleus and upper cervical nociceptive neurons (Biondi 2000; Piovesan et al. 2003; Bogduk 2004). Pressure-pain hyperalgesia has been found in the trigeminal region in patients with chronic neck pain, suggesting spreading of sensitization to the trigeminal region in this patient population (La Touche et al. 2010). TMD has also been associated with a higher prevalence of self-reported migraine headache and chronic fatigue (Dahan et al. 2016), and since migraine headaches have been associated with the presence of neck pain (Kaniecki 2002; Calhoun et al. 2010), the role of the cervical spine as a source of head and orofacial pain, mimicking migraine or a possible pathogenesis for migraine, cannot be ignored. Clinicians treating patients for TMD, headache, and orofacial pain must consider cervical spine dysfunction as a primary source of symptom generation or at least as a concurrent source of symptoms.

Neck pain and symptoms of TMD can be related (Ciancaglini et al. 1999). In some cases, cervical spine dysfunction or injury may precede the onset of TMD symptoms. A prospective 15-year follow-up study showed that individuals who experienced a cervical spine extension-flexion rear-end collision without any direct trauma to the head or neck had a higher prevalence of TMD symptoms over a 15-year period when compared to a control group over the same period of time (Sale et al. 2014). TMD has also been associated with a higher prevalence of self-reported migraine headache and chronic fatigue (Dahan et al. 2016), and since migraine headaches have been associated with the presence of neck pain (Kaniecki 2002; Calhoun et al. 2010), the role of the cervical spine in contributing to TMD cannot be ignored. There appears to be a strong relationship between neck disability and jaw disability in patients with orofacial pain (Olivo et al. 2010). The cervical spine may be a source of masticatory muscle hyperactivity resulting in MTrPs. Evidence has shown cervical spine mobility, and positioning influences the kinematics of the human mandible (Visscher et al. 2000). Biomechanically, a link exists between the stomatognathic system and the cervical spine in that normal mouth opening is accompanied by an initial extension at the cervical-cranial junction (Eriksson et al. 2000). Changes in head posture have been associated with changes in masticatory muscle activity (Funakoshi et al. 1976; Boyd et al. 1987; Yotsuya et al. 2009), resting mandibular position (McLean et al. 1973; Solow and Tallgren 1976; Moya et al. 1994; Gonzalez and Manns 1996), and movement of the condyle within the glenoid fossa (Visscher et al. 2000). Urbanowicz (1991) has suggested a physiological model to show how changes in mandibular posture, specifically an increase in vertical dimension when wearing an oral appliance of the mandible, may contribute to craniovertebral extension leading to suboccipital compression. Straightening of cervical posture may reduce superior and retrusive forces on the mandible, allowing the mandible to seek an improved rest position (Goldstein et al. 1984). An improved mandibular rest position would allow for improved joint mechanics during movement and reduced muscular stress. Abnormal head posture may also affect the path of jaw motion during chewing, talking, swallowing, and any contact of the teeth (Mohl 1976). The tonic neck reflex (TNR) is an important developmental reflex to orient the limbs in relationship to the head-body angle. The TNR can affect masticatory muscle tone through the trigeminal neck reflex, and there is an organized neurophysiologic reflex relationship between the TNR and trigeminal motor neuron activity (Funakoshi et al. 1976).

Kinematic connections between the mandible, occiput, and cervical spine and TNR influences may all play a role in increasing masticatory muscle activity. The expenditure of additional masticatory muscle activity compensating for the effects of head posture and abnormal mobility may lead to the development of MP and MTrPs. Cervical pain, tension, limited mobility, and abnormal posture may lead to the inability of the masticatory muscles to adapt to influences originating from the cervical spine as previously described, resulting in masticatory muscle pain and MTrPs. Insight into the relationship between the cervical spine (mobility and position) and masticatory muscle activity has been demonstrated in several ways. A single injection of 2% lidocaine solution to MTrPs in the upper trapezius muscle has been shown to reduce pain and electromyographic activity in the masseter in patients with facial pain (Carlson et al. 1993). In addition, experimental trapezius muscle pain has been shown to spread over a wide area and be accompanied by a temporary reduction of mouth opening (Komiyama et al. 2005). Postural reeducation has been used as part of a successful behavioral intervention program in patients with TMD who have limited mouth opening (Komiyama et al. 1996; Komiyama et al. 1999). A combination of manual therapy and exercise directed at the cervical spine has been shown to improve pain intensity and pressure pain sensitivity in patients with myofascial TMD (La Touche et al. 2009).

Physical therapy directed at treating the cervical component may have a positive impact on reducing headache and orofacial pain of cervical spine origin and masticatory MP. Physical therapy treatment may include manual therapy (Fig. 8.4), therapeutic exercise including stretching (Fig. 8.5),

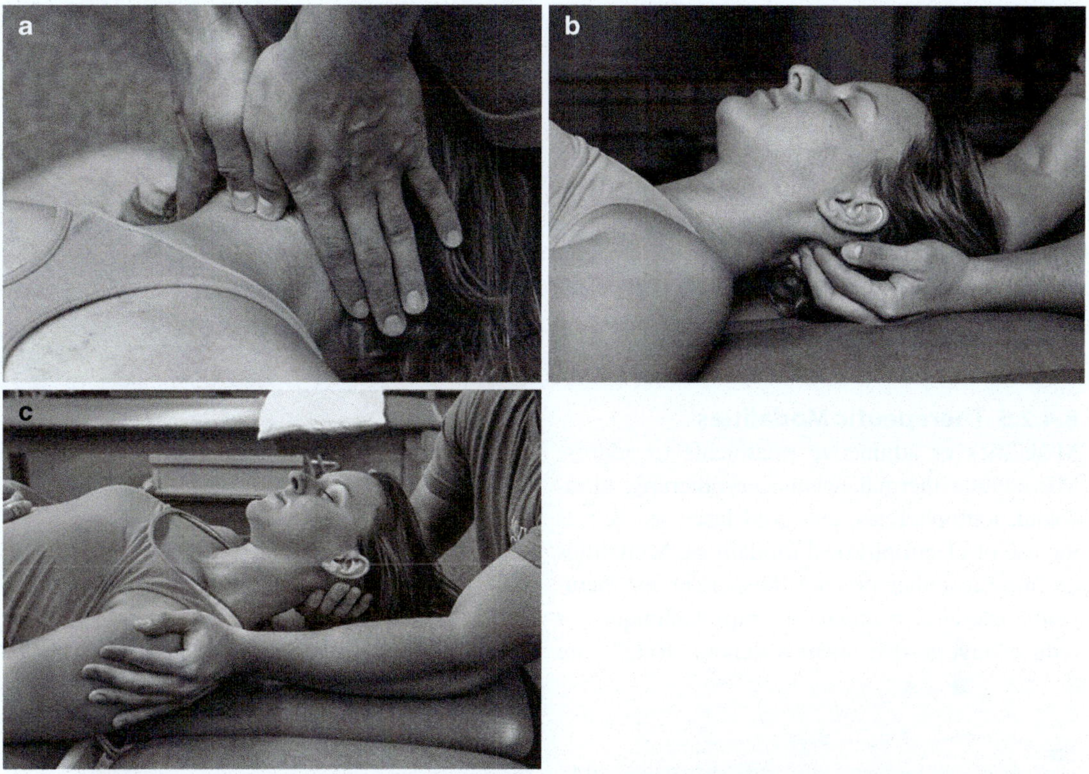

Fig. 8.4 Examples of physical therapy and manual therapy directed toward the cervical area

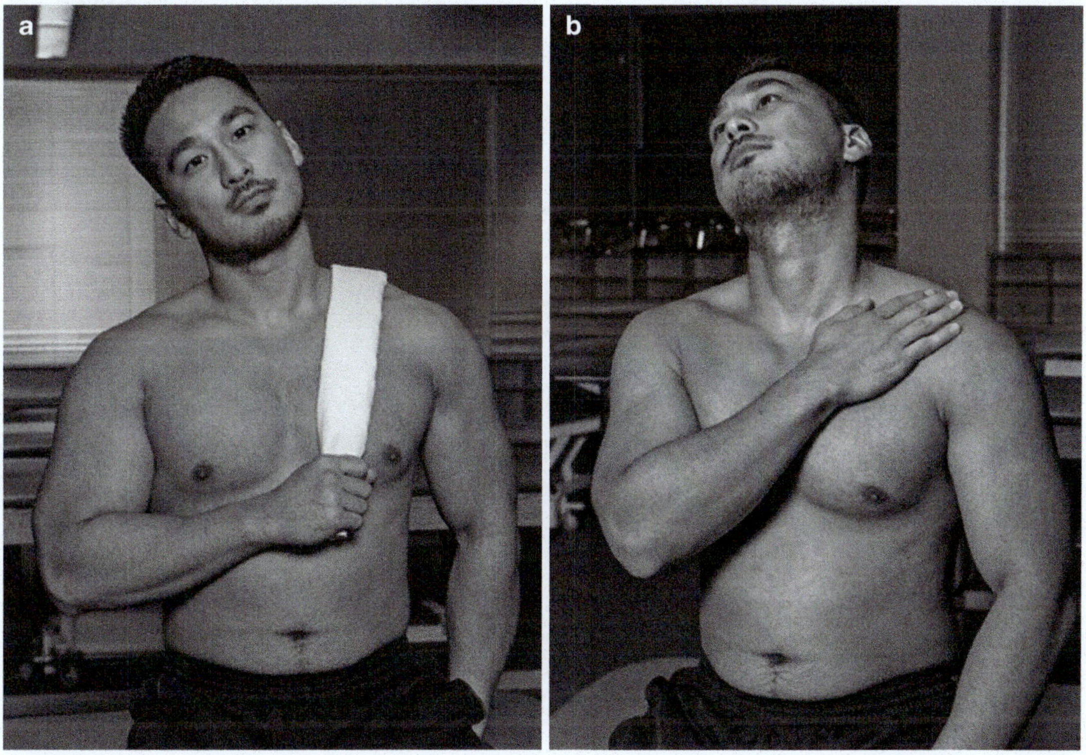

Fig. 8.5 Examples of cervical stretching exercises

dry needling, soft tissue mobilization, and postural correction activities (Fig. 8.6). Restoring cervical mobility is often a precursor to addressing postural dysfunction. Thrust and non-thrust joint mobilization can be used by the physical therapist to restore cervical spine segmental mobility, particularly in the upper cervical region. This is usually combined with activities aimed at increasing strength and endurance of the deep cervical flexor muscles (Fig. 8.7) to promote maintenance of appropriate head and neck posture (Jull et al. 2002, 2009).

8.4.2.5 Therapeutic Modalities

Modalities or adjunctive treatments to address MP include thermal agents, cryotherapy, ultrasound, iontophoresis, and cold laser, as well as the use of electrophysical modalities. Modalities are used to either prepare the patient for therapeutic exercise or manual therapy techniques or reduce any posttreatment soreness. Rarely are modalities used as the only form of treatment. The exception would be if a patient had recent acute pain due to trauma or extreme pain and disability contributing to hyperalgesia or allodynia. Thermal modalities such as heat and ultrasound

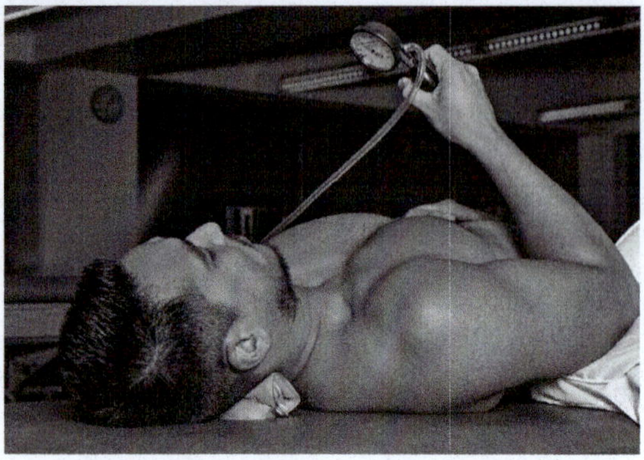

Fig. 8.7 Training of deep neck flexor muscle activation and endurance using biofeedback

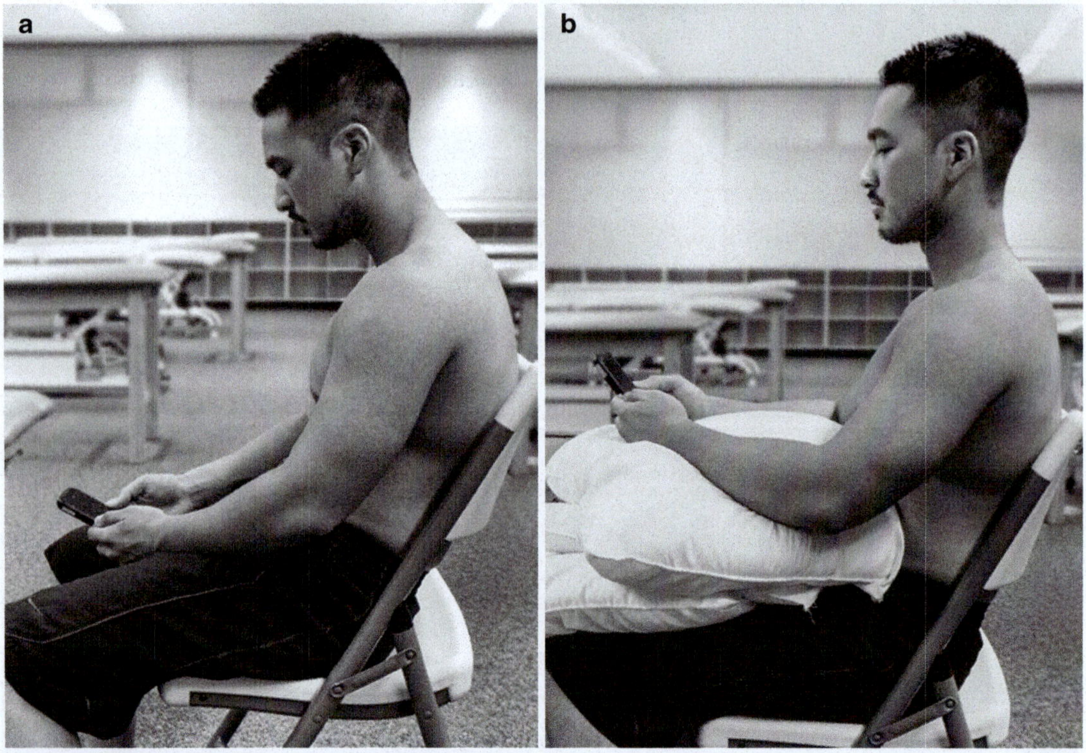

Fig. 8.6 Examples of prolonged abnormal sitting posture that can be corrected with patient education and the use of postural support for the arms

and electrophysical modalities such as iontophoresis and electric stimulation have similar goals of increasing circulation to help with ischemic muscle pain in patients with pain of muscular origin. In contrast, cold laser therapy is proposed to eliminate areas of increased muscle activity and MTrPs by increasing abnormally attenuated skin resistance to the level of the surrounding tissue (Snyder-Mackler et al. 1986). The application of heat over muscle tissue can promote reduced pain through stimulation of cutaneous thermal receptors and increased soft tissue extensibility (Cameron 2013) and lead to decreased tissue stiffness of MTrPs (Draper et al. 2010). Thermal modalities promote local vasodilation leading to increased blood flow in muscle tissue (Bickford and Duff 1953), although care should be taken when applying heat to the facial region given that pain intensity in the masseter muscle has been shown to increase when intramuscular tissue temperature is significantly elevated (Sato et al. 2015). The therapeutic effects of applying physical agents to the muscles of mastication, primarily the masseter and temporalis, can be combined with stretching exercises to promote increased muscle extensibility and jaw motion. In acute stages of muscle injury, however, the application of heat may be contraindicated, and cryotherapy or nonthermal ultrasound can be used instead to reduce inflammation and promote tissue healing. Ultrasound (Fig. 8.8) applied at intensities below a thermal level has been shown to increase intracellular calcium levels (Mortimer and Dyson 1988), increase the rate of protein synthesis by fibroblasts (Harvey et al. 1975), and increase blood flow in ischemic muscles (Barzelai et al. 2006). When ultrasound is used to promote transdermal delivery of pain-relieving and anti-inflammatory drugs such as indomethacin or hydrocortisone, this is called phonophoresis. Phonophoresis can be effective in helping to reduce pain at the TMJ (Wing 1982; Shin and Choi 1997), although its effectiveness on relieving pain due to masticatory muscle dysfunction has not been established.

Different forms of electrophysical modalities can also be used in the treatment of patients with myogenous forms of TMD. For example, transcutaneous electrical nerve stimulation (TENS) and interferential current (IFC) are typically used to modulate pain (Fig. 8.9), whereas neuromuscular electrical stimulation (NMES) is used to produce muscle contractions in innervated muscle. Pain control through the use of electrophysical modalities is achieved by different mechanisms depending on the parameters of stimulation used. For example, short-duration, high-frequency pulses can interfere with pain transmission at the spinal cord level (Melzack and Wall 1965). In contrast, lower pulse durations and higher current amplitudes can modulate pain by stimulating the production and release of endogenous opioids, endorphins, and enkepha-

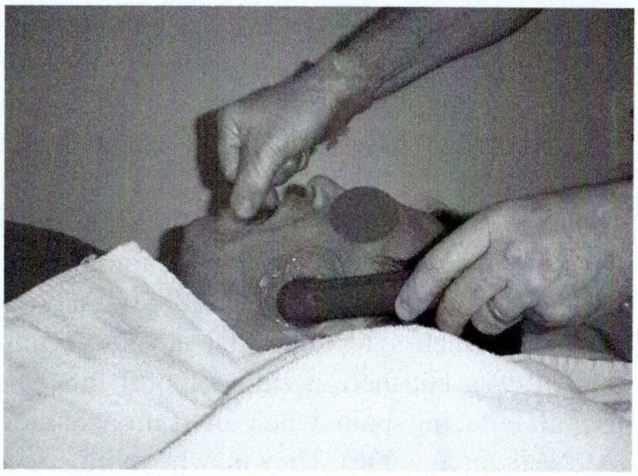

Fig. 8.8 Therapeutic ultrasound being delivered to the TMJ and masseter while applying a manual stretch to improve mouth opening

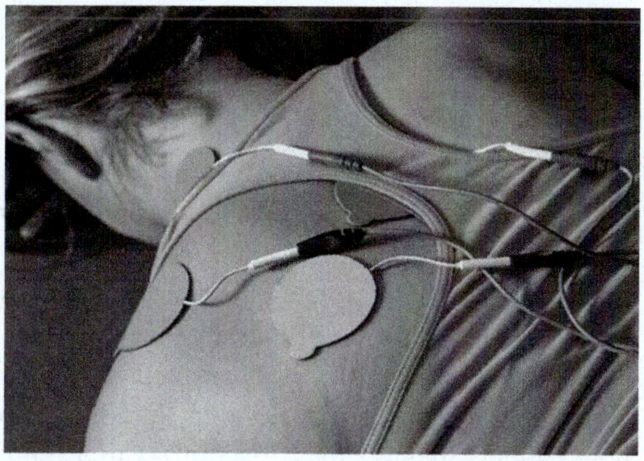

Fig. 8.9 Interferential stimulation being delivered to the trapezius area

lins (Sabino et al. 2008) and reduce painful muscle activity. Stimulation of muscle through NMES can promote increased blood flow which may accelerate tissue healing (Indergand and Morgan 1994).

The use of thermal, nonthermal, and electrophysical modalities to reduce myogenous pain or muscle tightness in patients with TMD may be beneficial when symptoms first develop (Gray et al. 1994), but there is little support for their use in reducing pain when used in isolation (McNeely et al. 2006). They may be more effective however when performed in conjunction with jaw mobility exercises or relaxation and awareness exercises to improve restricted mouth opening (Fig. 8.8).

8.4.3 Pharmacotherapy

The use of pharmacotherapy for the treatment of myogenous TMD pain may be as a monotherapy in some cases but is more often utilized in conjunction with other treatment options such as physiotherapy, behavioral therapy, or oral appliance therapy. The role of pharmacotherapy in TMD pain is typically to serve as an adjunct to help patients manage their discomfort to a point where it subsides or decreases to a level at which it no longer interferes with their daily activities. No one agent has been shown to be efficacious for the entire spectrum of TMD pain. Therefore, the effective use of pharmacotherapy relies on a good understanding as to the nature of pain of which the patient presents as well as a comprehensive knowledge of the agents contemplated for use. Mechanisms of action (MOA), potential adverse events (AEs), and possible interactions should all be considered in making the choice of agents to be prescribed. The prescriber should attempt to prescribe the most appropriate agent at the most appropriate dose utilizing the best route of administration for the individual being treated. As required for (PRN) dosing should be avoided in order to prevent persistent and breakthrough pain episodes (Sutters et al. 2010).

The evidence-based literature that supports the efficacy and safety of pharmacotherapy in the TMD population is limited (Cascos-Romero et al. 2009). Very few studies have evaluated specific pharmacological treatments for myogenous TMDs by well-controlled methods. In many clinical trials of TMD treatments, patients with myogenous pain are not distinguished from those who may have arthrogenous types of TMD (Goss et al. 1985). In addition, most reports that evaluate the pharmacological treatment of TMD pain are typically observational rather than randomized controlled trials (RTCs) (Dionne 1997). A recent review concluded that even the RTCs on this topic were of low quality (Graham et al. 2013). This section will discuss some of the more common agents as well as some newer pharmacological approaches utilized to treat muscle pain. Specific classes discussed will include analgesics, muscle relaxants, antidepressants, anticonvulsants, benzodiazepines, botulinum toxin, and the cannabinoids. A brief discussion of topical applications is also included.

8.4.3.1 Analgesics

Opioids

It has long been recognized that opioids are highly effective analgesics in both acute and chronic pain states. However, the use of opioids in chronic nonmalignant pain remains controversial due to the potential for dependence, abuse, and diversion. Prolonged use of opioids has also been linked to a potential for worsening of depression frequently seen in chronic pain patients (Graham et al. 2013). The phenomenon of opioid-induced hyperalgesia (OIH) was reported as early as 1870 in morphine-addicted patients (Albutt 1870). OIH is a paradoxical effect whereby patients who are exposed to opioids experience a decline in their pain thresholds and an increase in their pain sensitivity. OIH can occur with even brief durations of therapy. The pathophysiology of this phenomenon appears to be different from tolerance (Chu et al. 2008). However, tolerance to opioid agents may in fact be a consequence of OIH (Williams et al. 2013). Other studies have demonstrated that with persistent opioid exposure, cholecystokinin (CCK) is upregulated in the rostral ventromedial medulla

(RVM), which produces both anti-opioid and pro-nociceptive effects by activating descending RVM pain facilitation. This in turn increases pain transmission and produces hyperalgesia (Ossipov et al. 2004). Watkins and colleagues recently described the potential role that glial mechanisms may play in the pathophysiology of the pro-nociceptive sequela of opioids. Their work demonstrated the opioid-induced activation of glia by way of the toll-like receptor 4 (TLR4) and other receptors, resulting in inflammation and the release of neuroexcitatory substances (Watkins et al. 2009). Ultimately, the use of opioid analgesics in the myogenous pain patient should be limited to carefully screened individuals who have failed other, more proven, and conservative modalities. Patients prescribed opioids require careful monitoring to ensure compliance, patient safety, and efficacy of the prescribed dose.

Tramadol

Tramadol is a non-opioid analgesic that weakly binds to opioid receptors and functions as a weak mu-opioid agonist. Tramadol will also inhibit the uptake of both serotonin and norepinephrine in the dorsal horns of the spinal cord similar to the effect of tricyclic antidepressants (Stoops et al. 2012; Modi et al. 2013). There are no published studies to support the use of tramadol as a single agent in myofascial pain patient populations. However, three controlled trials have studied its efficacy in fibromyalgia and demonstrated an overall reduction in pain in this patient group (Biasi et al. 1998; Russell et al. 2000; Bennett et al. 2003). A recent study by Kaneko and colleagues demonstrated an improvement in experimentally induced neuropathic and myogenous pain in the rat model (Kaneko et al. 2014). Other studies would seem to support its use in chronic widespread pain, chronic low back pain, and osteoarthritis (Schnitzer et al. 2000; Wilder-Smith et al. 2001; Kean et al. 2009; Rosenberg 2009). The combination of tramadol with acetaminophen has also been demonstrated to be effective in the fibromyalgia patient population (Bennett et al. 2003; Bennett et al. 2005). While not considered a controlled substance in the United States, there is evidence to suggest potential for abuse and dependence with tramadol (Senay et al. 2003). However, abuse potential appears to be reduced relative to opioid agents (Stoops 2014).

NSAIDS

Nonsteroidal anti-inflammatory drugs (NSAIDs) have long been utilized in the management of acute and in some instances chronic pain. They are the most commonly used drugs for pain, largely due to their availability in both prescriptive and over-the-counter preparations. They are a class of structurally diverse agents with very similar effects. They are generally well tolerated but do include cardiovascular, gastrointestinal, and renal risks. The analgesic action of NSAIDs is via the inhibition of the cyclooxygenase 2 (COX 2) enzymes. The adverse gastrointestinal effects are a result of inhibition of the cyclooxygenase 1 (COX 1) enzyme. NSAIDs are generally classified as being nonselective COX inhibitors where they inhibit both COX 1 and COX 2 enzymes, semi-selective COX 2 inhibitors, or highly selective COX 2 inhibitors in which they are seven times or more selective in their COX 2 enzyme blocking activity (Hersh et al. 2005). Currently, literature to support the use of NSAIDs for muscle pain is lacking. Several studies have demonstrated the effectiveness of NSAIDs for chronic pain and fibromyalgia in combination with other medications, but the efficacy of oral NSAIDs as a stand-alone agent in myogenous pain remains to be demonstrated (Borg-Stein and Iaccarino 2014). Recently, the Food and Drug Administration (FDA) requested that manufacturers of all NSAIDs make labeling changes to their products. The changes are to include a boxed warning, highlighting the potential for increased risk of cardiovascular events as well as the potentially life-threatening gastrointestinal bleeding associated with their use (Health and Services 2015). Even with the lack of good evidence to support their routine use, NSAIDs are commonly recommended and prescribed for myogenous pain therapy due to being readily available and mostly inexpensive (Table 8.1). Also, many patients are comfortable utilizing these agents without a

Table 8.1 Classification of commonly prescribed NSAIDs and the usual oral adult dosing for nonspecific analgesia (Crofford 2013)

Class	Subclass	Generic drug (trade name available in the United States)	Usual adult oral dose for pain
Carboxylic acids	Salicylic acids	Acetylsalicylic acid (Aspirin)	325–650 mg PO q4h
		Diflunisal (Dolobid)	500 mg PO q12h
		Salsalate (Disalcid)	1500 mg PO bid
	Acetic acids		
		Diclofenac sodium (Voltaren-XR)	50 mg PO bid-tid
		Diclofenac potassium (Cataflam)	50 mg PO tid
		Diclofenac/misoprostol (Arthrotec)	50–75 mg PO bid-tid
		Diclofenac (Zorvolex)	18–35 mg PO tid
		Etodolac (Lodine)	200–400 mg PO q6-8 h
		Indomethacin (Indocin, Tivorbex)	25–50 mg PO bid-tid
		Sulindac (Clinoril)	150–200 mg Po bid
		Tolmetin (Tolectin)	200–600 mg PO tid
	Propionic acids	Flurbiprofen (Ansaid)	50–100 mg PO bid-tid
		Ketoprofen (Orudis)	50 mg PO q4-6 h
		Oxaprozin (Daypro)	1200 mg PO qd
		Ibuprofen (Motrin, Advil, etc.)	400 mg PO q4-6 h
		Naproxen sodium (Anaprox, Aleve, Naprelan, etc.)	220–550 PO q12h
		Naproxen (Naprosyn)	250–500 mg PO q12h
		Fenoprofen (Nalfon)	300–600 mg PO tid-qid
	Fenamic acids	Meclofenamate (Meclomen)	50–100 mg PO q4-6 h
Enolic acids	Oxicams	Piroxicam (Feldene)	20 mg PO qd
		Meloxicam (Mobic)	7.5–15 mg PO qd
		Meloxicam (Vivlodex)	5–10 mg PO qd
Nonacidic		Nabumetone	1000–2000 mg/day PO divided qd-bid
Cox 2 selective	Sulfonamide	Celecoxib (Celebrex)	200 mg PO bid

mg milligrams; *PO* (per os) by mouth; *q* (quaque) every, each; *h* (hora) hour; *bid* (bis in die) two times a day; tid (ter in die) three times a day

healthcare provider's input. NSAIDs are most commonly used as a single agent but may be formulated in combination with other agents such as opioids.

Corticosteroids

Corticosteroids are potent anti-inflammatory agents often used for acute pain and in some cases chronic pain. They reduce prostaglandin synthesis by inhibiting both phospholipase enzyme and COX 2 but have only a minor effect on COX 1 (Sapolsky et al. 2000; Rhen and Cidlowski 2005). In addition, they inhibit tumor necrosis factor alpha and interleukins 1 and 6 which are pro-inflammatory mediators (Holte and Kehlet 2002). The analgesic properties of corticosteroids have been shown primarily in surgical and osteoarthritic pain models and have not been well studied for muscular pain (Waldron et al. 2013; Abou-Raya et al. 2014). In a double-blinded crossover trial, Clark and colleagues found no benefit over placebo in patient diagnosed with what was known as fibrositis, a term previously used for fibromyalgia (Clark et al. 1985). Conversely, a study by Ernberg and colleagues demonstrated a positive response to the injection of methylprednisolone into localized areas of pain in the superficial masseter muscle (Ernberg et al. 1997). Another more recent study found that injection of a solution combining a local anesthetic with a corticosteroid provided relief of local muscle soreness a few days after injection and that there was less need for oral analgesics for the primary complaint (Venancio Rde et al. 2008). One of the primary concerns with the use of corticosteroids is the potential for endogenous adrenal suppression limiting the body's ability to respond normally to a stressful event. They can also cause a suppression of the immune response making patients more susceptible to a secondary infection. Prolonged use of corticosteroids can potentially increase the risk of a number of complications, including osteoporosis and avascular necrosis (Liu et al. 2013). Limiting the cumulative dose over the course of therapy appears to reduce the risk of adverse effects (Curtis et al. 2006). Caution or avoidance should be considered in patients with diabetes mellitus. Exogenous corticosteroids have been shown to cause elevated blood glucose levels via a decrease in glucose utilization, increased glucose production, inhibition of the effect of insulin on myocytes and adipocytes, and an increase in hepatic glucose release. Gurwitz and colleagues found that subjects receiving prednisone at a daily dose of 30 mg or more had a relative risk of 10.34 of developing diabetes as compared to controls not taking corticosteroids (Gurwitz et al. 1994). Caution or avoidance is also advised if corticosteroids are contemplated for patients with an infective process. As corticosteroids can prevent or decrease the inflammatory response to multiple mechanisms, their use in the presence of infection may mask the underlying pathological process involved. For the above-described reasons, the course of treatment with corticosteroids should be limited to the shortest duration possible and preferably for only episodic use.

Acetaminophen

Acetaminophen, known as paracetamol outside of the United States, is a non-opioid analgesic that, like the NSAIDs, may be used as a single agent or in combination with other agents such as opioids. In contrast to NSAIDs, acetaminophen is not known to be associated with myocardial infarction or gastrointestinal bleeding and is usually better tolerated (Graham et al. 2013). While it is usually considered a weaker analgesic than the NSAIDs, when acetaminophen is combined with an NSAID, the efficacy exceeds either agent used alone (Graham et al. 2013). Acetaminophen also differs from the majority of NSAIDs in that it lacks significant anti-inflammatory activity. The analgesic mechanism of action of acetaminophen has not been fully described but may be due to the inhibition of central prostaglandin synthesis and an elevation of the pain threshold (Graham et al. 2013). Other potential mechanisms of action may include the facilitation of the serotonergic descending inhibitory pathways and activation of cannabinoid receptors (Smith 2009). Hepatotoxicity is the most serious potential adverse effect associated with the use of acetaminophen, even at the recommended doses of a maximum of 4 g per day (Gupta and Jakobsson 2014). A recent recommendation from the FDA asks that providers not prescribe or dispense combination analgesic agents containing more than 325 mg of acetaminophen due to this potential for life-threatening hepatotoxicity (Mitka 2014).

Local Anesthetics

The use of local anesthetics for myogenous pain is generally reserved for times when a myofascial trigger point or a well-defined area of discomfort in the muscle can be identified. The usual route of administration is via injection, but topical preparations (transdermal) may be used as well. This application will be discussed later in this section. Trigger point injections (TPIs) have been utilized to treat a variety of painful musculoskeletal and neurological disorders for years (Ashkenazi et al. 2010). One percent lidocaine or 0.5% of bupivacaine is usually appropriate for most muscle injections (Robbins et al. 2014). To avoid ischemia and potential tissue necrosis, it is advisable to use a local anesthetic preparation without a vasoconstrictor. The MOA of local anesthetic is to decrease the permeability of ion channels to sodium ions. Trigger point injections are most often utilized to facilitate physical therapy modalities such as mobilization and stretching but may also serve as a modality to quickly relieve pain. Some debate exists as to the benefit of using local anesthetics in TPIs. Hameroff and colleagues found that based on patient's subjective report of pain relief, TPIs with bupivacaine and etidocaine were preferred over saline injections (Hameroff et al. 1981). Conversely, a 2001 review determined that TPIs using local anesthetics proved to be no more beneficial than injecting saline or using the needle alone (Cummings and White 2001). Another more recent meta-analysis of 12 studies showed no significant difference in pain reduction for trigger point injections using local anesthetics compared with control treatments consisting of saline injections, oral analgesics, or other nonpharmacological interventions (Mosshammer et al. 2013). Other studies have suggested that dry needling alone may be as effective for inactivating trigger points as utilizing a local anesthetic (Jaeger 1987; Hong 1994). It does appear that the use of a local anesthetic significantly reduces post-procedure soreness (Hong 1994). Finally, a 2008 meta-analysis examining the effectiveness of injection therapy for low back pain concluded that evidence to support or refute the use of injection therapy is currently lacking (Staal et al. 2008).

8.4.3.2 Muscle Relaxants

Muscle relaxants comprise a group of pharmacological agents with varying MOAs that appear to act on the central nervous system (CNS) to disrupt nociceptive signaling. The specific MOA of these agents is still poorly understood. Sedation is potentially a useful benefit for this class of drugs in the TMD population (Manfredini et al. 2004). Muscle relaxants appear to be more efficacious in acute muscle pain as opposed to chronic (McQuay et al. 1995). A recent Cochrane review was able to only identify one study evaluating the efficacy of a muscle relaxant on TMD pain (Mujakperuo et al. 2010). The conclusion was that the agent cyclobenzaprine was statistically superior to placebo when combined with a self-care program for jaw pain at awakening (Herman et al. 2002). Cyclobenzaprine appears to have no direct activity on skeletal muscle. Its MOA has not been fully described but is thought to be due primarily to its sedative effects (Kruidering-Hall and Campbell 2015). Of note, cyclobenzaprine is a tricyclic amine, structurally similar to amitriptyline, with ventricular dysrhythmia as a possible adverse event (Hessler 2006).

Other common agents utilized in this class include carisoprodol, metaxalone, methocarbamol, baclofen, and tizanidine (Table 8.2). Carisoprodol undergoes hepatic biotransformation to three primary metabolites: hydroxycarisoprodol, hydroxymeprobamate, and meprobamate. Meprobamate is a potent anxiolytic with significant abuse and dependency issues (Toth and Urtis 2004). Withdrawal from extended use of meprobamate may result in severe reactions including seizures and coma. The MOA of metaxalone has not yet been fully elucidated. A direct effect on skeletal muscles or nerve fibers has not been established, but CNS depression may be responsible for its effects. Compared with other muscle relaxants, metaxalone has a relatively low risk of drowsiness or cognitive defects (Milanov and Georgiev 1994). Methocarbamol is a centrally acting agent that is a derivative of guaifenesin (Kruidering-Hall and Campbell 2015). The MOA of methocarbamol is mostly unknown but is thought to be due to sedation. A fairly unique AE of this agent is the production of brown or green urine discoloration. Baclofen is a natural analog

Table 8.2 Commonly prescribed muscle relaxants (Lo and Alan 2015)

Drug (generic/trade name)	Common dosing
Cyclobenzaprine (Flexeril, Amrix, Fexmid)	5–10 mg PO qd/tid
	Maximum 40 mg/day
Chlorzoxazone (Lorzone)	250–500 mg PO tid/qid
	Maximum 750 mg/dose
Carisoprodol (Soma)	250–350 mg tid or qhs
Metaxalone (Skelaxin)	800 mg PO tid/qid
Methocarbamol (Robaxin)	1000 mg PO qid
	Maximum 8000 mg/day
Orphenadrine citrate	100 mg PO bid
Tizanidine (Zanaflex)	2–8 mg tid/qid
	Maximum 12 mg/dose, 24 mg/day
Dantrolene (Dantrium)	100 mg PO tid/qid
	Maximum 400 mg/day for 3 weeks
Baclofen	20–80 mg/day divided tid/qid

mg milligrams; *PO* (per os) by mouth; *q* (quaque) every; *d* (die) day, each; *h* (hora) hour; *bid* (bis in die) two times a day; tid (ter in die) three times a day; *qid* (quater in die) four times a day

of gamma-aminobutyric acid (GABA) that binds to GABA B receptors. It appears to act presynaptically as well as postsynaptically to inhibit spinal reflexes (Kruidering-Hall and Campbell 2015). Baclofen is available as an oral preparation, as an intrathecal injection, or for use in an intrathecal pump. This later form of administration is typically reserved for cases of severe spasticity. Common AEs include dry mouth and transient sedation that tend to subside with prolonged use. Withdrawal symptoms have been reported following abrupt discontinuation of baclofen (Terrence and Fromm 1981). These may include auditory and visual hallucinations, agitation, delirium, anxiety, fever, tremors, tachycardia, and, in some cases, seizures. As with most muscle relaxants, the precise mechanism of action of tizanidine has not been fully described but may be linked to its central alpha 2-adrenoceptor agonist properties (Kaddar et al. 2012). Therefore, caution is advised when prescribing this agent to patients with impaired renal/liver function or who may have cardiac disease. Tizanidine appears to inhibit presynaptic release of excitatory neurotransmitters, reducing the excitability of postsynaptic α motor neurons. In addition, it has been demonstrated to reduce abnormal co-contractions of opposing muscle groups (Milanov and Georgiev 1994).

8.4.3.3 Antidepressants

This class of medication is typically used in the management of depressive conditions; however, due to their inhibition of the reuptake of serotonin and norepinephrine, antidepressants are commonly used for many painful conditions (Verdu et al. 2008). Antidepressants can be grouped into four main categories: the tricyclic antidepressants (TCAs), the monoamine oxidase inhibitors (MAOIs), the selective serotonin reuptake inhibitors (SSRIs), and the dual selective norepinephrine and serotonin reuptake inhibitors (SNRIs). The SNRIs demonstrate similar properties to those of the older TCAs. The TCAs and the SNRIs have both been shown to have the greatest efficacy of the antidepressants in chronic pain conditions (Mico et al. 2006). While depression is often comorbid with chronic pain, the TCAs imipramine and amitriptyline have both demonstrated efficacy in the depressed and nondepressed subjects (Alcoff et al. 1982; Watson et al. 1982). This would seem to suggest that a unique MOA other than the antidepressant qualities is responsible for their efficacy in painful conditions. In addition, the analgesic effect of these agents is typically seen to occur more rapidly than the mood-stabilizing effect, and the required dosages for pain management have been shown to be much less than those required for mood disorders (Arnold et al. 2005; Goldstein et al. 2005). While not specific to TMD myogenous pain, several trials have explored the efficacy of amitriptyline in patients with TMD. In fact, two studies have shown a clinically significant reduction in pain utilizing amitriptyline as compared to placebo (Plesh et al. 2000; Rizzatti-Barbosa et al. 2003). Common side effects of TCAs and SNRIs include nausea, sedation, psychomotor impairment, xerostomia, and constipation (Plesh et al. 2000). These agents should be avoided in patients taking MAOIs and any other serotonergic drugs as the combination may lead to serotonin syndrome which is hallmarked by confusion, fever, shivering, diaphoresis, ataxia, myoclonus, and severe hypertension (Sporer 1995). Also of note, the prescribed dosage for pain management should be well below that required for the management of depression.

8.4.3.4 Anticonvulsants

Traditionally in the facial pain patient population, the anticonvulsant class of drugs has been utilized primarily for neuropathic pain presentations. However, as TMD pain persists, CNS changes may occur which include a sensitization similar to that seen in other chronic pain disorders such as fibromyalgia (Sessle 1995). The most commonly prescribed anticonvulsants in the orofacial pain population are carbamazepine, oxcarbazepine, gabapentin, and pregabalin. The MOA of the anticonvulsants in orofacial pain appears to be via a reduction in neurogenic inflammation and central trigeminal activation as well as an augmentation of antinociceptive activity in the CNS (Soderpalm 2002). A recent trial utilizing gabapentin for masticatory muscle pain found it to be clinically and statistically superior to placebo in reducing the subject's report of pain and muscle hyperalgesia as well as reducing the impact of pain on their day-to-day functioning (Kimos et al. 2007). Gabapentin and the structurally similar pregabalin are possible considerations due to the relative low occurrence of side effects as compared to other agents in this class and their proven efficacy in trials involving various chronic pain syndromes (Pandey et al. 2005; Arnold et al. 2007; Tassone et al. 2007). It is important to note that in 2008, the FDA announced that all anticonvulsant drugs must display a clear warning that their use increases risk of suicidal thoughts and behaviors.

8.4.3.5 Benzodiazepines

Benzodiazepines are neuropsychoactive agents utilized primarily for their anxiolytic, sedative-hypnotic, muscle relaxant, and anticonvulsant properties. These agents produce their primary therapeutic effects through their interaction with the GABA A receptors, the major inhibitory receptors in the brain. Benzodiazepines could be considered as an alternative to the more traditional skeletal muscle relaxants, albeit with limited evidence of efficacy and potential for abuse (Chou et al. 2007). In one study of 20 TMD patients with both joint and muscle pain, clonazepam was found to be significantly more effective than placebo (Harkins et al. 1991). A larger study in patients with fibromyalgia found a decrease in the subject's rating of their symptoms after 6 weeks of receiving a combination of alprazolam and ibuprofen (Russell et al. 1991). While most would agree that benzodiazepine use should be limited to low doses over a short duration, Schenck and colleagues found that long-term, nightly use of clonazepam for the treatment of what was described as injurious parasomnias proved to have sustained efficacy with a low risk of dosage tolerance, adverse events, or even abuse (Schenck and Mahowald 1996). New data suggest that benzodiazepine use is associated with an increased risk of Alzheimer's disease as well as other dementias (de Gage et al. 2014). However, other recent reports would seem to dispute these conclusions (Imfeld et al. 2015).

8.4.3.6 Botulinum Toxin

Botulinum toxin (BTX) is a neurotoxin that when injected intramuscularly will temporarily prevent the release of acetylcholine at the neuromuscular junction resulting in a generalized decrease in muscle contraction strength. It has traditionally been utilized for the treatment of movement disorders such as spasticity and dystonia and autonomic disorders associated with cholinergic overactivity, such as hyperhidrosis and sialorrhea. In the TMD patient population, a randomized clinical trial using double-blinding and placebo control to discern its efficacy for myofascial pain found improvements in both the objective and subjective outcome variables as compared to placebo (Guarda-Nardini et al. 2008). A more recent review concluded that BTX was no more effective to treat TMD myofascial pain than other more conventional and established therapies (Dall'Antonia et al. 2013). In a recent updated Cochrane review looking at BTX for myofascial pain syndromes (MPS), the authors concluded that there is inconclusive evidence to support the use of BTX based on the data from four studies with a total of 233 participants (Soares et al. 2014). This is in agreement with their previous review (Soares et al. 2012). Another recent review by Gerwin and colleagues emphasized the need for better evidence to determine the true efficacy of BTX for MPS (Gerwin 2012). Standardization of dosing and injection site protocols will most likely prove beneficial going forward. It has recently been revealed that BTX possesses MOAs independent of its effect on muscle contractions such as the inhibition of mechanical nociception in peripheral trigeminovascular neurons (Burstein et al. 2014). The BTX molecule has been shown to inhibit the release of serotonin, dopamine, noradrenaline, glutamate, gamma-aminobutyric acid (GABA), enkephalin, glycine, substance P, ATP, calcitonin gene-related peptide (CGRP), somatostatin, and neuronal nitric oxide synthase which could partially explain its analgesic effect (Pavone and Luvisetto 2010). It should be noted that due to the reduction of contractile strength seen when BTX is injected intramuscularly, there appears to be a risk for a reduction in bone mineral density or osteopenic changes even after a single injection (Tsai et al. 2011; Raphael et al. 2014; Matthys et al. 2015).To date, this occurrence has been primarily demonstrated in the animal model with only one small pilot study appearing to replicate the effect in the human subject (Raphael et al. 2014). Further trials are needed with larger sample sizes followed over a longer duration. However, for this reason and due to the limited evidence of efficacy, it would seem reasonable to reserve the use of BTX for the more refractory cases until further data can be accumulated.

8.4.3.7 Cannabinoids

Cannabinoids have been used for medical purposes for many years. The cannabinoid (CB) receptors have emerged as a therapeutic target of interest in pain management in recent years particularly in patients where conventional therapies have failed. The antinociceptive effect of CBs can be mediated by either the CB1 receptor or the CB2 receptors depending on the type of pain. CB1 receptors are expressed at high levels in the CNS and to a degree in the spinal cord, the dorsal root ganglion, and in the periphery (Herkenham 1995). CB2 analgesia is related to peripheral mechanisms without apparent CNS effects (Zogopoulos et al. 2013). CB1 appears to be more involved with acute pain, whereas with chronic pain, it appears to be mediated by both CB1 and CB2 (Cox et al. 2007). As a whole, CBs appear to be better suited for chronic pain conditions (Beaulieu and Ware 2007). However, a recent report from Bagues and colleagues found that tetrahydrocannabinol (THC), a cannabinoid natural derivative with therapeutic use in humans, reduced the nociceptive behaviors in two models of acute muscle pain in rats (Bagues et al. 2014). While it is encouraging that some studies on the use of CBs for multiple sclerosis and spasticity-related pain (Svendsen et al. 2004; Wissel et al. 2006) report positive outcomes, overall, robust evidence for routine use in acute or chronic myogenous condition pain is still lacking. Future research and utilization of CBs in pain management will most certainly be affected at least in part by the legal climate.

8.4.3.8 Topical Applications

Topical (transdermal) medications allow for the distribution of a pharmacological agent in a very concentrated delivery area. There are some patients averse to taking oral medications that may be more agreeable to a topical preparation. Topical applications are also advantageous in patients taking multiple other medications where there is concern of drug interactions or other adverse events. Topical preparations may be used in conjunction with the systemic analog of the same agent thereby reducing the systemic dose needed and decreasing the incidence of AEs. Topical agents for pain management typically involve a local anesthetic agent and/or an analgesic but may include other pharmacological agents. Topical NSAIDs have been demonstrated to be effective in relieving muscle pain with a low incidence of adverse effects (Derry et al. 2015). Specifically, diclofenac, ibuprofen, ketoprofen, piroxicam, and indomethacin proved to be significantly more effective than placebo where subjects reported at least a 50% decrease in their pain scores (Derry et al. 2015). Topicals are usually prepared as a cream, ointment, and gel or in a patch (reservoir design) and must have the ability to penetrate the skin. Factors that may influence the ability of the preparation to penetrate the skin include the integrity of the skin, the patient's age, and the presence of any dermatologic disorders or disease. The ability of the preparation to absorb effectively is augmented by the use of carrier agents that are highly lipid soluble. Topical preparations should be avoided in individuals with broken skin, skin lesions, or atrophy or who have a known sensitivity to any of the ingredients of the agents being utilized. It is beneficial for the clinician to work with a qualified compounding pharmacist in order to ensure that the most appropriate agents are correctly prepared and utilized for the problem being addressed.

8.4.4 The Role of Occlusion and Occlusal Oriented Treatments

Over the years, there has been much controversy and debate as to the role of occlusion in the etiology and/or maintenance of TMDs. For many years, dentists have utilized occlusal therapies for the treatment and prevention of TMDs. However, recent evidence suggests that the role of occlusion in TMDs is much less important than once believed (Turp and Schindler 2012). In fact, a recent review concluded that static occlusal factors had no significant association with TMD (Cruz et al. 2015). Yet, in the same review, dynamic occlusal factors including the absence of canine guidance, laterotrusive interferences, and a shift of ≥2 mm from the retruded contact position (RCP) to maximum intercuspation (MI) demonstrated a recognizable impact. Another recent study found that some occlusal features may play a small role (10.8%) in myogenous TMDs, namely, a mediotrusive interference and RCP-MI slide of ≥2 mm (Landi et al. 2004). The following sections will briefly look at occlusal factors pertaining to orthodontics, occlusal therapy, and oral appliances from a therapeutic viewpoint.

8.4.4.1 Orthodontics

Orthodontic therapy is a well-proven modality for the correction of occlusal discrepancies in both the growing and adult population. Given that the role of occlusal factors in TMDs is limited at best (Turp and Schindler 2012), the correction of occlusal discrepancies solely to treat a TMD should be viewed with caution. In fact, orthodontic therapy for the treatment of TMDs is not supported by the evidence (Macfarlane et al. 2009). A recent Cochrane review concluded there is no evidence from randomized controlled trials (RTCs) to support the notion that orthodontic treatment can prevent or treat TMDs (Luther et al. 2010). It should also be noted that orthodontic treatment carries with it the risk of destabilizing the stomatognathic system during the course of therapy (Greene 1982).

8.4.4.2 Occlusal Therapy

Many dental practitioners continue to believe that occlusal factors are causative or at the very least a significant perpetuating factor for TMDs and subsequently utilize occlusal adjustment as an initial treatment for these disorders, in spite of evidence to the contrary (Koh and Robinson 2004). Occlusal therapy (OT) can be a subtractive, additive, or combination procedure with the goal being to adjust the dentition in such a way as to allow the upper and lower arches to occlude in the most stable manner as possible. Occlusal therapy can also be performed to remove undesirable tooth contacts in functional movements such as nonworking side contacts allowing for cuspid-guided or group function in lateral excursive movements. It has long been thought that guidance on the anterior teeth in lateral excursive movements with the absence of posterior tooth contact resulted in a reduction of masticatory muscle electromyography (EMG) activity (Williamson and Lundquist 1983). However, these early reports mostly measured EMG activity utilizing occlusal splints as opposed to the natural dentition. In one small study of nine healthy and asymptomatic subjects, those without nonworking side contacts demonstrated a more uniform signal of the masticatory muscle EMG than those with the working side contacts (Nishigawa et al. 1997). However, it remains to be proven if these EMG patterns have any relationship to myogenous TMD. Treatment outcomes are often used as proof of concept, but to date, most studies of occlusal adjustment involve case series with a lack of control groups or placebo interventions for comparison. With the growing appreciation for evidence-based dentistry/medicine, it recognized that studies that rely on clinical observation and expert opinion can lead to strongly biased and nonsupported conclusions about treatment effects (Richards and Lawrence 1995; Raphael and Marbach 1997). Even as early as 1976, Goodman and colleagues showed that there was no difference in pain outcomes in patients treated with occlusal adjustments as compared with mock adjustments (Goodman et al. 1976). In another study, Tsolka and colleagues found no difference in treatment outcomes after real and mock occlusal adjustment (Tsolka et al. 1992). Their group attributed the positive effects of the supposed intervention to be primarily a placebo response. Given the irreversible nature of occlusal adjustments combined with the lack of evidence as to its efficacy for the treatment of myogenous facial pain, this approach cannot be recommended (Stohler 2008).

8.4.5 Oral Appliances

A 1993 survey of members of the American Dental Association found that the oral appliance (OA) was the most commonly prescribed therapy for the treatment of TMDs by both general dentists and specialists (Glass et al. 1993). Oral appliances may be soft or hard and may be made to cover a full or partial dental arch. There are a number of theories as to how OAs may benefit the patient with myogenous TMD pain, yet debate persists as to the validity of these theories (Klasser et al. 2010). There is some evidence to suggest that an OA will, at least for the short term, reduce sleep-time masticatory muscle activity (Dube et al. 2004). However, a recent review found that a hard acrylic OA, termed a stabilization splint, does not demonstrate better clinical outcomes than a non-occluding palatal appliance, a soft OA, or other conservative therapies such as physical therapy or acupuncture (Turp et al. 2004). A stabilization splint has been described as a hard acrylic OA that provides a temporary, so-called, ideal occlusion (Al-Ani et al. 2005). In contrast to Turp and colleagues, a 10-week RCT found that the stabilization appliance was more effective in alleviating symptoms of myogenous TMD pain than a palatal, non-occluding appliance (Ekberg et al. 2003). In a more recent review and meta-analysis, what was described as a properly adjusted, hard stabilization appliance demonstrated "good evidence of modest efficacy" in the treatment of TMD pain as "compared to non-occluding appliances and no treatment" (Fricton et al. 2010). Interestingly, several recent short-term studies have demonstrated a reduction in sleep bruxism with the use of a mandibular advancement type OA (Landry et al. 2006; Landry-Schonbeck et al. 2009). However, the relationship between sleep bruxism and myogenous TMD pain is debated in the literature (Raphael et al. 2012). When the existing literature on oral appliance therapy is reviewed, it becomes clear that there is a need for more RCTs looking at subjects over a longer period of time. It would also prove beneficial to standardize the trials in ways such as OA design, material used, and patterns of use. While even part-time use of an OA can lead to unwanted permanent bite changes, it is generally recommended that their use be limited to sleep or part-time wear only (Magdaleno and Ginestal 2010). As with any therapy, careful patient selection and compliance monitoring will decrease the incidence of adverse events.

References

Abou-Raya A, Abou-Raya S, Khadrawi T, Helmii M. Effect of low-dose oral prednisolone on symptoms and systemic inflammation in older adults with moderate to severe knee osteoarthritis: a randomized placebo-controlled trial. J Rheumatol. 2014;41(1):53–9.

Aggarwal VR, Tickle M, Javidi H, Peters S. Reviewing the evidence: can cognitive behavioral therapy improve outcomes for patients with chronic orofacial pain? J Orofac Pain. 2010;24(2):163–71.

Al-Ani Z, Gray RJ, Davies SJ, Sloan P, Glenny AM. Stabilization splint therapy for the treatment of temporomandibular myofascial pain: a systematic review. J Dent Edu. 2005;69(11):1242–50.

Albutt C. On the abuse of hypodermic injections of morphia. Practitioner. 1870;3:327–30.

Alcoff J, Jones E, Rust P, Newman R. Controlled trial of imipramine for chronic low back pain. J Fam Pract. 1982;14(5):841–6.

American Academy of Orofacial Pain. In: de Leeuw R, Klasser GD, editors. Orofacial pain guidelines for assessment, diagnosis, and management. Hanover Park, IL: Quintessence Publishing Co, Inc; 2013.

American Association of Dental Research (Adopted 1996, revised 2010). Policy Statement on Tempromandibular Disorders, American Association of Dental Research.

American Physical Therapy Association. Description of Dry Needling In Clinical Practice: An Educational Resource Paper, APTA Public Policy, Practice, and Professional Affairs Unit. 2013.

Andersen LL, Jay K, Andersen CH, Jakobsen MD, Sundstrup E, Topp R, Behm DG. Acute effects of massage or active exercise in relieving muscle soreness: randomized controlled trial. J Strength Cond Res. 2013;27(12):3352–9.

Ariji Y, Katsumata A, Hiraiwa Y, Izumi M, Sakuma S, Shimizu M, Kurita K, Ariji E. Masseter muscle sonographic features as indices for evaluating efficacy of massage treatment. Oral Surg Oral Med Oral Pathol Oral Radiol Endod. 2010;110(4):517–26.

Armijo-Olivo S, Pitance L, Singh V, Neto F, Thie N, Michelotti A. Effectiveness of manual therapy and therapeutic exercise for temporomandibular disorders: systematic review and meta-analysis. Phys Ther. 2016;96(1):9–25.

Arnold LM, Goldenberg DL, Stanford SB, Lalonde JK, Sandhu HS, Keck PE Jr, Welge JA, Bishop F, Stanford

KE, Hess EV, Hudson JI. Gabapentin in the treatment of fibromyalgia: a randomized, double-blind, placebo-controlled, multicenter trial. Arthritis Rheum. 2007;56(4):1336–44.

Arnold LM, Rosen A, Pritchett YL, D'Souza DN, Goldstein DJ, Iyengar S, Wernicke JF. A randomized, double-blind, placebo-controlled trial of duloxetine in the treatment of women with fibromyalgia with or without major depressive disorder. Pain. 2005;119(1–3):5–15.

Ashkenazi A, Blumenfeld A, Napchan U, Narouze S, Grosberg B, Nett R, DePalma T, Rosenthal B, Tepper S, Lipton RB, Interventional Procedures Special Interest Section of the American. Peripheral nerve blocks and trigger point injections in headache management - a systematic review and suggestions for future research. Headache. 2010;50(6):943–52.

Ay S, Evcik D, Tur BS. Comparison of injection methods in myofascial pain syndrome: a randomized controlled trial. Clin Rheumatol. 2010;29(1):19–23.

Bagues A, Martin MI, Sanchez-Robles EM. Involvement of central and peripheral cannabinoid receptors on antinociceptive effect of tetrahydrocannabinol in muscle pain. Eur J Pharmacol. 2014;745:69–75.

Barzelai S, Sharabani-Yosef O, Holbova R, Castel D, Walden R, Engelberg S, Scheinowitz M. Low-intensity ultrasound induces angiogenesis in rat hind-limb ischemia. Ultrasound Med Biol. 2006;32(1):139–45.

Beaulieu P, Ware M. Reassessment of the role of cannabinoids in the management of pain. Curr Opin Anaesthesiol. 2007;20(5):473–7.

Bennett RM, Kamin M, Karim R, Rosenthal N. Tramadol and acetaminophen combination tablets in the treatment of fibromyalgia pain: a double-blind, randomized, placebo-controlled study. Am J Med. 2003;114(7):537–45.

Bennett RM, Schein J, Kosinski MR, Hewitt DJ, Jordan DM, Rosenthal NR. Impact of fibromyalgia pain on health-related quality of life before and after treatment with tramadol/acetaminophen. Arthritis Rheum. 2005;53(4):519–27.

Bialosky JE, Bishop MD, Price DD, Robinson ME, George SZ. The mechanisms of manual therapy in the treatment of musculoskeletal pain: a comprehensive model. Man Ther. 2009;14(5):531–8.

Biasi G, Manca S, Manganelli S, Marcolongo R. Tramadol in the fibromyalgia syndrome: a controlled clinical trial versus placebo. Int J Clin Pharmacol res. 1998;18(1):13–9.

Bickford RH, Duff RS. Influence of ultrasonic irradiation on temperature and blood flow in human skeletal muscle. Circ Res. 1953;1(6):534–8.

Biondi DM. Cervicogenic headache: mechanisms, evaluation, and treatment strategies. J Am Osteopath Assoc. 2000;100(9 Suppl):S7–14.

Bogduk N. The neck and headaches. Neurol Clin. 2004;22(1):151–71, vii.

Bonathan CJ, Zakrzewska JM, Love J, Williams AC. Beliefs and distress about orofacial pain: patient journey through a specialist pain consultation. J Oral Facial Pain Headache. 2014;28(3):223–32.

Borg-Stein J, Iaccarino MA. Myofascial pain syndrome treatments. Phys Med Rehabil Clin N Am. 2014;25(2):357–74.

Boyd CH, Slagle WF, Boyd CM, Bryant RW, Wiygul JP. The effect of head position on electromyographic evaluations of representative mandibular positioning muscle groups. Cranio. 1987;5(1):50–4.

Burstein R, Zhang X, Levy D, Aoki KR, Brin MF. Selective inhibition of meningeal nociceptors by botulinum neurotoxin type a: therapeutic implications for migraine and other pains. Cephalalgia. 2014;34(11):853–69.

Calhoun AH, Ford S, Millen C, Finkel AG, Truong Y, Nie Y. The prevalence of neck pain in migraine. Headache. 2010;50(8):1273–7.

Calixtre LB, Moreira RF, Franchini GH, Alburquerque-Sendin F, Oliveira AB. Manual therapy for the management of pain and limited range of motion in subjects with signs and symptoms of temporomandibular disorder: a systematic review of randomised controlled trials. J Oral Rehabil. 2015;42(11):847–61.

Cameron MH. Physical agents in rehabilitation from research to practice. St Louis, MO: Elsevier Saunders; 2013.

Carlson CR, Okeson JP, Falace DA, Nitz AJ, Lindroth JE. Reduction of pain and EMG activity in the masseter region by trapezius trigger point injection. Pain. 1993;55(3):397–400.

Carlsson GE. Critical commentary 1: the etiology of temporomandibular disorders: implications for treatment. J Orofac Pain. 2001;15:106–8.

Cascos-Romero J, Vazquez-Delgado E, Vazquez-Rodriguez E, Gay-Escoda C. The use of tricyclic antidepressants in the treatment of temporomandibular joint disorders: systematic review of the literature of the last 20 years. Med Oral Patol Oral Cir Bucal. 2009;14(1):E3–7.

Celik D, Mutlu EK. Clinical implication of latent myofascial trigger point. Curr Pain Headache Rep. 2013;17(8):353.

Chen Q, Bensamoun S, Basford JR, Thompson JM, An KN. Identification and quantification of myofascial taut bands with magnetic resonance elastography. Arch Phys Med Rehabil. 2007;88(12):1658–61.

Chen Q, Wang HJ, Gay RE, Thompson JM, Manduca A, An KN, Ehman RE, Basford JR. Quantification of myofascial taut bands. Arch Phys Med Rehabil. 2016;97(1):67–73.

Chou R, Qaseem A, Snow V, Casey D, Cross JT Jr, Shekelle P, Owens DK, Clinical Efficacy Assessment Subcommittee of the American College of, Physicians; American College of and Physicians; American Pain Society Low Back Pain Guidelines. Diagnosis and treatment of low back pain: a joint clinical practice guideline from the American College of Physicians and the American Pain Society. Ann Int Med. 2007;147(7):478–91.

Chu LF, Angst MS, Clark D. Opioid-induced hyperalgesia in humans: molecular mechanisms and clinical considerations. Clin J Pain. 2008;24(6):479–96.

Ciancaglini R, Testa M, Radaelli G. Association of neck pain with symptoms of temporomandibular dysfunction in the general adult population. Scand J Rehabil Med. 1999;31(1):17–22.

Cioffi I, Landino D, Donnarumma V, Castroflorio T, Lobbezoo F, Michelotti A. Frequency of daytime tooth clenching episodes in individuals affected by masticatory muscle pain and pain-free controls during standardized ability tasks. Clin Oral Investig. 2016;21(4):1139–48.

Clark S, Tindall E, Bennett RM. A double blind crossover trial of prednisone versus placebo in the treatment of fibrositis. J Rheumatol. 1985;12(5):980–3.

Coppola G, Di Lorenzo C, Schoenen J, Pierelli F. Habituation and sensitization in primary headaches. J Headache Pain. 2013;14:65.

Costen JB. A syndrome of ear and sinus symptoms dependent upon disturbed function of the temporomandibular joint. Ann Otol Rhinol Laryngol. 1934;43:1–15.

Cox ML, Haller VL, Welch SP. The antinociceptive effect of Delta9-tetrahydrocannabinol in the arthritic rat involves the CB(2) cannabinoid receptor. Eur J Pharmacol. 2007;570(1–3):50–6.

Crofford LJ. Use of NSAIDs in treating patients with arthritis. Arthritis Res Ther. 2013;15(Suppl 3):S2.

Cruz CL, Lee KC, Park JH, Zavras A. Malocclusion characteristics as risk factors for temporomandibular disorders: lessons learned from a meta-analysis. J Oral Dis. 2015:1–11.

Cummings TM, White AR. Needling therapies in the management of myofascial trigger point pain: a systematic review. Arch Phys Med Rehabil. 2001;82(7):986–92.

Curtis JR, Westfall AO, Allison J, Bijlsma JW, Freeman A, George V, Kovac SH, Spettell CM, Saag KG. Population-based assessment of adverse events associated with long-term glucocorticoid use. Arthritis Rheum. 2006;55(3):420–6.

Dahan H, Shir Y, Nicolau B, Keith D, Allison P. Self-reported migraine and chronic fatigue syndrome are more prevalent in people with myofascial vs nonmyofascial temporomandibular disorders. J Oral Facial Pain Headache. 2016;30(1):7–13.

Dall'Antonia M, et al. Jaw muscles myofascial pain and botulinum toxin. Revista Dor. 2013;14.1:52–7.

De Felicio CM, Ferreira CL, Medeiros AP, Rodrigues Da Silva MA, Tartaglia GM, Sforza C. Electromyographic indices, orofacial myofunctional status and temporomandibular disorders severity: a correlation study. J Electromyogr Kinesiol. 2012;22(2):266–72.

de Gage SB, et al. Benzodiazepine use and risk of Alzheimer's disease: case-control study. BMJ. 2014;349:g5205.

De Laat A, Stappaerts K, Papy S. Counseling and physical therapy as treatment for myofascial pain of the masticatory system. J Orofac Pain. 2003;17(1):42–9.

Derry S, Moore RA, Gaskell H, McIntyre M, Wiffen PJ. Topical NSAIDs for acute musculoskeletal pain in adults. Cochrane Database Syst rev. 2015;6:CD007402.

Dionne RA. Pharmacologic treatments for temporomandibular disorders. Oral Surg Oral Med Oral Pathol Oral Radiol Endod. 1997;83(1):134–42.

Dommerholt J, Gerwin RD. A critical evaluation of Quintner et al: missing the point. J Bodyw Mov Ther. 2015;19(2):193–204.

Draper DO, Mahaffey C, Kaiser D, Eggett D, Jarmin J. Thermal ultrasound decreases tissue stiffness of trigger points in upper trapezius muscles. Physiother Theory Pract. 2010;26(3):167–72.

Dube C, Rompre PH, Manzini C, Guitard F, de Grandmont P, Lavigne GJ. Quantitative polygraphic controlled study on efficacy and safety of oral splint devices in tooth-grinding subjects. J Dent Res. 2004;83(5):398–403.

Ekberg E, Vallon D, Nilner M. The efficacy of appliance therapy in patients with temporomandibular disorders of mainly myogenous origin. A randomized, controlled, short-term trial. J Orofac Pain. 2003;17(2):133–9.

Eriksson PO, Haggman-Henrikson B, Nordh E, Zafar H. Co-ordinated mandibular and head-neck movements during rhythmic jaw activities in man. J Dent Res. 2000;79(6):1378–84.

Ernberg M, Hedenberg-Magnusson B, Alstergren P, Kopp S. Short-term effect of glucocorticoid injection into the superficial masseter muscle of patients with chronic myalgia: a comparison between fibromyalgia and localized myalgia. J Orofac Pain. 1997;11(3):249–57.

Fernandes G, Franco-Micheloni AL, Siqueira JT, Goncalves DA, Camparis CM. Parafunctional habits are associated cumulatively to painful temporomandibular disorders in adolescents. Braz Oral Res. 2016;30

Fernandez-Carnero J, La Touche R, Ortega-Santiago R, Galan-del-Rio F, Pesquera J, Ge HY, Fernandez-de-Las-Penas C. Short-term effects of dry needling of active myofascial trigger points in the masseter muscle in patients with temporomandibular disorders. J Orofac Pain. 2010;24(1):106–12.

Ferreira CL, Machado BC, Borges CG, Rodrigues Da Silva MA, Sforza C, De Felicio CM. Impaired orofacial motor functions on chronic temporomandibular disorders. J Electromyogr Kinesiol. 2014;24(4):565–71.

Feu D, Catharino F, Quintao CC, Almeida MA. A systematic review of etiological and risk factors associated with bruxism. J Orthod. 2013;40(2):163–71.

Fricton J, Heir GM. History of temporomandibular disorders and orofacial pain in the United States. The past, present and future of temporomandibular disorders and orofacial pain. C. a. Friction, Shinhung International; 2006.

Fricton J, Look JO, Wright E, Alencar FG Jr, Chen H, Lang M, Ouyang W, Velly AM. Systematic review and meta-analysis of randomized controlled trials evaluating intraoral orthopedic appliances for temporomandibular disorders. J Orofac Pain. 2010;24(3):237–54.

Fricton JR, Auvinen MD, Dykstra D, Schiffman E. Myofascial pain syndrome: electromyographic changes associated with local twitch response. Arch Phys Med Rehabil. 1985;66(5):314–7.

Funakoshi M, Fujita N, Takehana S. Relations between occlusal interference and jaw muscle activities in response to changes in head position. J Dent res. 1976;55(4):684–90.

Ge HY, Monterde S, Graven-Nielsen T, Arendt-Nielsen L. Latent myofascial trigger points are associated with an increased intramuscular electromyographic activity during synergistic muscle activation. J Pain. 2014; 15(2):181–7.

Gerwin R. Botulinum toxin treatment of myofascial pain: a critical review of the literature. Curr Pain Headache Rep. 2012;16(5):413–22.

Giesecke T, Gracely RH, Williams DA, Geisser ME, Petzke FW, Clauw DJ. The relationship between depression, clinical pain, and experimental pain in a chronic pain cohort. Arthritis Rheum. 2005;52(5):1577–84.

Glass EG, Glaros AG, McGlynn FD. Myofascial pain dysfunction: treatments used by ADA members. Cranio. 1993;11(1):25–9.

Goldstein DF, Kraus SL, Williams WB, Glasheen-Wray M. Influence of cervical posture on mandibular movement. J Prosthet Dent. 1984;52(3):421–6.

Goldstein DJ, Lu Y, Detke MJ, Lee TC, Iyengar S. Duloxetine vs. placebo in patients with painful diabetic neuropathy. Pain. 2005;116(1–2):109–18.

Gonzalez HE, Manns A. Forward head posture: its structural and functional influence on the stomatognathic system, a conceptual study. Cranio. 1996;14(1):71–80.

Goodman P, Greene CS, Laskin DM. Response of patients with myofascial pain-dysfunction syndrome to mock equilibration. J Am Dent Assoc. 1976;92(4):755–8.

Goss AN, Speculand B, Hallet E. Diagnosis of temporomandibular joint pain in patients seen at a pain clinic. J Oral Maxillofac Surg. 1985;43(2):110–4.

Graham GG, Davies MJ, Day RO, Mohamudally A, Scott KF. The modern pharmacology of paracetamol: therapeutic actions, mechanism of action, metabolism, toxicity and recent pharmacological findings. Inflammopharmacology. 2013;21(3):201–32.

Gray RJ, Quayle AA, Hall CA, Schofield MA. Physiotherapy in the treatment of temporomandibular joint disorders: a comparative study of four treatment methods. Br Dent J. 1994;176(7):257–61.

Greene CS. Orthodontics and the temporomandibular joint. Angle Orthod. 1982;52(2):166–72.

Greene CS. The etiology of temporomandibular disorders: implications for treatment. J Orofac Pain. 2001;15(2):93–105; discussion 106–116.

Guarda-Nardini L, Manfredini D, Salamone M, Salmaso L, Tonello S, Ferronato G. Efficacy of botulinum toxin in treating myofascial pain in bruxers: a controlled placebo pilot study. Cranio. 2008;26(2):126–35.

Gupta A, Jakobsson J. Acetaminophen, nonsteroidal antiinflammatory drugs, and cyclooxygenase-2 selective inhibitors: an update. Plast Reconstr Surg. 2014;134(4 Suppl 2):24S–31S.

Gurwitz JH, Field TS, Glynn RJ, Manson JE, Avorn J, Taylor JO, Hennekens CH. Risk factors for non-insulin-dependent diabetes mellitus requiring treatment in the elderly. J Am Geriatr Soc. 1994;42(12):1235–40.

Hameroff SR, Crago BR, Blitt CD, Womble J, Kanel J. Comparison of bupivacaine, etidocaine, and saline for trigger-point therapy. Anesth Analg. 1981;60(10): 752–5.

Harkins S, Linford J, Cohen J, Kramer T, Cueva L. Administration of clonazepam in the treatment of TMD and associated myofascial pain: a double-blind pilot study. J Craniomandib Disord. 1991;5(3):179–86.

Harvey W, Dyson M, Pond JB, Grahame R. The stimulation of protein synthesis in human fibroblasts by therapeutic ultrasound. Rheumatol Rehabil. 1975;14(4):237.

Health and Services. FDA drug safety communication: FDA strengthens warning that non-aspirin nonsteroidal anti-inflammatory drugs (NSAIDs) can cause heart attacks or strokes. 2015. Accessed25

Herkenham M. Localization of cannabinoid receptors in the brain and periphery. In: Pertwee RG, editor. Cannabinoid Receptors. London: Academic Press; 1995. p. 145–66.

Herman CR, Schiffman EL, Look JO, Rindal DB. The effectiveness of adding pharmacologic treatment with clonazepam or cyclobenzaprine to patient education and self-care for the treatment of jaw pain upon awakening: a randomized clinical trial. J Orofac Pain. 2002;16(1):64–70.

Hersh EV, Lally ET, Moore PA. Update on cyclooxygenase inhibitors: has a third COX isoform entered the fray? Curr Med Res Opin. 2005;21(8):1217–26.

Hessler RA. Cardiovascular principles. In: Goldfrank LR, Flomenbaum N, editors. Goldfrank's toxicologic emergencies. New York: McGraw-Hill, Medical Pub; 2006. Division: 364–79.

Holte K, Kehlet H. Perioperative single-dose glucocorticoid administration: pathophysiologic effects and clinical implications. J Am Coll Surg. 2002;195(5):694–712.

Hong CZ. Lidocaine injection versus dry needling to myofascial trigger point. The importance of the local twitch response. Am J Phys Med Rehabil. 1994;73(4):256–63.

Hong CZ, Simons DG. Pathophysiologic and electrophysiologic mechanisms of myofascial trigger points. Arch Phys Med Rehabil. 1998;79(7):863–72.

Imfeld P, Bodmer M, Jick SS, Meier CR. Benzodiazepine use and risk of developing Alzheimer's disease or vascular dementia: a case-control analysis. Drug Saf. 2015;38(10):909–19.

Indergand HJ, Morgan BJ. Effects of high-frequency transcutaneous electrical nerve stimulation on limb blood flow in healthy humans. Phys Ther. 1994;74(4):361–7.

International Association for the Study of Pain. Classification of chronic pain. Descriptions of chronic pain syndromes and definitions of pain terms. Prepared by the International Association for the Study of Pain, subcommittee on taxonomy. Pain Suppl. 1986;3:S1–226.

Jaeger B. Double blind, controlled study of different myofacial trigger point injection techniques. Pain. 1987;4(Suppl):S292.

Jafri MS. Mechanisms of myofascial pain. Int Sch Res Notices. 2014;2014

Jull G, Trott P, Potter H, Zito G, Niere K, Shirley D, Emberson J, Marschner I, Richardson C. A random-

ized controlled trial of exercise and manipulative therapy for cervicogenic headache. Spine (Phila Pa 1976). 2002;27(17):1835–43; discussion 1843.
Jull GA, Falla D, Vicenzino B, Hodges PW. The effect of therapeutic exercise on activation of the deep cervical flexor muscles in people with chronic neck pain. Man Ther. 2009;14(6):696–701.
Kaddar N, Vigneault P, Pilote S, Patoine D, Simard C, Drolet B. Tizanidine (Zanaflex): a muscle relaxant that may prolong the QT interval by blocking IKr. J Cardiovasc Pharmacol Ther. 2012;17(1):102–9.
Kaneko K, Umehara M, Homan T, Okamoto K, Oka M, Oyama T. The analgesic effect of tramadol in animal models of neuropathic pain and fibromyalgia. Neurosci Lett. 2014;562:28–33.
Kaniecki RG. Migraine and tension-type headache: an assessment of challenges in diagnosis. Neurology. 2002;58(9 Suppl 6):S15–20.
Karlsson L, Gerdle B, Ghafouri B, Backryd E, Olausson P, Ghafouri N, Larsson B. Intramuscular pain modulatory substances before and after exercise in women with chronic neck pain. Eur J Pain. 2015;19(8):1075–85.
Kean WF, Bouchard S, Roderich Gossen E. Women with pain due to osteoarthritis: the efficacy and safety of a once-daily formulation of tramadol. Pain med. 2009;10(6):1001–11.
Kimos P, Biggs C, Mah J, Heo G, Rashiq S, Thie NM, Major PW. Analgesic action of gabapentin on chronic pain in the masticatory muscles: a randomized controlled trial. Pain. 2007;127(1–2):151–60.
Klasser GD, Greene CS. Predoctoral teaching of temporomandibular disorders: a survey of U.S. and Canadian dental schools. J Am Dent Assoc. 2007;138(2):231–7.
Klasser GD, Greene CS. The changing field of temporomandibular disorders: what dentists need to know. J Can Dent Assoc. 2009;75(1):49–53.
Klasser GD, Greene CS, Lavigne GJ. Oral appliances and the management of sleep bruxism in adults: a century of clinical applications and search for mechanisms. Int J Prosthodont. 2010;23(5):453–62.
Klasser GD, Rei N, Lavigne GJ. Sleep bruxism etiology: the evolution of a changing paradigm. J Can Dent Assoc. 2015;81:f2.
Koh H, Robinson PG. Occlusal adjustment for treating and preventing temporomandibular joint disorders. J Oral Rehabil. 2004;31(4):287–92.
Komiyama O, Arai M, Kawara M, Kobayashi K, De Laat A. Pain patterns and mandibular dysfunction following experimental trapezius muscle pain. J Orofac Pain. 2005;19(2):119–26.
Komiyama O, Arai M, Kitamura M, Kawara M, Kobayashi K. Effect of posture correction in patients with painful limited mouth opening. J Dent Res. 1996;75(Special issue):434.
Komiyama O, Kawara M, Arai M, Asano T, Kobayashi K. Posture correction as part of behavioural therapy in treatment of myofascial pain with limited opening. J Oral Rehabil. 1999;26(5):428–35.
Korr IM, editor. The Neurobiologic mechanisms in manipulative therapy. New York: Plunum Press; 1978.
Kostopoulos D, Rizopoulos K. Effect of topical aerosol skin refrigerant (spray and stretch technique) on passive and active stretching. J Bodyw Mov Ther. 2008;12(2):96–104.
Kotiranta U, Suvinen T, Kauko T, Le Bell Y, Kemppainen P, Suni J, Forssell H. Subtyping patients with temporomandibular disorders in a primary health care setting on the basis of the research diagnostic criteria for temporomandibular disorders axis II pain-related disability: a step toward tailored treatment planning? J Oral Facial Pain Headache. 2015;29(2):126–34.
Kraus SL, editor. Clinics in physical therapy. Temporomandibualr disorders. New York, NY: Chruchill Livingstone Inc; 1994.
Kraus SL. Physical therapy management of temporomandibular disorders. In: Fonseca RJ, editor. Oral and maxillofacial surgery: temporomandibular disorders, vol. 4: WB Saunders Company; 2000. p. 161–93.
Kraus SL. Characteristics of 511 patients with temporomandibular disorders referred for physical therapy. Oral Surg Oral Med Oral Pathol Oral Radiol. 2014;118(4):432–9.
Kruidering-Hall M, Campbell L. Skeletal muscle relaxants. In: Katzung BG, Trevor AJ, editors. Basic & clinical pharmacology, vol. 13. New York, NY: McGraw-Hill; 2015.
La Touche R, Fernandez-de-Las-Penas C, Fernandez-Carnero J, Diaz-Parreno S, Paris-Alemany A, Arendt-Nielsen L. Bilateral mechanical-pain sensitivity over the trigeminal region in patients with chronic mechanical neck pain. J Pain. 2010;11(3):256–63.
La Touche R, Fernandez-de-las-Penas C, Fernandez-Carnero J, Escalante K, Angulo-Diaz-Parreno S, Paris-Alemany A, Cleland JA. The effects of manual therapy and exercise directed at the cervical spine on pain and pressure pain sensitivity in patients with myofascial temporomandibular disorders. J Oral Rehabil. 2009;36(9):644–52.
Landi N, Manfredini D, Tognini F, Romagnoli M, Bosco M. Quantification of the relative risk of multiple occlusal variables for muscle disorders of the stomatognathic system. J Prosthet Dent. 2004;92(2):190–5.
Landry-Schonbeck A, de Grandmont P, Rompre PH, Lavigne GJ. Effect of an adjustable mandibular advancement appliance on sleep bruxism: a crossover sleep laboratory study. Int J Prosthodont. 2009;22(3):251–9.
Landry ML, Rompre PH, Manzini C, Guitard F, de Grandmont P, Lavigne GJ. Reduction of sleep bruxism using a mandibular advancement device: an experimental controlled study. Int J Prosthodont. 2006;19(6):549–56.
Liu D, Ahmet A, Ward L, Krishnamoorthy P, Mandelcorn ED, Leigh R, Brown JP, Cohen A, Kim H. A practical guide to the monitoring and management of the complications of systemic corticosteroid therapy. Allergy Asthma Clin Immunol. 2013;9(1):30.
Lo JC, Alan DK. Benzodiazepines and muscle relaxants. New York: Springer; 2015. p. 167–78.

Luther F, Layton S, McDonald F. Orthodontics for treating temporomandibular joint (TMJ) disorders. Cochrane Database Syst Rev. 2010;7:CD006541.
Macfarlane TV, Kenealy P, Kingdon HA, Mohlin BO, Pilley JR, Richmond S, Shaw WC. Twenty-year cohort study of health gain from orthodontic treatment: temporomandibular disorders. Am J Orthod Dentofacial Orthop. 2009;135(6.): 692 e691–8; discussion 692–693.
Magdaleno F, Ginestal E. Side effects of stabilization occlusal splints: a report of three cases and literature review. Cranio. 2010;28(2):128–35.
Manfredini D, Arveda N, Guarda-Nardini L, Segu M, Collesano V. Distribution of diagnoses in a population of patients with temporomandibular disorders. Oral Surg Oral Med Oral Pathol Oral Radiol. 2012;114(5):e35–41.
Manfredini D, Landi N, Tognini F, Orlando B, Bosco M. Muscle relaxants in the treatment of myofascial face pain. A literature review. Minerva Stomatol. 2004;53(6):305–13.
Manolopoulos L, Vlastarakos PV, Georgiou L, Giotakis I, Loizos A, Nikolopoulos TP. Myofascial pain syndromes in the maxillofacial area: a common but underdiagnosed cause of head and neck pain. Int J Oral Maxillofac Surg. 2008;37(11):975–84.
Martins WR, Blasczyk JC, Aparecida Furlan de Oliveira M, Lagoa Goncalves KF, Bonini-Rocha AC, Dugailly PM, de Oliveira RJ. Efficacy of musculoskeletal manual approach in the treatment of temporomandibular joint disorder: a systematic review with meta-analysis. Man Ther. 2015;21:10–17.
Matthys T, Ho Dang HA, Rafferty KL, Herring SW. Bone and cartilage changes in rabbit mandibular condyles after 1 injection of botulinum toxin. Am J Orthod Dentofac Orthop. 2015;148(6):999–1009.
McLean LF, Brenman HS, Friedman MG. Effects of changing body position on dental occlusion. J Dent Res. 1973;52(5):1041–5.
McNeely ML, Armijo Olivo S, Magee DJ. A systematic review of the effectiveness of physical therapy interventions for temporomandibular disorders. Phys Ther. 2006;86(5):710–25.
McQuay H, Carroll D, Jadad AR, Wiffen P, Moore A. Anticonvulsant drugs for management of pain: a systematic review. BMJ. 1995;311(7012):1047–52.
Medlicott MS, Harris SR. A systematic review of the effectiveness of exercise, manual therapy, electrotherapy, relaxation training, and biofeedback in the management of temporomandibular disorder. Phys Ther. 2006;86(7):955–73.
Melzack R, Wall PD. Pain mechanisms: a new theory. Science. 1965;150(3699):971–9.
Mico JA, Berrocoso E, Ortega-Alvaro A, Gibert-Rahola J, Rojas-Corrales MO. The role of 5-HT1A receptors in research strategy for extensive pain treatment. Curr Top Med Chem. 2006;6(18):1997–2003.
Milanov I, Georgiev D. Mechanisms of tizanidine action on spasticity. Acta Neurol Scand. 1994;89(4):274–9.
Mitka M. FDA asks physicians to stop prescribing high-dose acetaminophen products. JAMA. 2014;311(6):563.
Modi H, Mazumdar B, Bhatt J. Study of interaction of tramadol with amlodipine in mice. Indian J Pharm. 2013;45(1):76–9.
Mohl ND. Head posture and its role in occlusion. N Y State Dent J. 1976;42(1):17–23.
Mortimer AJ, Dyson M. The effect of therapeutic ultrasound on calcium uptake in fibroblasts. Ultrasound Med Biol. 1988;14(6):499–506.
Mosshammer D, Mayer B, Joos S. Local anesthetics injection therapy for musculoskeletal disorders: a systematic review and meta-analysis. Clin J Pain. 2013;29(6):540–50.
Moya H, Miralles R, Zuniga C, Carvajal R, Rocabado M, Santander H. Influence of stabilization occlusal splint on craniocervical relationships. Part I: cephalometric analysis. Cranio. 1994;12(1):47–51.
Mujakperuo HR, Watson M, Morrison R, Macfarlane TV. Pharmacological interventions for pain in patients with temporomandibular disorders. Cochrane Database Syst Rev. 2010;10:CD004715.
Newham DJ, Edwards RHT, Mills KR. Skeletal muscle pain. In: Melzack R, Wall PD, editors. Textbook of pain. Edinburgh: Churchill Livingstone; 1994. p. 423–40.
Nicolakis P, Erdogmus B, Kopf A, Nicolakis M, Piehslinger E, Fialka-Moser V. Effectiveness of exercise therapy in patients with myofascial pain dysfunction syndrome. J Oral Rehabil. 2002;29(4):362–8.
Nilsson N. The prevalence of cervicogenic headache in a random population sample of 20-59 year olds. Spine (Phila Pa 1976). 1995;20(17):1884–8.
Nishigawa K, Nakano M, Bando E. Study of jaw movement and masticatory muscle activity during unilateral chewing with and without balancing side molar contacts. J Oral Rehabil. 1997;24(9):691–6.
Olivo SA, Fuentes J, Major PW, Warren S, Thie NMR, Magee DJ. The association between neck disability and jaw disability. J Oral Rehabil. 2010;37(9):670–9.
Ossipov MH, Lai J, King T, Vanderah TW, Malan TP Jr, Hruby VJ, Porreca F. Antinociceptive and nociceptive actions of opioids. J Neurobiol. 2004;61(1):126–48.
Pandey CK, Raza M, Tripathi M, Navkar DV, Kumar A, Singh UK. The comparative evaluation of gabapentin and carbamazepine for pain management in Guillain-Barre syndrome patients in the intensive care unit. Anesth Analg. 2005;101(1):220–5, table of contents.
Pavone F, Luvisetto S. Botulinum neurotoxin for pain management: insights from animal models. Toxins (Basel). 2010;2(12):2890–913.
Pierson MJ. Changes in temporomandibular joint dysfunction symptoms following massage therapy: a case report. Int J Ther Massage Bodywork. 2011;4(4):37–47.
Piovesan EJ, Kowacs PA, Oshinsky ML. Convergence of cervical and trigeminal sensory afferents. Curr Pain Headache Rep. 2003;7(5):377–83.
Plesh O, Curtis D, Levine J, McCall WD Jr. Amitriptyline treatment of chronic pain in patients with temporomandibular disorders. J Oral Rehabil. 2000;27(10):834–41.
Quartana PJ, Finan PH, Smith MT. Evidence for sustained mechanical pain sensitization in women with chronic

temporomandibular disorder versus healthy female participants. J Pain. 2015;16(11):1127–35.
Quintner JL, Bove GM, Cohen ML. A critical evaluation of the trigger point phenomenon. Rheumatology (Oxford). 2015;54(3):392–9.
Raphael K, Marbach JJ. Evidence-based care of musculoskeletal facial pain: implications for the clinical science of dentistry. J Am Dent Assoc. 1997;128(1):73–9.
Raphael KG, Sirois DA, Janal MN, Wigren PE, Dubrovsky B, Nemelivsky LV, Klausner JJ, Krieger AC, Lavigne GJ. Sleep bruxism and myofascial temporomandibular disorders: a laboratory-based polysomnographic investigation. J Am Dent Assoc. 2012;143(11):1223–31.
Raphael KG, Tadinada A, Bradshaw JM, Janal MN, Sirois DA, Chan KC, Lurie AG. Osteopenic consequences of botulinum toxin injections in the masticatory muscles: a pilot study. J Oral Rehabil. 2014;41(8):555–63.
Restrepo CC, Vasquez LM, Alvarez M, Valencia I. Personality traits and temporomandibular disorders in a group of children with bruxing behaviour. J Oral Rehabil. 2008;35(8):585–93.
Rhen T, Cidlowski JA. Antiinflammatory action of glucocorticoids--new mechanisms for old drugs. N Engl J Med. 2005;353(16):1711–23.
Richards D, Lawrence A. Evidence based dentistry. Br Dent J. 1995;179(7):270–3.
Rizzatti-Barbosa CM, Nogueira MT, de Andrade ED, Ambrosano GM, de Barbosa JR. Clinical evaluation of amitriptyline for the control of chronic pain caused by temporomandibular joint disorders. Cranio. 2003;21(3):221–5.
Robbins MS, Kuruvilla D, Blumenfeld A, Charleston L, Sorrell M, Robertson CE, Grosberg BM, Bender SD, Napchan U, Ashkenazi A. Trigger point injections for headache disorders: expert consensus methodology and narrative review. Headache. 2014;54(9):1441–59.
Rosenberg MT. The role of tramadol ER in the treatment of chronic pain. Int J Clin Pract. 2009;63(10):1531–43.
Russell IJ, Fletcher EM, Michalek JE, McBroom PC, Hester GG. Treatment of primary fibrositis/fibromyalgia syndrome with ibuprofen and alprazolam. A double-blind, placebo-controlled study. Arthritis Rheum. 1991;34(5):552–60.
Russell IJ, Kamin M, Bennett RM, Schnitzer TJ, Green JA, Katz WA. Efficacy of tramadol in treatment of pain in fibromyalgia. J Clin Rheumatol. 2000;6(5):250–7.
Sabino GS, Santos CM, Francischi JN, de Resende MA. Release of endogenous opioids following transcutaneous electric nerve stimulation in an experimental model of acute inflammatory pain. J Pain. 2008;9(2):157–63.
Sale H, Bryndahl F, Isberg A. A 15-year follow-up of temporomandibular joint symptoms and magnetic resonance imaging findings in whiplash patients: a prospective, controlled study. Oral Surg Oral Med Oral Pathol Oral Radiol. 2014;117(4):522–32.
Santana-Mora U, Martinez-Insua A, Santana-Penin U, del Palomar AP, Banzo JC, Mora MJ. Muscular activity during isometric incisal biting. J Biomech. 2014;47(16):3891–7.
Sapolsky RM, Romero LM, Munck AU. How do glucocorticoids influence stress responses? Integrating permissive, suppressive, stimulatory, and preparative actions. Endocr Rev. 2000;21(1):55–89.
Sato H, Castrillon EE, Cairns BE, Bendixen KH, Wang K, Nakagawa T, Wajima K, Svensson P. Intramuscular temperature modulates glutamate-evoked masseter muscle pain intensity in humans. J Oral Facial Pain Headache. 2015;29(2):158–67.
Schenck CH, Mahowald MW. Long-term, nightly benzodiazepine treatment of injurious parasomnias and other disorders of disrupted nocturnal sleep in 170 adults. Am J med. 1996;100(3):333–7.
Schiffman E, Ohrbach R, Truelove E, Look J, Anderson G, Goulet JP, List T, Svensson P, Gonzalez Y, Lobbezoo F, Michelotti A, Brooks SL, Ceusters W, Drangsholt M, Ettlin D, Gaul C, Goldberg LJ, Haythornthwaite JA, Hollender L, Jensen R, John MT, De Laat A, de Leeuw R, Maixner W, van der Meulen M, Murray GM, Nixdorf DR, Palla S, Petersson A, Pionchon P, Smith B, Visscher CM, Zakrzewska J, Dworkin SF. Diagnostic criteria for temporomandibular disorders (DC/TMD) for clinical and research applications: recommendations of the international RDC/TMD consortium network* and orofacial pain special interest groupdagger. J Oral Facial Pain Headache. 2014;28(1):6–27.
Schnitzer TJ, Gray WL, Paster RZ, Kamin M. Efficacy of tramadol in treatment of chronic low back pain. J Rheumatol. 2000;27(3):772–8.
Senay EC, Adams EH, Geller A, Inciardi JA, Munoz A, Schnoll SH, Woody GE, Cicero TJ. Physical dependence on Ultram (tramadol hydrochloride): both opioid-like and atypical withdrawal symptoms occur. Drug Alcohol Depend. 2003;69(3):233–41.
Sessle B. Masticatory muscle disorders: a basic science perspective. In: Sessle B, Bryant P, Dionne R, editors. Temporomandibular disorders and related pain conditions, vol. 4. Seattle, WA: IASP Press; 1995.
Sessle BJ. Peripheral and central mechanisms of orofacial inflammatory pain. Int Rev Neurobiol. 2011;97:179–206.
Shah JP, Phillips TM, Danoff JV, Gerber LH. An in vivo microanalytical technique for measuring the local biochemical milieu of human skeletal muscle. J Appl Physiol (1985). 2005;99(5):1977–84.
Shin SM, Choi JK. Effect of indomethacin phonophoresis on the relief of temporomandibular joint pain. Cranio. 1997;15(4):345–8.
Sikdar S, Ortiz R, Gebreab T, Gerber LH, Shah JP. Understanding the vascular environment of myofascial trigger points using ultrasonic imaging and computational modeling. Conf Proc IEEE Eng Med Biol Soc. 2010;2010:5302–5.
Sikdar S, Shah JP, Gebreab T, Yen RH, Gilliams E, Danoff J, Gerber LH. Novel applications of ultrasound technology to visualize and characterize myofascial trigger points and surrounding soft tissue. Arch Phys Med Rehabil. 2009;90(11):1829–38.
Simons DG, Mense S. Understanding and measurement of muscle tone as related to clinical muscle pain. Pain. 1998;75(1):1–17.

Simons DG, Travell JG, Simons LS. Travell and Simons' myofacial pain and dysfunction. The trigger point manual. Volume 1. Upper half of body. Baltimore, MD: Lippincott Williams & Wilkins; 1999.

Smith HS. Potential analgesic mechanisms of acetaminophen. Pain Phys. 2009;12(1):269–80.

Snyder-Mackler L, Bork C, Bourbon B, Trumbore D. Effect of helium-neon laser on musculoskeletal trigger points. Phys Ther. 1986;66(7):1087–90.

Soares A, Andriolo RB, Atallah AN, da Silva EM. Botulinum toxin for myofascial pain syndromes in adults. Cochrane Database Syst Rev. 2012;4:CD007533.

Soares A, Andriolo RB, Atallah AN, da Silva EM. Botulinum toxin for myofascial pain syndromes in adults. Cochrane Database Syst Rev. 2014;7:CD007533.

Soderpalm B. Anticonvulsants: aspects of their mechanisms of action. Eur J Pain. 2002;6(Suppl A):3–9.

Solow B, Tallgren A. Head posture and craniofacial morphology. Am J Phys Anthropol. 1976;44(3):417–35.

Sporer KA. The serotonin syndrome. Implicated drugs, pathophysiology and management. Drug Saf. 1995;13(2):94–104.

Staal JB, de Bie R, de Vet HC, Hildebrandt J, Nelemans P. Injection therapy for subacute and chronic low-back pain. Cochrane Database Syst Rev. 2008;3:CD001824.

Stohler CS. Management of persistent orofacial pain. In: Sessle BJ, Lavigne GJ, Lund JP, Dubner R, editors. Orofacial pain: from basic science to clinical management. Chicago, IL: Quintessence; 2008. p. 153–60.

Stoops WW. Abuse potential of tapentadol compared to tramadol and hydromorphone in recreational opioid users. Drug Alcohol Depend. 2014;140:e217–8.

Stoops WW, Lofwall MR, Nuzzo PA, Craig LB, Siegel AJ, Walsh SL. Pharmacodynamic profile of tramadol in humans: influence of naltrexone pretreatment. Psychopharmacology. 2012;223(4):427–38.

Sturdivant J, Fricton JR. Physical therapy for temporomandibular disorders and orofacial pain. Curr Opin Dent. 1991;1(4):485–96.

Sutters KA, Miaskowski C, Holdridge-Zeuner D, Waite S, Paul SM, Savedra MC, Lanier B, Mahoney K. A randomized clinical trial of the efficacy of scheduled dosing of acetaminophen and hydrocodone for the management of postoperative pain in children after tonsillectomy. Clin J Pain. 2010;26(2):95–103.

Svendsen KB, Jensen TS, Bach FW. Does the cannabinoid dronabinol reduce central pain in multiple sclerosis? Randomised double blind placebo controlled crossover trial. BMJ. 2004;329(7460):253.

Tassone DM, Boyce E, Guyer J, Nuzum D. Pregabalin: a novel gamma-aminobutyric acid analogue in the treatment of neuropathic pain, partial-onset seizures, and anxiety disorders. Clin Ther. 2007;29(1):26–48.

Tekin L, Akarsu S, Durmus O, Cakar E, Dincer U, Kiralp MZ. The effect of dry needling in the treatment of myofascial pain syndrome: a randomized double-blinded placebo-controlled trial. Clin Rheumatol. 2013;32(3):309–15.

Terrence CF, Fromm GH. Complications of baclofen withdrawal. Arch Neurol. 1981;38(9):588–9.

Tosato Jde P, Caria PH, Gomes CA, Berzin F, Politti F, Gonzalez Tde O, Biasotto-Gonzalez DA. Correlation of stress and muscle activity of patients with different degrees of temporomandibular disorder. J Phys Ther Sci. 2015;27(4):1227–31.

Toth PP, Urtis J. Commonly used muscle relaxant therapies for acute low back pain: a review of carisoprodol, cyclobenzaprine hydrochloride, and metaxalone. Clin Ther. 2004;26(9):1355–67.

Treacy K. Awareness/relaxation training and transcutaneous electrical neural stimulation in the treatment of bruxism. J Oral Rehabil. 1999;26(4):280–7.

Tsai CY, Shyr YM, Chiu WC, Lee CM. Bone changes in the mandible following botulinum neurotoxin injections. Eur J Orthod. 2011;33(2):132–8.

Tsolka P, Morris RW, Preiskel HW. Occlusal adjustment therapy for craniomandibular disorders: a clinical assessment by a double-blind method. J Prosthet Dent. 1992;68(6):957–64.

Turp JC, Komine F, Hugger A. Efficacy of stabilization splints for the management of patients with masticatory muscle pain: a qualitative systematic review. Clin Oral Investig. 2004;8(4):179–95.

Turp JC, Schindler H. The dental occlusion as a suspected cause for TMDs: epidemiological and etiological considerations. J Oral Rehabil. 2012;39(7):502–12.

Urbanowicz M. Alteration of vertical dimension and its effect on head and neck posture. Cranio. 1991;9(2):174–9.

van Selms MK, Visscher CM, Naeije M, Lobbezoo F. Bruxism and associated factors among Dutch adolescents. Community Dent Oral Epidemiol. 2013;41(4):353–63.

Venancio Rde A, Alencar FG Jr, Zamperini C. Botulinum toxin, lidocaine, and dry-needling injections in patients with myofascial pain and headaches. Cranio. 2009;27(1):46–53.

Venancio Rde A, Alencar FG, Zamperini C. Different substances and dry-needling injections in patients with myofascial pain and headaches. Cranio. 2008;26(2):96–103.

Verdu B, Decosterd I, Buclin T, Stiefel F, Berney A. Antidepressants for the treatment of chronic pain. Drugs. 2008;68(18):2611–32.

Visscher CM, Huddleston Slater JJ, Lobbezoo F, Naeije M. Kinematics of the human mandible for different head postures. J Oral Rehabil. 2000;27(4):299–305.

Waldron NH, Jones CA, Gan TJ, Allen TK, Habib AS. Impact of perioperative dexamethasone on postoperative analgesia and side-effects: systematic review and meta-analysis. Br J Anaesth. 2013;110(2):191–200.

Watkins LR, Hutchinson MR, Rice KC, Maier SF. The "toll" of opioid-induced glial activation: improving the clinical efficacy of opioids by targeting glia. Trends Pharmacol Sci. 2009;30(11):581–91.

Watson CP, Evans RJ, Reed K, Merskey H, Goldsmith L, Warsh J. Amitriptyline versus placebo in postherpetic neuralgia. Neurology. 1982;32(6):671–3.

Wilder-Smith CH, Hill L, Spargo K, Kalla A. Treatment of severe pain from osteoarthritis with slow-release tramadol or dihydrocodeine in combination with NSAID's: a randomised study comparing analgesia, antinociception and gastrointestinal effects. Pain. 2001;91(1–2):23–31.

Williams JT, Ingram SL, Henderson G, Chavkin C, von Zastrow M, Schulz S, Koch T, Evans CJ, Christie MJ. Regulation of mu-opioid receptors: desensitization, phosphorylation, internalization, and tolerance. Pharmacol Rev. 2013;65(1):223–54.

Williamson EH, Lundquist DO. Anterior guidance: its effect on electromyographic activity of the temporal and masseter muscles. J Prosthet Dent. 1983;49(6):816–23.

Wing M. Phonophoresis with hydrocortisone in the treatment of temporomandibular joint dysfunction. Phys Ther. 1982;62(1):32–3.

Wirianski A, Deall S, Whittle T, Wong M, Murray GM, Peck CC. Isotonic resistance jaw exercise alters jaw muscle coordination during jaw movements. J Oral Rehabil. 2014;41(5):353–66.

Wissel J, Haydn T, Muller J, Brenneis C, Berger T, Poewe W, Schelosky LD. Low dose treatment with the synthetic cannabinoid Nabilone significantly reduces spasticity-related pain: a double-blind placebo-controlled cross-over trial. J Neurol. 2006;253(10):1337–41.

Wong D, Dzemidzic M, Talavage TM, Romito LM, Byrd KE. Motor control of jaw movements: an fMRI study of parafunctional clench and grind behavior. Brain Res. 2011;1383:206–17.

Xu YM, Ge HY, Arendt-Nielsen L. Sustained nociceptive mechanical stimulation of latent myofascial trigger point induces central sensitization in healthy subjects. J Pain. 2010;11(12):1348–55.

Yotsuya M, Sato T, Kawamura S, Furuya E, Saito F, Hisanaga R, Onodera K. Electromyographic response in inferior head of human lateral pterygoid muscle to anteroposterior postural change during opening and closing of mouth. Bull Tokyo Dent Coll. 2009;50(4):191–8.

Zogopoulos P, Vasileiou I, Patsouris E, Theocharis SE. The role of endocannabinoids in pain modulation. Fundam Clin Pharmacol. 2013;27(1):64–80.

9 Temporomandibular Joints

Christopher J. Spencer and John P. Neary

Abstract

The management of temporomandibular joint (TMJ) conditions has changed dramatically since the 1970s as more advanced knowledge regarding the physiology, pathology, and evidence base has developed. One of the main barriers for this progression was the lack of specific definitions for different diagnoses associated with temporomandibular (TMD) conditions. The most recent DC/TMD guidelines have refined the different diagnoses so that clinicians can apply these criteria during the examination, diagnosis, and management of TMD patients. Historically, management strategies for articular disc displacements were aimed at surgically repositioning the articular disc or utilizing an oral appliance to advance the mandible to a point where the condyle was repositioned on the articular disc. These early management approaches often failed to produce the reduction of the pain and dysfunction that both the health-care provider and patient desired. Over time management strategies have evolved into less invasive, more patient centered, and more multidisciplinary as the multifactorial nature of TMD conditions, and specifically those related to the TMJ became evident. This chapter reviews the specific DC/TMD diagnoses and the evidence base for the utilization of different management strategies based upon a patient-centered approach. This is followed with a discussion for the implementation of various interventions such as oral appliances, physical therapy, clinical psychology, pharmacotherapy, and surgical management.

9.1 Introduction

This chapter begins with the assumption that muscular and other causes of temporomandibular joint (TMJ) pain or dysfunction have been ruled out or treated. This discussion is based on the premise

C.J. Spencer (✉) • J.P. Neary
LSU Health New Orleans School of Dentistry,
1100 Florida Ave, New Orleans, LA 70119, USA
e-mail: cspen4@lsuhsc.edu; jneary@lsuhsc.edu

© Springer International Publishing AG 2018
H.A. Gremillion, G.D. Klasser (eds.), *Temporomandibular Disorders*,
https://doi.org/10.1007/978-3-319-57247-5_9

that the patient's concern is intracapsular in origin. Nonsurgical management of these conditions has until recent times been treatment by trial and error. Theories for the cause of the painful syndromes have been developed, and treatment based on theories of the cause rather than evidence-based treatments have been proposed. From a historical perspective, there was a general lack of understanding of the causes of the pain emanating from the TMJ or the area around it. In many cases, irreversible occlusal treatments (Forssell et al. 1999; Kopp 1979) or oral appliances with various designs were used by practitioners resulting in varying degrees of success (Bush 1984; Tsukiyama et al. 2001). In the 1970s TMJ arthrography techniques were developed (Bronstein 1989). Arthrography images revealed changes in TMJ structures (Murakami et al. 1986; Murakami and Segami 1993) associated with various TMJ diseases or dysfunctional syndromes (Kurita et al. 1989). In many cases, an anterior displacement of the articular disc was present along with bony and articular surface cartilaginous degeneration. At the time, it seemed reasonable that the anterior disc displacement now visualized was the etiological basis for the degenerative changes and the pain, even though this theory was not tested or studied with controls. The result, however, was that anterior displacement of the disc became "universally adopted as the mechanism which helped explain the pain, clicking, and joint locking experienced in patients diagnosed with internal derangement" (Dimitroulis 2005). Consequentially, it also made sense to recommend surgical repositioning of the disc (Dolwick and Nitzan 1994) or, in the cases of significant discal integrity compromise, disc removal (Eriksson and Westesson 1985; Eriksson and Westesson 2001; Bjornland and Larheim 2003; Holmlund et al. 2013) and replacement by various autologous or alloplastic materials (Feinerman and Piecuch 1993; Ryan 1989). Although the goal was resolution of the pain and dysfunction, the original premise was not definitively correlated to the clinical presentation. Therefore, the focus was directed to disc repositioning or determination as to the material best suited to serve as a disc replacement. Unfortunately, many patients had incorrect or unnecessary procedures performed yet their pain and dysfunction remained (Abramowicz et al. 2008). It was also recognized that disc position was not the only factor important for joint health. Currently, these procedures are less commonly employed giving greater consideration to more minimally invasive surgical interventions (Sanders and Buoncristiani 1993; Hall et al. 2005).

This is not to say that those approaches were in vain. Importantly, a better understanding of when surgery is appropriate and when it is of questionable benefit became more evident. This led surgeons to further define the indications for surgery and the type of surgery indicated. The evolution of TMJ disorder management is not unlike the treatment of many other medical conditions that have undergone their own evolution over time and experience. Perhaps the greatest revelation is the need for evidence-based surgical treatment of TMJ disorders rather than treatment based upon anecdotal perspectives. Further refinements to the previous methodology of treatment occurred when scientific studies demonstrated that the incidence, within the general population, of disc displacement was greater than originally thought and that many individuals with "displaced discs" were asymptomatic (Dolwick 1995). It has been further established that TMJ sounds are rather common and generally asymptomatic. Studies revealed that approximately one-third of the US population displays disc displacement with minimal pain or dysfunction (Dolwick 1995). Furthermore, research has begun to elucidate the properties of synovial fluid (Bouloux 2009) and some of the biochemical characteristics (Cai et al. 2006) of a symptomatic or inflamed joint (De Sotillo et al. 2011) and the inherent adaptive capacity in most TMJs. Anterior displacement of the disc is no longer viewed as the main etiology of pathologic changes in the TMJ but possibly as a comorbid condition. It has also been elucidated that the long-term prognosis for articular disc dysfunction is likely good with the expectation of low pain impairment (Manfredini et al. 2013).

Notwithstanding, there are multiple disease processes where surgery is unquestionably indicated. Those processes include neoplastic disease both benign and malignant, congenital deformity, ankylosis, trauma severe enough to destroy the anatomy and integrity of the TMJ, and rheumatologic disease associated with severe pain and dysfunction. Additional situations where surgical intervention may be indicated are chronic dislocation and posttraumatic injuries resulting in pain or dysfunction severe enough to impact the patient's life. The most common TMJ disease process, TMJ biomechanical compromise, often requires a multidisciplinary approach and, at times, may involve surgical intervention. In these cases, surgery is only indicated after a proper complex protocol is followed allowing for complete evaluation, prior to less than satisfactory outcomes from nonsurgical management, and careful discussions with the patient on the risks, benefits, and potential complications of the planned surgical intervention.

9.2 Evaluation of a Patient with TMJ Pain and/or Dysfunction

The ideal situation for the majority of patients with TMJ disorders is for them to be evaluated by a team which includes a practitioner skilled in the nonsurgical management of the TMJ patient as well as an experienced surgeon with a track record of positive results. The basic information needed from an initial exam is a detailed history of the problem from the patient, possibly a panoramic radiograph to screen for neoplastic pathology, an exam of the function of the masticatory system to include palpation and auscultation of the joint, and evaluation of the patient's occlusion.

It is incumbent on the practitioner whom is evaluating the TMJ patient to assure that there is not a neoplastic process present. More definitive imaging (CT or MRI) assessment may be necessary in questionable situations (Kaneyama et al. 2010; Kaplan et al. 1987). Detailed radiographic and clinical exam revealing a neoplastic process such as chondroma, synovial chondroma, chondrosarcoma, odontogenic tumor, or other erosive lesion would necessitate a more complex surgical intervention. Recognizing that neoplasm of the TMJ is rare, it should always be a consideration in the patient presenting with TMJ complaints.

Acute TMJ conditions, for example, trauma or acute painful capsulitis, reflect acute inflammation that is likely monofactorial. This is usually seen following an injury and is usually associated with a short duration, resolving with time and supportive care. In most circumstances, the use of anti-inflammatories/analgesics, diet modification, and oral appliance therapy may be indicated.

9.3 Evaluation of the Patient with Nonspecific TMJ Dysfunction

This is not to imply that patients without a specific neoplasm or congenital or traumatic deformity do not have a disease process. In fact, there is a disease process; however, it is just not as easy to associate this nonspecific TMJ dysfunction with one causative agent or process. Most likely the etiology is multifactorial in nature thereby requiring an extensive evaluation, a differential diagnosis to include all known contributing factors, and a multidisciplinary team which can stage and coordinate appropriate management strategies. If the patient has failed conservative management, the following general algorithm may be applicable. After obtaining the history of the process and the physical exam, a decision on advanced imaging is made. Factors that would suggest a need for advanced imaging are history or clinical findings that are not conclusive, very limited opening, loud joint noises, knowledge or suspicion of a rheumatologic disease, and a history of significant trauma.

If an MRI is contemplated, utilization of a strong magnet (3.0 Tesla) with a surface coil is recommended. Open and closed mouth views in the sagittal and coronal plane, with a preference for dynamic (cinematic) imaging, should be prescribed. An open MRI is not recommended as open MRI studies with the magnet further from the patient have not demonstrated images with quality image resolution. The stronger and closer the magnet to the patient, the greater the resolution of the images. One should consider this expensive modality only if it will truly aid in enhanced diagnosis and improved management for the patient.

The most appropriate management strategy for chronic TMJ conditions, prior to surgical intervention, is patient education as to their disease process and the effect that chronic pain conditions may have on all aspects of their life. Topics to be discussed include anxiety, depression, sleep disturbance, decreased libido, and generalized decreased quality of life. If the patient understands the disease process, the ability to implement strategies to help provide their own supportive care will be easier. Self-management strategies can be utilized alone or as a range of management options associated with a multidisciplinary approach to care. The arsenal of management options for a patient with intra-articular disease is limited as far as conservative options go. They include range of motion exercises, self-behavioral modification, stress management, relaxation techniques, and nutritional supplementation. The most efficacious nonsurgical modality is oral appliance therapy. Certainly the most commonly used modality, the oral appliance and its specific design need to be patient specific, diagnosis based, and part of an overall management plan.

9.4 Management Strategies

9.4.1 Oral Appliances

9.4.1.1 Use of Oral Appliances

Oral appliances can be utilized in articular disc displacement with or without reduction. Chang and colleagues, after evaluating patients at 3- and 12-month intervals, reported a significant reduction in pain and increase in maximum opening in a multidisciplinary treatment (physical therapy, moist heat, NSAIDS, and muscle relaxants) that included a maxillary flat plane oral appliance as compared to the group with the same multidisciplinary treatment but without the oral appliance. An additional finding was that participants in the study with the oral appliances demonstrated a significant difference in the number that were pain free after 1 year as compared to the group without (Chang et al. 2010). A randomized clinical trial compared two types of oral appliances for the diagnosis of articular disc displacement without reduction. One appliance was a "centric appliance" designed with bilateral contacts in the posterior region of equal intensity upon biting with immediate canine disclusion of posterior teeth in excursive movements. The other "distraction" appliance had predominately bilateral posterior contacts on the first and second molars with immediate canine disclusion. The clinical trial reported that both oral appliances reduced the overall pain level and increased the range of motion over 9 months. The "centric" appliance significantly reduced overall pain and increased the overall range of motion (active mouth opening) (Schmitter et al. 2005). Oral appliances can be utilized for TMJ pain due to disc displacements (Niemela et al. 2012) and often with joints presenting with degenerative joint disease (Dalla-Bona et al. 2015; Ebrahim et al. 2012).

9.4.1.2 Types of Oral Appliances

The most reported oral appliance in the literature is the stabilization flat plane splint—usually placed on the maxillary arch (the Michigan splint). There is only a small base of literature employing randomized control trials, masked clinicians, and patients that reports advantages or disadvantages of different oral appliance designs (Truelove et al. 2006). One randomized controlled clinical trial describes the provided oral appliance as a hard heat-processed acrylic flat-plane maxillary oral appliance. This hard acrylic oral appliance was compared to a soft thermoplastic vinyl athletic mouth guard provided with dentist supervision and direction. Both appliances were part of a self-care protocol, which included mandibular stretching exercises, nonsteroidal anti-inflammatory drugs, relaxation, reduction of parafunction, stress reduction, and thermal packs. The results were that the authors observed no significant differences in pain levels or TMD symptoms between the two types of appliances with the same self-care protocols. A shortcoming of this study was that minimal information about oral appliance design was provided; therefore, the results may be somewhat circumspect as it would be very difficult to understand the exact types of oral appliances actually compared (Truelove et al. 2006). Systematic literature reviews do not support specific designs of oral appliances (Fricton 2006). Notwithstanding, there are many different types of oral appliances discussed in the literature such as anterior positioning oral appliances, soft oral appliances, and anterior bite plane oral appliances (Fricton 2006). Over-the-counter (OTC) oral appliances are available commercially as well. In Great Britain, one study reported more than 20 different brands commercially available with various designs (Wassell et al. 2014). One major oversight in the literature regarding oral appliances is that the majority of studies provide little detail as to the design or level of adjustment performed with the oral appliance being investigated. Interestingly, one study provided the "mean time" for adjusting the stabilization splint as 17 min and another segmental anterior appliance, the Nociceptive Trigeminal Inhibition or NTI as 27 min. This suggests that there was little time spent adjusting a full arch appliance that would seemingly require a lengthier adjustment period as compared to a very small anterior only device (Magnusson et al. 2004).

9.4.1.3 Response to Oral Appliances

One study (Chang et al. 2010) compared two groups of individuals with a painful clicking TMJ exposed to different management modalities. Group A utilized moist heat, massage, a muscle relaxant for 1 week, and a maxillary oral appliance which was adjusted every 2 weeks for 90 days. Group B received exactly the same management without the maxillary oral appliance. At 90 days, a significant increase in maximum opening and complete remission of symptoms were associated with Group A (included the maxillary oral appliance) as compared to Group B. At 1 year, Group A demonstrated a significant remission of symptoms of 61.3% compared to 20.6% for Group B. A systematic review reports that anterior repositioning oral appliances are not more effective in treating TMJ clicking and locking as compared to a flat-plane stabilization oral appliance. The exception would be an acute case likely following trauma (Schmitter et al. 2005). Anterior bite plane oral appliances do not have sufficient evidence to establish efficacy for the use in managing TM joint pathology. Nitzan demonstrated that a full arch oral appliance can alter intra-articular pressure inside the functioning TM joint. The mean decrease in pressure in the synovial fluid was 81.2% with the placement of an oral appliance (Nitzan 1994; Casares et al. 2014).

9.4.1.4 Potential Side Effects

Overall, oral appliances are considered reversible conservative treatment for TM joint conditions. However, this is not always the case as a number of case reports demonstrate that risks exist for occlusal changes. One of the main risks appears to be utilization of oral appliances that do not cover an entire arch. One case report demonstrates the risk of leaving second molars uncovered by an oral appliance, which resulted in overeruption of these same second molars (Chate and Falconer 2011). Significant side effects have been reported with utilization of the NTIss appliance (occludes on the anterior teeth but lacks posterior tooth coverage). The development of an altered occlusion including the development of an anterior open bite, sensitive and intruded maxillary incisors and/or mandibular incisors, swallowing and aspiration of the device, and mobility of incisors have all been documented (Stapelmann and Turp 2008). There are also reports of significant side effects associated with OTC appliances. Patients have experienced intraoral burns from boil and bite types of appliances. Other reports include soreness to teeth and gingiva including mucosal irritation and soreness. Often these appliances display a poor fit thereby impacting patient compliance, comfort, and speech (Gawlak et al. 2016). Appliances have been reported to have been broken and even partially swallowed (Wassell et al. 2014). Animal (rabbit and pig) models using oral appliance testing have shown degenerative changes in both osseous and subchondral cartilage of the condyles (Hendersen et al. 2015; Sindelar and Alonzo 2003). Oral appliances can be very safe and effective if utilized for the appropriate diagnoses within a multidisciplinary treatment plan including the self-management protocols and periodically monitored by the oral health-care provider.

9.4.2 Physical Therapy

Physical therapy has been utilized for the treatment of TM joint conditions. Physical therapy has been shown to increase the range of motion, to increase the range of pain-free opening, and to decrease pain intensity. A systematic review and meta-analysis reviewed the evidence basis for the effectiveness of manual therapy and home physical therapy for TMD. The conclusions from this review were that there is poor evidence for the above claims because of unclear or high risk of bias. The most robust evidence in this study was for the combination of home exercises with manual therapy (Armijo-Olivo et al. 2016). In a randomized controlled trial of TMD (including disc displacement with reduction) patients, manual therapy combined with home physical therapy has been shown to be more effective than home physical therapy alone (Tuncer et al. 2013). The types of physical therapy modalities applicable for the management of TM joint conditions are presented in Table 9.1 (Martins et al. 2016; Kraus 2014; Kraus 2007).

9.4.3 Clinical Psychology

Patients with TMJ conditions associated with chronic pain demonstrate comorbidity with depression, anxiety, and posttraumatic stress disorder (de Leeuw et al. 2005; Reiter et al. 2015). It has been shown that these psychological conditions will often influence the examination findings of patients with TMJ conditions (Koutris et al. 2013). The presence of other chronic pain conditions or psychological conditions is often associated with increased pain sensitivity and lower pain thresholds. This in turn can lead to palpation tests in the masticatory system with severe responses that may or may not be due to local etiology. In other words, the examination could lead to false-positive findings resulting in inaccurate diagnoses and the provision of inappropriate

Table 9.1 Physical therapy related to temporomandibular management: Modality, Indication, Description

Physical therapy modalities		
Treatment provided	Indication	Specifics of treatment
Education	All temporomandibular joint diagnoses	Education: In the physiology of the diagnosis, prognosis, and management options
Self-physical therapy Training of patients	All temporomandibular joint diagnoses	Range of motion exercises to increase opening (Haketa et al. 2010) Decrease harmful habits to decrease load on the temporomandibular joint
Manual therapy (Sault et al. 2016) (Kraus 2014)	Disc displacement with reduction with limited opening Partial fibrous ankylosis or adhesions limiting the range of motion	Distraction of TM joint to help mobilize closed lock Lateral glide maneuvers while patient is opening to increase the range of motion
Iontophoresis	Temporomandibular joint pain	Application of nonsteroidal anti-inflammatory medications, local anesthetic, or corticosteroids to the temporomandibular joint through the skin to provide anti-inflammatory action and analgesia
Treat contributing factors	Myofascial pain, with spreading or pain referral	Mobilization of tight muscles, stretching, and release of taught bands to increase range of motion

interventions. One aid in determining whether the pain response is due to a TMJ (or muscle in other diagnoses) is to utilize the term "familiar pain" as part of the patient response questioning. "Is the pain you feel in this palpation, a familiar pain or related to your chief concern?" (Koutris et al. 2013). This question can help the patient provide accurate information as it relates to their chief concern.

Chronic TMJ conditions affect the quality of patient's lives which is part of the "pain" experience. Patients with comorbid psychological conditions report that their chronic pain condition affects their lives to a greater degree than other patients (Turner et al. 2001). These patients are much more apt to report being disabled by their pain. This in turn suggests that a multidisciplinary model for management will be more likely to provide patients with an improvement in their life, if psychological factors are included (Carrió et al. 2004). Whether conditions such as depression, anxiety, posttraumatic stress disorder, or elevated emotional distress are comorbid conditions directly related to the patient's chief concern, they still negatively affect the patient's ability to cope with daily chronic pain in the TM joint (Velly et al. 2011). Dysfunctional coping mechanisms such as an inability to self-distract, pessimistic outlook, and catastrophization interfere with the patient's ability to comply with management strategies. Not surprisingly, patients with these characteristics are less likely to respond successfully to interventions (Litt and Porto 2013). Clinical psychology management strategies (see Chap. 10) have been shown to help patient coping skills.

9.4.4 Pharmacological Management

Many dentists and primary care physicians are not prepared to maintain patients on narcotics, benzodiazepines, anticonvulsants, or psychoactive medications long term. Pharmacotherapy for chronic pain follows the same needs and complexities as other management modalities. Medication management requires a multidisciplinary approach. "With ongoing chronic pain, it is unusual for a single medication to result in satisfactory pain relief in a unimodal, stand-alone fashion" (Dale and Stacey 2016). The operative concept is "satisfactory" as compared to "complete" pain relief. Different medications that affect different "targets" offer a combined additive effect. Medications offer potential efficacy but also the potential for serious side effects. Each new medication requires an adjustment period for the patient to determine efficacy and demonstrate acceptable adverse effects and compatibility with existing medications. This process is called titration and is best accomplished in a slow gradual process (Jose et al. 2007). A medication may be effective, but if the initial dose is too high, a patient may reject it because of the side effects. In a randomized controlled trial of gabapentin, different rates of titration were evaluated. It was found that for gabapentin, dizziness occurred more frequently in the rapid titration group as compared to the slow titration group (Fisher et al. 2001).

9.4.4.1 Nonsteroidal Anti-inflammatory Drugs and Analgesics (NSAIDs)

Most TMJ pain is associated with inflammation. Therefore, NSAIDs are often the pharmacotherapeutic treatment of choice for painful TMJ (Table 9.2). NSAIDSs are able to decrease tenderness in the TMJ to palpation often within 1 week and also improve function associated with range of motion and chewing (Mejersjo and Wenneberg 2008). There is the possibility that specific NSAIDS (meloxicam, naproxen) may provide some protection from early breakdown of cartilaginous structures (Chu et al. 2008). Other studies show no significant improvement of pain or range of motion as compared to palliative care (Minakuchi et al. 2001). It has been shown that most NSAIDs are able to decrease pro-inflammatory synovial proteins called cytokines (interleukin-6 and tumor necrosis factor-alpha) that are part of the induction of inflammation in human joints. One study demonstrated that there was no significant difference over a 14-day period of the decrease of these inflammatory proteins with utilization of ibuprofen, diclofenac, and celecoxib

Table 9.2 NSAIDs used in the management of intra-articular disorders

NSAIDs	Dosage regimen	Evidence
Diclofenac sodium	18–35 mg three times/day	Reduces pain associated with jaw movement and palpation of the TMJ in 1 week (Mejersjo and Wenneberg 2008). One of the most commonly prescribed NSAIDs for osteoarthritis and as effective as any of the other NSAIDS (Pavelka 2012)
Meloxicam	7.5–15 mg once per day	Reportedly effective for TMJ pain with fewer gastrointestinal adverse effects as compared to other NSAIDs (Zeidler et al. 2002; Argoff 2011). Meloxicam displays greater affinity for inflamed synovium as compared to non-inflamed synovium (Lapicque et al. 2000)
Celecoxib	100–200 mg twice per day	Decreased efficacy for analgesia in TMJ pain as compared to non-selective Cox inhibitors (Ta and Dionne 2004). Fewer gastrointestinal adverse effects (Gallelli et al. 2013)
Ketoprofen	75 mg three times per day orally or as topical transdermal application	Utilized in topical gel formulations that have shown efficacy for osteoarthritis. Studies also report that the gel carrier itself provides relief. Cochrane review reports 63% subjects received 50% or more improvement with ketoprofen gel (ketoprofen concentration did effect efficacy), while 48% of subjects received the same benefit with just the gel (Derry et al. 2016)
Ibuprofen	600–800 mg three to four times per day	1800 mg per day significantly more effective in reducing inflammatory cytokines in synovial fluid as compared to 1200 mg per day (Gallelli et al. 2013). The increased dosage also poses a greater risk for systemic bleeding (Gallelli et al. 2013)

NSAIDS nonsteroidal anti-inflammatory drugs, *TMJ* temporomandibular joint

(Gallelli et al. 2013). The one finding that was significant was that the higher therapeutic dosage of these three NSAIDs was more effective than the lower dose as compared to which NSAID was utilized for reducing pro-inflammatory proteins. For example, 150 mg of diclofenac significantly reduced cytokine levels as compared to 75 mg of diclofenac. This was true for ibuprofen and celecoxib as well (Gallelli et al. 2013). However, the same study reports that as the dosage regimen increases, the risks of systemic bleeding also increase.

9.4.5 Corticosteroids

It is well known that either systemic corticosteroids or intra-articular corticosteroids will suppress the inflammatory response. Intra-articular injections of corticosteroids may pose a risk for impedance of growth in juvenile TMJ (Stoustrup et al. 2013). Dexamethasone 8 mg as part of an arthrocentesis procedure (Tabrizi et al. 2014) was deemed safe, but literature reports no difference with/without dexamethasone for decrease in stiffness or pain (Huddleston Slater et al. 2012).

9.4.5.1 Transdermal Medications

Most medications such as NSAIDS, neuropathic medications, and local anesthetics can be utilized as transdermal medications formulated by a compounding pharmacy (Haribabu et al. 2013). Transdermal medications are comprised of a vehicle such as pluronic lecithin organogel and active medication(s). The vehicle helps transport the active medication through the skin into the TMJ to provide a local therapeutic effect with minimal systemic effects (Senve et al. 2012). There are clinical trials of transdermal NSAIDS prior to joint surgery (Sekiya et al. 2010) which compared oral ketoprofen to transdermal ketoprofen in muscle, tendon, and plasma over a 12-h period. The transdermal ketoprofen produced a more rapid concentration in tissues after 1 h compared to oral ketoprofen. The transdermal ketoprofen reached its peak tissue concentration at 6 h. At 14 h, the transdermal and oral ketoprofen were very similar, but the plasma concentration of the transdermal ketoprofen was only 1/17 of the oral ketoprofen. NSAIDS employed utilized with a transdermal approach primarily include diclofenac and ketoprofen (Plaza-Villegas et al. 2012). In older adults, both topical diclofenac and ketoprofen can provide pain relief of approximately 10% more than the inert vehicle alone. In elderly patients with a greater proclivity to adverse effects, transdermal NSAIDs should be considered before oral NSAIDs are utilized (Derry et al. 2016). Neuropathic medications such as gabapentin and pregabalin have been shown to penetrate the dermis effectively as well (Bassani and Banov 2016).

9.4.5.2 Neuropathic Medication

Medication(s) commonly used for the management of neuropathic may also be considered for the TMJ when some TMJ conditions that are not primarily associated with inflammatory pain are present. Mandibular surgery including TMJ surgery can sometimes be associated with postoperative neuropathic pain (Kirchheimer et al. 2013; Bergi 2002). Medications (gabapentinoids) are sometimes the main therapeutic management intervention in addition to patient education. It has been shown that gabapentin and pregabalin are utilized with efficacy for overall chronic pain due to its association with the process of central sensitization (Tuchman et al. 2010).

9.4.5.3 Antidepressants

Chronic TMJ conditions associated with chronic pain, like any other chronic condition, respond differently than acute TMJ pain. Therefore, this requires a different pharmacotherapeutic management strategy as previously discussed. Medication classes such as the tricyclic antidepressants (amitriptyline, nortriptyline) are often a consideration (Plesh et al. 2000). The serotonin-norepinephrine reuptake medication class with examples of venlafaxine or duloxetine may also have benefit (Beal and Wallace 2016).

9.4.5.4 Opioids

For acute pain conditions, the opioid class of medications is routinely utilized postsurgery. Opioid medications are also utilized for chronic pain conditions, when other medications and approaches have failed to provide adequate pain relief. However, pain management with opioids is fraught with many difficulties and may involve physiological and psychological consequences (Swift and Roszkowski 1998). Adverse effects are common and include nausea, constipation, sedation, mood disturbance, sleep disturbance, respiratory depression, etc. (Bouloux 2011). One underappreciated adverse effect is ototoxicity and irreversible sensorineural hearing loss (Kaye et al. 2013). Most patients utilizing opioids will require escalation of the necessary dose to manage pain. This may be caused by the well-known development of tolerance to the analgesic, but opioid-induced hyperalgesia (heightened sensitivity to pain associated with utilization of an opioid analgesic) is another factor to be addressed for decreased analgesic response (Martins et al. 2016). Opioid-induced hyperalgesia occurs in the following manner: as opioid doses increase, the pain increases as well (as opposed to the development of tolerance) without any exacerbation of the underlying condition. The opioid which originally was an effective analgesic now creates more pain (Yi and Pryzbylkowski 2015). Opioid-induced hyperalgesia pain is likely different (though it might be difficult to tease out in the history) from the original pain. It is likely more ill-defined or general as compared to focal pain associated with a particular structure. This is likely due to the central sensitization of the pain process. It is worth noting that in a double-blind placebo-controlled study, tolerance was found to be the main reason for increased opioid dosage (Chu et al. 2012).

9.4.6 Medical Specialties for Consultation, Medication Management, and Patient Coping Skills

Multidisciplinary management of complex TMJ conditions often requires referral to medical specialists for several reasons. A consult may be necessary to rule out possible diagnoses. Under certain circumstances, a medical practitioner may be the most appropriate health-care provider to manage the overall condition. For example, TMJ rheumatoid arthritis would require referral to a rheumatologist (Lin et al. 2007) but would still require care from a dentist to provide palliative care as the degenerative changes cause pain in the joints and also affect the occlusion as well as function (Aliko et al. 2011). Primary headaches are significantly more common in patients with TMD, and pain in the TMJ may exacerbate both the intensity and frequency of headaches (Tomaz-Morales et al. 2015). Therefore, it would be important to work collaboratively with a neurologist, when appropriate, to manage the multifactorial nature of the patient's pain concerns. The following medical disciplines may be important referral sources and consultants and may provide management for medications on a long-term basis: internal medicine, otolaryngology, pain management, behavioral medicine (psychiatry, psychology) (Aggarwal et al. 2010), neurology (Dahan et al. 2016), rheumatology, and physical medicine and rehabilitation.

9.5 Sequencing of Management Strategies

9.5.1 Patient Education and Self-management

Patients need to understand that TMJ pain is often related to inflammation and is exacerbated due to function. Palliative care involving education should begin with the concept of engaging in a soft diet (minimize foods with a tough consistency) thus avoiding undo excessive loading of their joints. It is very important that they maintain function and range of motion as compared to restricting joint movement. Therefore, range of motion exercises would be very appropriate (Yoshida et al. 2010) as soon as possible in conjunction with an NSAID (Table 9.2). If the patient is clenching during the day, self-behavioral modification would need implementation to keep their teeth apart while awake (Motghare et al. 2015). An over-the-counter non-pharmacologic supplement option to consider is the use of glucosamine (Giordano et al. 2009) in conjunction with chondroitin sulfate and methylsulfonylmethane (MSM). While the available evidence for the utilization for these nutritional supplements is not of the highest level, there are very few reported side effects (Anderson et al. 2005), and there is a continued record of safety in self-administration (Reginster et al. 2001; Yang et al. 2015). Undoubtedly, patient self-management is the first stage of overall management strategies (De Freitas et al. 2013).

9.5.2 Intervention

The inflammation is best treated with an NSAID for likely duration of 30 days with reevaluation. In addition to inflammation management, excessive load or force applied to the TMJ must be managed that would be associated with sleep bruxism. An oral appliance that provides posterior support with bilateral even contacts should be considered. Any distalizing contacts on the appliance that would force the mandible and therefore the condyles in a posterior direction must be eliminated from the anterior ramp of the appliance as this direction of force may further irritate the TMJ. The appliance should be adjusted to allow the patient to move freely as possible. If the patient improves rapidly in the first month, then no new levels of management need to be added. The patient would be titrated off of the NSAID unless another flare of their pain occurred. The oral appliance would need to be adjusted occasionally to maintain the posterior contacts and to make sure no distalizing contacts occur as well as to review the integrity of the occlusal platform. The patient would continue to wear the occlusal appliance as long as they are receiving benefit.

9.5.3 Staging Treatment

If the first line of patient management and intervention is not progressively producing comfort and reducing the patient's pain associated with function, then additional imaging (CBCT, MRI), as previously indicated, should be considered to investigate whether there are additional pathologies present that could be causing pain and dysfunction (Helenius et al. 2005). These could range from joint effusion associated with inflammatory fluids in the TMJ spaces, to masses or tumors, to calcifications within the capsular area. If any of these findings are present, an immediate referral to an oral surgeon would be in order.

9.6 Diagnosis: Specific Management Considerations

9.6.1 Capsulitis, Synovitis, or Retrodiscitis

These three painful diagnoses are all closely related and are all associated with inflammation. The staging of treatment is similar to TMJ arthritis. The inflammation should be addressed with NSAIDs likely for 1 month with reevaluation. Likewise, orthopedic overload which requires management with use of an oral appliance should be a consideration. A corticosteroid such as prednisolone or methylprednisolone may be utilized if the inflammation and pain levels are moderate/severe. The patient would likely require an alternative to a NSAID analgesic if corticosteroids are prescribed to avoid gastrointestinal adverse effects (Masclee et al. 2014). If pain is reduced progressively, the NSAIDs may be reduced and tapered off. The oral appliance would likely be needed long term if parafunctional habits are present during sleep. If the pain remains with minimal abatement, further investigation and diagnostic testing such as additional imaging needs to be considered.

9.6.2 Disc Displacement

9.6.2.1 Disc Displacement with Reduction

This diagnosis is very common as it exists in approximately 30% of the general population, and in the majority of cases, it requires no treatment unless pain or dysfunction is present (Larheim et al. 2001; Schiffman et al. 1990). However, patient education and reassurance regarding the relatively benign nature of this condition are still needed. The long-term prognosis is excellent, and most patients do not progress to a painful TMJ diagnosis (de Leeuw et al. 1994). Even with the evidence that most patients with disc displacement with reduction do not need treatment, a small subset of patients do present with discomfort or even significant pain. They may complain of their joint sounds as annoying, and the movement of their mandible may interfere with everyday function. Foremost, as health-care professionals, we must not cause them harm but provide supportive care appropriate for their condition. During dental appointments, patients can be provided with periods of rest so that they can rest their jaws. Unilateral rubber bite blocks should be avoided and never wedged or forced into place. The pain is likely associated with inflammation and would be treated as previously discussed. An oral appliance may be considered to provide protection from excessive orthopedic load.

In certain individuals, there may be a progression of the condition from a reducing articular disc to a nonreducing articular disc with limitation in opening. The risk of this progression and its predictability is unknown (Kalaykova et al. 2010). But it must be remembered that the level of mandibular pain or dysfunction is not necessarily related to the position of the articular disc, the presence of joint sounds, or the presence of an internal derangement (Schiffman et al. 1992) and that most patients with an internal derangement do not seek care (Schiffman et al. 1990).

9.6.2.2 Disc Displacement Without Reduction and Without Limited Opening

Most patients with this diagnosis require no treatment unless signs or symptoms of pain and dysfunction are present. The prevalence of this diagnosis is unknown, but the condition is likely of long duration without signs or symptoms. It is primarily diagnosed by history of previous intracapsular sounds (clicking or popping which may or may not be asymptomatic) that is no longer present and also associated with a period of time when there was either a partial or complete sensation of being "locked." Furthermore, there would be a report of significant decrease in range of motion and deviation upon opening to the side of the affected TMJ which decreased over time.

9.6.2.3 Disc Displacement Without Reduction and with Limited Opening

This is a case of an "acute closed lock" in which the articular disc is recently changed from reducing to nonreducing. The patient requires immediate care initially with an attempt to manually reduce the articular disc (Camino et al. 2015). If pain is present, an auriculotemporal nerve block to the affected TMJ may be provided to assist with the aforementioned procedure. Then with gloved and protected thumbs positioned upon the mandibular molars, the clinician depresses the mandible in order to try a distraction movement upon the affected TMJ to see if the condyle is now able to translate and reduce or move back onto the articular disc. In the event that a manual reduction is unsuccessful, the patient may be referred to an oral surgeon for additional interventions. Once the patient's range of motion is restored, then self-management, an oral appliance, and potential assistance from physical therapy may be helpful to maintain the range of motion and function. This same conservative approach may be even trialed prior to involving an oral surgical approach. With time, pain and range of motion may naturally improve (Schiffman et al. 2014).

9.6.3 Degenerative Joint Disease

Chronic degenerative joint disease (DJD) may be self-limiting and therefore not require any management as it is (Schiffman et al. 1990) often asymptomatic and without dysfunction other than an annoying intracapsular sound (often crepitus). If pain occurs, the management would likely involve the use of anti-inflammatory medications and/or intra-articular injections. The most likely consequence of DJD would be morphological alterations to the condyles such as flattening, beaking, and reduction in posterior vertical ramus height, with irregular articular surfaces present on imaging (Helenius et al. 2006). The changes to the masticatory system will depend upon the rate of change in condylar height and whether the degeneration is unilateral or bilateral. As condylar height decreases, the pressure on posterior teeth increases. If condylar degeneration is more rapid than tooth attrition, then an open bite will occur in the contralateral side or if the condition is bilateral, the open bite will be more symmetrical presenting as an anterior open bite. These occlusal changes may affect the patient's ability to function both in chewing and speaking. Management would likely involve supportive care with an oral appliance to provide tooth contact on the acrylic occlusal platform for comfort. Once the degenerative changes have stabilized, an orthodontic consult may be considered to determine possible treatment options.

9.6.4 Systemic Arthritides

Systemic arthritides are a group of conditions that affect not only the musculoskeletal system, primarily synovial and cartilage cells of joints, but also multiple other "extra-articular disease" sites that include pulmonary, ocular, vascular, cardiac, neurological, and cutaneous sites. Inflammation in the different sites is caused by the rheumatoid factor or autoantibody associated with several different inflammatory cascades (Scott et al. 2010). The result can be severe tissue damage virtually anywhere in the body. This patient will need to be referred to a rheumatologist. The rheumatologist will provide the direction for medical management of the disease including the oversight of pharmacotherapy as well. The dentist will likely be a part of the health-care team and provide management for TMJ dysfunction and possible associated occlusal changes.

9.7 Surgical Intervention of the Nonspecific TMJ Dysfunction Patient

If the patient has no discernable pathology and has failed conservative management, an initial option is an arthrocentesis (Alpasian et al. 2003). Arthrocentesis involves conscious sedation of the patient, providing local anesthesia to the TMJ area, placement of an inflow port (generally an 18 gauge needle), and an outflow port (also an 18 gauge needle) (Chandrashekhar et al. 2015). The joint is irrigated with intravenous (IV) lactated ringers or saline solution. The hydrostatic pressure and the "flushing" of the joint can release adhesions and flush the biochemical pain mediators from the joint space (Nitzan and Price 2001). After the flushing is complete, and after removal of the outflow port, the joint space can be filled with hyaluronic acid (HA, normally produced by the synovium of healthy joints) or corticosteroid. The HA serves as a moderator of inflammation and a joint lubricant. Corticosteroids, although powerful moderators of inflammation, provide no lubrication and have side effects, most notably erosion of articular surfaces (Lavelle et al. 2007).

Another potential material that could be placed into the joint space is platelet-rich plasma. This can be performed with or without arthrocentesis and/or HA (Hegab et al. 2015; Cömert Kiliç et al. 2015). This has not been well studied but is gaining popularity especially in the specialty of orthopedics. Theoretically, the platelet-derived growth factors may have a positive influence on a dysfunctional joint (Kütük et al. 2014).

The next step up in the treatment option tree is an arthroscopic arthroplasty (Indresano and Bradrick 1993). The arthroscopic arthroplasty provides all of the same benefits of an arthrocentesis with the addition of placing two 2 mm probes into the joint allowing for greater flow through the joint space (Fridrich et al. 1996). Additionally, fibrous adhesions, some disc deformities, and inflamed tissue can be treated under direct vision (Sanders and Buoncristiani 1993). Temporomandibular joint arthroscopic arthroplasty is technically challenging to perform and is certainly an invasive procedure with inherent risks (Wilkes 1991). However, many TMJ pathologies can be successfully treated in this manner, especially new onset joint pathology like an acute closed lock (Murakami et al. 1996). Although TMJ arthroscopic surgery is considered a mainstay of surgical management of the TMJ, a study published in the New England Journal of Medicine may call arthrocentesis and arthroscopy in general into question. In this landmark orthopedic study (Mosely et al. 2002) of the treatment of DJD of the knee, 180 patients were divided into 3 groups. One group received traditional knee arthroscopy, another group received knee arthrocentesis with arthroscopy incisions, and the last group only received sham incisions with nothing done inside the joint. The results showed that there was no difference in outcomes in the three groups, indicating that someone undergoing arthroscopy or arthrocentesis fared no better than someone who only thought they had something done. Is should be noted this study was performed in the knee and not the TMJ. This controversial study has its group of detractors questioning its validity, but with the lack of quality randomized controlled studies involving surgical management of the TMJ, there currently does not exist the scientific evidence that would make surgical choices easier.

There are those that are of the belief that there are only two procedures recommended for the TMJ surgeon, that being TMJ arthroscopic arthroplasty and total joint replacement. There is actually no consensus on any of the surgeries considered between these two. There is, however, the open arthroplasty, with disc plication with a Mitek anchor or plication of the disc to periosteum (Gocmen et al. 2013). This procedure is based on the notion that TMJ pathology is due to disc displacement. Based on multiple studies indicating that up to 30–40% of the general population has asymptomatic disc displacement and other studies that show that repaired discs return to their displaced location postsurgery, this surgery is falling out of favor. If a surgery less than total joint replacement is contemplated, then discectomy with placement of a fat autograft or placement of nothing may be a consideration. Discectomy has been successfully preformed since the early 1900s with good results (Tolvanen and Oikarinenvj 1988) as related to lessened pain and improved function (Bowman 1947). The chief concerns of this surgery are the resulting joint noise and the theory that the occlusion will be affected (Silver 1984). Surgeons in the 1970s felt that if the disc was removed and nothing placed, the occlusion would be altered and theoretically result in problems for the patient. Since 1970, a search has been for made for a disc replacement material. No material has proven superiority over the other, and alloplastic materials have proven to be harmful as they frequently degrade under the load of the joint.

The only TMJ surgical procedure with acceptable scientific data to promote its use in the proper situations is total joint replacement. The TMJ Concepts joint now has 27 years of data supporting its use in the correct situations (Wolford et al. 2015). This is not to say that all patients with TMJ dysfunction should go directly to a total joint prosthesis. Many caveats bear discussing. In regard to decreasing pain, the fewer number of surgical procedures performed on a patient, the less likely they are to end up with uncontrolled pain. For example, the TMJ dysfunction patients who have the best outcomes are those with a rheumatologic condition that has a deformed joint, and the patient goes directly to total joint replacement. Those patients who undergo multiple procedures before total joint replacement often end up with adequate function but continue to experience chronic pain. Theoretically, this phenomenon occurs as every surgery causes micro-injury to nerves and lymphatics in an area of the anatomy that has an abundance of motor, sensory, sympathetic, and parasympathetic nerves. Postsurgical result may be less than satisfactory and associated with the complex pain syndromes seen in multiply-operated patients. Thus, the goal is to relieve pain and dysfunction involving as few procedures as possible and not utilizing the most invasive procedure as first-line treatment.

Perhaps the most difficult task in TMJ dysfunction surgery is determining the correlation of patient pain with dysfunction and both pain and dysfunction with anatomical abnormalities. What we do know is that pain alone is not an indication for surgery. We also know that a displaced disc or joint sounds alone are not indications for surgery. The indications become more focused when there is a combination of pain and dysfunction along with a correctable anatomic abnormality. It must be recognized that a patient who has pain, dysfunction, and anatomic abnormality but has had multiple previous surgeries may be able to regain function. However, the likelihood of continued pain remains as previously outlined. This is most commonly manifest in the ankylosed patient with multiple previous surgeries.

Certainly, a patient with little or no opening may be ankylosed. If bony or fibrous ankylosis is diagnosed, surgery would be the only likely curative procedure. Release of ankylosis surgery is one of the most challenging TMJ surgeries as frequently the abnormal bone over growth is near major arteries and nerves. After the release of the ankylosis, the reconstruction is most reliably performed using a custom-fitted total joint replacement (Christensen 1963; Wolford et al. 2003; Mercuri et al. 2007). Other choices are stock total joints or costochondral rib grafts. Typically any reconstructive method following ankylosis release incorporates a graft of the patient's fat around the condyle. Recurrent ankylosis sometimes requires low dose radiation to the area to reduce the likelihood of bone regrowth.

TMJ deformities that result from trauma or rheumatologic disease that are causing pain or dysfunction will require TMJ reconstruction. In the case of trauma, a residual condylar fragment will need to be removed and the damaged disc repaired or removed. The condyle can be replaced with a costochondral rib graft or a total joint replacement. These disease processes that result in patient pain and/or dysfunction represent the noncontroversial aspects of when to perform TMJ surgery. Although the surgery itself may be difficult, the decision of whether to perform surgery or not is relatively a straightforward decision.

Another category of TMJ dysfunction patients are those with chronic dislocation. Some of these patients will present to emergency rooms multiple times with their mandible dislocated being unable to relocate the mandible (open lock). A possible cause for this condition may be due to the anatomy associated with a steep articular eminence. Effective surgical treatment may involve either arthroscopic or open eminectomy. This procedure can actually be done outside of the capsule, minimizing degenerative changes caused by surgical intervention.

9.8 Summary

Management of TMJ conditions has many facets for a successful outcome. This process begins with an accurate and complete diagnosis and, if possible, determining cause and effect. It must be recognized that surgery is one component of an overall plan of care; therefore, it is important that the management team include someone well skilled in nonsurgical management. Additionally, it is equally important that the patient be educated as to the nature of their problem and the discussed management plan including realistic expectations.

References

Abramowicz S, Dolwick MF, Lewis SB, Dolce C. Temporomandibular joint reconstruction after failed teflon-propast implant: case report and literature review. Int J Oral Maxillofac Surg. 2008;39(8):763–7.

Aggarwal VR, Tickle M, Javidi H, Peters S. Reviewing the evidence: can cognitive behavioral therapy improve the outcomes for patients with chronic orofacial pain? J Orofac Pain. 2010;24(2):163–71.

Aliko A, Ciancaglini A, Alushi A, Tafaj A, Ruci D. Temporomandibular joint involvement in rheumatoid arthritis, systemic lupus erythematosus and systemic sclerosis. Int J Oral Maxillofac Surg. 2011; 40:704–9.

Alpasian C, Dolwick MF, Heft MW. Five-year retrospective evaluation of temporomandibular joint arthrocentesis. Int J Oral Maxillofac Surg. 2003;32:263–7.

Anderson JW, Nicolosi RJ, Borzelleca JF. Glucosamine effects in humans: a review of effects on glucose metabolism, side effects, safety consideratins and efficacy. Food Chem Toxicol. 2005;43:187–201.

Argoff CE. Recent developments in the treatment of osteoarthritis with NSAIDs. Curr Med Res Opin. 2011;27(7):1315–27.

Armijo-Olivo S, Pitance L, Singh V, Neto F, Thie N, Michelotti A. Effectiveness of manual therapy and therapeutic exercise for temporomandibular disorders: systematic review and meta-analysis. Phys Ther. 2016;96(1):9–25.

Bassani AS, Banov D. Evaluation of the percutaneous absorption of ketamine HCL, gabapentin, clonidine HCL, and baclofen, in compounded transdermal pain formulations, using the Franz finite dose model. Pain Med. 2016;17:230–8.

Beal BR, Wallace MS. An overview of pharmacologic Management of Chronic Pain. Med Clin North Am. 2016;100:65–79.

Bergi TI. Incidence of chronic neuropathic pain subsequent to surgical removal of impacted third molars. Acta Odontol. 2002;60(2):108–12.

Bjornland T, Larheim TA. Discectomy of the temporomandibular joint: three year follow-up as a predictor of the ten year outcome. J Oral Maxillofac Surg. 2003;61(1):55–60.

Bouloux GF. Temporomandibular joint pain and synovial fluid analysis: a review of the literature. J Oral Maxillofac Surg. 2009;67:2497–504.

Bouloux GF. Use of opioids in long-term management of temporomandibular joint dysfunction. J Oral Maxillofac Surg. 2011;69(7):1885–189.

Bowman K. Temporomandibular joint arthrosis and its treatment by extirpation of the disc. Acta Chir Scand. 1947;95(Suppl 1):18–156.

Bronstein S. Diagnostic and operative arthrography. Oral Maxillofac Surg Clin North Am. 1989;1:59–68.

Bush FM. Occlusal therapy in management of chronic orofacial pain. Anesth Prog. 1984;31(1):10–6.

Cai HX, Luo JM, Long X, Li XD, Cheng Y. Free-radical oxidation and superoxide dismutase activity in synovial fluid of patients with temporomandibular disorders. J Orofac Pain. 2006;20(1):53–8.

Camino R, Manzi RM, de Carvalho MF, Luz JG, Pimentel AC, Deboni MCZ. Manual reduction of articular disc after traumatic extraction of mandibular third molar a case report. Dental Press J Orthod. 2015;20(5):101–7.

Carrió F, Suchman AL, Epstein RM. The biopsychosocial model 25 years later: principles, practice, and scientific inquiry. Ann Fam Med. 2004;2(6):576–82.

Casares G, Thomas A, Carmona J, Acero J, Vila CV. Influence of oral stabilization appliances in intra-articular pressure of the temporomandibular joint. Cranio. 2014;32(3):219–23.

Chandrashekhar VK, Kenchappa U, Chinnannavar SN, Sing S. Arthrocentesis a minimally invasive method for TMJ disc disorders – a prospective study. J Clinic Diag Res 2015;9(10):zc59–62.

Chang SW, Chuang CY, Li JR, Lin CY, Chiu CT. Treatment effects of maxillary flat occlusal spints for painful clicking of the temporomandibular joint. Kaohsiung J Med Sci. 2010;26:299–307.

Chate RA, Falconer DT. Dental appliances with inadequate occlusal coverage: a case report. Br Dent J. 2011;210(3):109–10.

Christensen RW. The correction of mandibular ankylosis by arthroplasty and insertion of a cast vital lium glenoid fossa. Am J Orthrop. 1963;48:16–24.

Chu SC, Yang SF, Lue KH, Hsieh YS, Li TJ, KH L. Naproxen, meloxicam and methylprednisolone inhibit urokinase plasminogen activator and inhibitor and gelatinases expression during the early stage of osteoarthritis. Clin Chim Acta. 2008;387:90–6.

Chu LF, D'Arcy N, Brady C, et al. Analgesic tolerance without demonstrable opioid-induced hyperalgesia: a double-blinded, randomized, placebo-controlled trial of sustained-release morphine for treatment of chronic nonradicular low-back pain. Pain. 2012;153:1583–92.

Cömert Kiliç S, Güngörmüş M, Sümbüllü MA. Is arthrocentesis plus platelet-rich plasma superior to arthrocentesis alone in the treatment of temporomandibular joint osteoarthritis? A randomized clinical trial. J Oral Maxillofac Surg. 2015;73(8):1473–83.

Dahan H, Shir U, Nicolau B, Keith D, Allison P. Self-reported migraine and chronic fatiigue syndrome are more prevalent I people with myofascial vs nonmyofascial temporomandibular disorders. J Oral Facial Pain Headaches. 2016;30(1):7–13.

Dale R, Stacey B. Multimodal treatment of chronic pain. Med Clin North Am. 2016;100:55–64.

Dalla-Bona D, Shackleton T, Clark G, Ram S. Unilateral ear fullness and temporary hearing loss diagnosed and successfully managed as a temporomandibular disorder. J Am Dent Assoc. 2015;146(3):192–4.

De Freitas RF, Ferreira MA, Barbosa GA, Calderon PS. Counseling and self-management therapies for temporomandibular disorders: a systematic review. J Oral Rehab. 2013;40:864–74.

de Leeuw R, Boering G, Stegenga B, de Bont LG. Clinical signs of TMJ osteoarthrosis and internal derangement 30 years after nonsurgical treatment. J Orofac Pain. 1994;8(1):18–24.

de Leeuw R, Bertoli E, Schmidt JE, Carlson CR. Prevalence of post-traumatic stress disorder in orofacial pain patients. Oral Surg Oral Med Oral Pathol Oral Radical Endod. 2005;99(5):558–68.

Derry S, Conaghan P, Da Silva JAP, Wiffen PJ, Moore RA. Topical NSAIDS for chronic musculoskeletal pain in adults (review). Cochrane Database Syst Rev. 2016;4:1–113.

De Sotillo RD, Velly AM, Hadley M, Fricton JR. Evidence of oxidative stress in temporomandibular disorders. J Oral Rehabil. 2011;38(10):722–8.

Dimitroulis G. The role of surgery in the management of disorders of the temporomandibular joint: a critical review of the literature. Part 1. Int J Oral Maxillofac Surg. 2005;34(2):107–13.

Dolwick MF, Nitzan DW. The role of disc-repositioning surgery for internal derangements of the temporomandibular joint. Oral Maxillofacial Surg Clin North Am. 1994;6:271–5.

Dolwick MF. Intra-articular disc displacement part I: it's questionable role in temporomandibular joint pathology. J Oral Maxillofac Surg. 1995;53:1069–72.

Ebrahim S, Montoya L, Busse JW, Carrasco-Labra A, Guyatt GH. The effectiveness of splint therapy in patients with temporomandibular disorders: a systematic review and meta-analysis. J Am Dent Assoc. 2012;143(8):847–57.

Eriksson L, Westesson PL. Long-term evaluation of meniscectomy of the temporomandibular joint. J Oral Maxillofac Surg. 1985;43(4):263–9.

Eriksson L, Westesson PL. Discectomy as an effective treatment for painful temporomandibular joint internal derangement: a five year clinical and radiographic follow-up. J Oral Maxillofac Surg. 2001;59(7):750–8.

Feinerman DM, Piecuch JF. Long-term retrospective analysis of twenty-three proplast-teflon temporomandibular joint interpositional implants. Int J Oral Maxillofac Surg. 1993;22(1):11–6.

Fisher RS, Sachdeo RC, Pellock J, Penovich PE, Magnus L, Bernstein P. Rapid initiation of gabapentin. A randomized controlled trial. Neurology. 2001;56:743–8.

Forssell H, Kalso E, Koskela P, Vehmanen R, Puukka P, Alanen P. Occlusal treatments in temporomandibular disorders: a qualitative systematic review of randomized controlled trials. Pain. 1999;83(3):549–60.

Fridrich KL, Wise JM, Zeitler DL. Prospective comparison of arthroscopy and arthocentesis for temporomandibular joint disorders. J Oral Maxillofac Surg. 1996;54:816–20.

Fricton J. Current evidence providing clarity in Management of Temporomandibular Disorders: summary of a systematic review of randomized clinical trials for intro-oral appliances and occlusal therapies. J Evid Base Dent Pract. 2006;6:48–52.

Gallelli L, Galasso O, Falcone D, et al. The effects of non-steroidal anti-inflammatory drugs on clinical outcomes, synovial fluid cytokine concentration and signal transduction pathways in knee osteoarthritis. A randomized open label trial. Osteoarthr Cartil. 2013;21:1400–8.

Gawlak D, Manka-Malara K, Kaminski T, Luniewska M, Mierzwinska-Nastalska E. Comparative evaluation of custom and standard boil and bite (self-adapted)mouthguards and their effect on the functioning of the oral cavity. Dent Traumatol. 2016;32(5):416–20.

Giordano N, Fioravanti A, Papakostas P, Montella A, Giorgi G, Nuti R. The efficacy and tolerability of glucosamine sulfate in the treatment of knee-osteoarthritis: a randomized double-blind placebo-controlled trial. Curr Ther Res. 2009;70(3):185–96.

Gocmen G, Varol A, Karatas B, Basa S. Evaluation of temporomandibular joint disc-repositioning surgery with Mitek mini-anchors. Natl J Maxillofac Surg. 2013;4(2):188–92.

Hall HD, Indresano AT, Kirk WS, et al. Prospective multicenter comparison of 4 temporomandibular joint operations. J Oral Maxillofac Surg. 2005;63(8):1174–9.

Haketa T, Kino K, Sugisaki M, Takaoka M, Ohata T. Randomized clinical trial of treatment for TMJ disc displacement. J Dent Res. 2010;89(11):1259–63.

Haribabu PK, Eliav E, Heir GM. Topical medications for the effective management of neuropathic orofacial pain. J Am Dent Assoc. 2013;144(6):612–4.

Hegab AF, Ali HE, Elmasry M, Khallaf MG. Platelet-rich plasma injection as an effective treatment for temporomandibular joint osteoarthritis. J Oral Maxillofac Surg. 2015;73(9):1706–13.

Helenius ML, Hallikainen D, Helenius I, et al. Clinical and radiographic findings of the temporomandibular joint in patients with various rheumatic diseases. A case control study. Oral Surg Oral Med Oral Pathol Oral Radical. 2005;99:455–63.

Helenius ML, Tervahatiala P, Helenius I, Al-Sukhn J et al. (2006) Clinical, radiographic and MRI findings of the temporomandibular joint in patients with different rheumatic diseases. Int J Oral Maxillofac Surg 35(1):983-989.

Hendersen SE, Tudares MA, Gold MS, Almarza AJ. Temporomandibular joint fibrocartilage degeneration from unilateral dental splints. Arch Oral Biol. 2015;60(1):1–11.

Holmlund A, Lund B, Weiner CK. Discectomy without replacement for the treatment of painful reciprocal clicking or catching and chronic closed lock of the temporomandibular joint: a clinical follow-up audit. Br J Oral Maxillofac Surg. 2013;51(8):E211–4.

Huddleston Slater JJ, Vos LM, Story LP, Stegenga B. Randomized trial of the effectiveness of dexamethasone in TMJ arthrocentesis. J Dent Res. 2012; 91(2):173–8.

Indresano AT, Bradrick J. Arthroscopic laser procedures. In: Clark G, Sanders B, Bertolami C, editors. Advances in diagnostic and surgical arthroscopy of the temporomandibular joint. Philadelphia: WB Saunders; 1993. p. 129–37.

Jose VM, Bhonasali A, Hota D, Pandhi P. Randomized double-blind study comparing efficacy and safety of lamotrigine and amitriptyline in painful diabetic neuropathy. Diabet Med. 2007;24(4):377–83.

Kalaykova S, Lobbezoo F, Naeije M. Two-year natural course of anterior disc displacement with reduction. J Orofac Pain. 2010;24(4):373–8.

Kaneyama K, Segami N, Yoshimura H, Honjo M, Demura N. Increased levels of soluble cytokine receptors in the synovial fluid of temporomandibular joint disorders in relation to joint effusion on magnetic resonance images. J Oral Maxillofac Surg. 2010;68:1088–93.

Kaplan PA, HK T, Williams SM, Lydiatt DD. The normal temporomandibular joint: MR and arthrographic correlation. Radiology. 1987;165(1):177–8.

Kaye AM, Kaye AD, Lofton EC. Basic Concepts in opioid prescribing and current concepts of opioid-mediated effects on driving. Ochsner J. 2013;13:525–32.

Kirchheimer S, Sainuddin S, Bojanic S, Saeed NR. Simultaneous custom-made replacement of the temporomandibular joint and cranioplasty. Brit. J Oral Maxillofac Surg. 2013;51:e70–1.

Kopp S. Short term evaluation of counseling and occlusal adjustment in patients with mandibular dysfunction involving the temporomandibular joint. J Oral Rehabil. 1979;6(2):101–9.

Koutris M, Visscher CM, Lobbezoo F, Naeije M. Comorbidity negatively influences the outcomes of diagnostic tests for musculoskeletal pain in the orofacial region. Pain. 2013;154(6):927–32.

Kraus SL. Temporomandibular disorders, head and orofacial pain: cervical spine considerations. Dent Clin North Am. 2007;51:161–93.

Kraus SL. Characteristics of 511 patients with temporomandibular disorders referred for physical therapy. Oral Surg Oral Med Oral Pathol Oral Radical. 2014;118(4):432–9.

Kurita K, Bronstein SL, Westesson PL, et al. Arthroscopic diagnosis or perforation and adhesions of the temporomandibular joint: correlation with post mortem morphology. Oral Surg Oral Med Oral Pathol. 1989;68(2):130–4.

Kütük N, Baş B, Soylu E, Gönen ZB, Yilmaz C, Balcioğlu E, Özdamar S, Alkan A. Effect of platelet-rich plasma on fibrocartilage, cartilage, and bone repair in temporomandibular joint. J Oral Maxillofac Surg. 2014;72(2):277–84.

Lapicque F, Vergne P, Jouzeau JY, et al. Articular diffusion of meloxicam after a single oral dose: relationship to cyclo-oxygenase inhibition in synovial cells. Clin Pharmacokinet. 2000;39(5):369–82.

Larheim TA, Westesson PL, Sano T. Temporomandibular joint disc displacement: comparison in asymptomatic volunteers and patients. Radiology. 2001;218:428–32.

Lavelle W, Lavell ED, Lavelle L. Intra-articular injections. Med Clin North Am. 2007;91(2):241–50.

Lin YC, Hsu ML, Yang JS, Liang TH, Chou SL, Lin HY. Temporomandibular joint disorders in patients with rheumatoid arthritis. J Chin Med Assoc. 2007;70(12):527–34.

Litt MD, Porto FB. Determinants of pain treatment response and non-response: identification of TMD patient subgroups. J Pain. 2013;14(11):1–16.

Magnusson T, Adielis AM, Nilsson HL, Helkimo M. Treatment effect on signs and symptoms of temporomandibular disorders – comparison between stabilization splint and a new type of splint (NTI). A pilot study. Swed Dent J. 2004;28(1):11–20.

Manfredini D, Favero L, Gregorini G, Cocilovo F, Guardanardini L. Natural course of temporomandibular disorders with low pain-related impairment: a 2-to-3 year follow-up study. J Oral Rehab. 2013;40:436–42.

Martins WR, Blasczyk JC, Furlan de Oliveira MA, et al. Efficacy of musculoskeletal manual approach in the treatment of temporomandibular joint disorder: a systematic review with meta-analysis. Man Ther. 2016;21:10–7.

Masclee GM, Balkhoff VE, Coloma PM, et al. Risk of upper gastrointestinal bleeding from different drug combinations. Gastroenterology. 2014;147(4):784–92.

Mejersjo C, Wenneberg B. Diclofenac sodium and occlusal splint therapy in TMJ osteoarthritis: a randomized controlled trial. J Oral Rehab. 2008;35:729–38.

Mercuri LG, Edibam NR, Giobbie-Hurder A. Fourteen-year follow-up of a patient-fitted Total temporomandibular joint reconstruction system. Am Assoc Oral Maxillofac Surg. 2007;65(6):1140–8.

Minakuchi H, Kuboki T, Matsuka Y, Maikawa K, Yatani H, Yamashita A. Randomized controlled evaluation of non-surgical treatments for temporomandibular joint anterior disc displacement without reduction. J Dent Res. 2001;80(3):924–8.

Mosely JB, O'Malley K, Petersen NJ, et al. (2002) A controlled trial of arthroscopic surgery for osteoarthritis of the knee. N Engl J Med 347(2):81-88.

Motghare V, Kumar J, Kamate S, Kushwaha S, Anand R, Gupta N, Gupta B, Singh I. Association between harmful oral habits and sign and symptoms of temporomandibular joint disorders among adolescents. J Clin Diagn Res. 2015;9(8):ZC45–8.

Murakami KL, Iizluka T, Matsuki M, et al. Diagnostic arthroscopy of the TMJ: differential diagnoses in patients with limited jaw opening. Cranio. 1986;4(2):117–26.
Murakami K, Segami N. Intra-articular adhesions of the temporomandibular joint: arthroscopic views and clinical perspectives. In: Clark G, Sanders B, Bertolami C, editors. Advances in diagnostic and surgical arthroscopy of the temporomandibular joint. Philadelphia: WB Saunders; 1993. p. 15–21.
Murakami K, Moriya Y, Goto K, Segami N. Four-year follow-up study of temporomandibular joint arthroscopic surgery for advanced stage internal derangements. J Oral Maxillofac Surg. 1996;54(3):285–90.
Niemela K, Korpela M, Raustia A, Ylostalo P, Sipila K. Efficacy of stabilization splint treatment on temporomandibular disorders. J Oral Rehab. 2012;39:799–804.
Nitzan DW. Intraarticular pressure in the functioning human temporomandibular joint and it's alteration by uniform elevation of the occlusal plane. J Oral Maxillofac Surg. 1994;52(7):671–9.
Nitzan DW, Price A. The use of arthrocentesis for treatment of osteoarthritic temporomandibular joints. J Oral Maxillofac Surg. 2001;59:1154–9.
Pavelka K. A comparison of the therapeutic efficacy of diclofenac in osteoarthritis: a systemic review of randomized controlled trials. Curr Med Res Opin. 2012;28(1):163–78.
Plaza-Villegas F, Heir G, Markham, et al. (2012) Topical pregabilin and diclofenac for treatment of neuropathic pain in rats. Oral Surg Oral Med Oral Pathol Oral Radical 114(4):449-456.
Plesh O, Curtis D, Levine J, McCall WD. Amitriptyline treatment of chronic pain in patients with temporomandibular disorders. J Oral Rehab. 2000;27:834–41.
Reginster JY, Deroisy R, Rovati LC, et al. Long-term effects of glucosamine sulphate on osteoarthritis progression: a randomized, placebo-controlled clinical trial. Lancet. 2001;357:251–6.
Reiter S, Emodi-Perlman A, Goldsmith C, Friedman-Rubin P, Winocur E. Comorbidity between depression and anxiety in patients with temporomandibular disorders according to the research diagnostic criteria for temporomandibular disorders. J Oral Facial Pain Headache. 2015;29(2):135–43.
Ryan DE. Alloplastic implants in the temporomandibular joint. Oral Maxillofac Surg Clin North Am. 1989;1:427–41.
Sanders B, Buoncristiani R. A 5-year experience with arthroscopic lysis and lavage for treatment of painful temporomandibular joint hypomobility. In: Clark G, Sanders B, Bertolami C, editors. Advances in diagnostic and surgical arthroscopy of the temporomandibular joint. Philadelphia: WB Saunders; 1993. p. 31–24.
Sault JD, Emerson Kavhchak AJ, Tow N, Courtney CA. Regional effects of orthopedic manual physical therapy in the successful management of chronic jaw pain. Cranio. 2016;34(4):124–32.
Schiffman EL, Fricton JR, Haley DP, Shapiro BL. The prevalence and treatment needs of subjects with temporomandibular disorders. J Am Dent Assoc. 1990;120(3):295–303.
Schiffman EL, Anderson GC, Fricton JR, Lindgren BR. The relationship between level of mandibular pain and dysfunction and stage of temporomandibular joint internal derangement. J Dent Res. 1992;19(3):1812–5.
Schiffman E, Ohrbach R, Truelove E, et al. Diagnostic criteria for temporomandibular disorders (DC/TMD) for clinical and research applications: recommendations of the international RDC/TMD consortium network and orofacial pain special interest group. J Oral Facial Pain Headache. 2014;28(1):6–27.
Schmitter M, Zahran M, Phu Duc JM, Henschel V, Rammelsburg P. Conservative therapy in patients with anterior disc displacement without reduction using 2 common splints: a randomized clinical trial. J Oral Maxillofac Surg. 2005;63:1295–303.
Scott DL, Wolfe F, Huizinga TWJ. Rheumatoid arthritis. Lancet. 2010;376:1094–108.
Sekiya I, Morito T, Hara K, et al. Ketoprofen absorption by muscle and tendon after topical or oral administration in patients undergoing anterior cruciated ligament reconstruction. AAPS Pharm Sci Tech. 2010;11(1):154–8.
Senve M, Mir CF, Morton S, Thie NM. Topical nonsteriodal anti-inflamatory drugs for treatment of temporomandibular joint degenerative pain: a systematic review. J Orofac Pain. 2012;26(1):26–32.
Silver CM. Long-term results of meniscectomy of the temporomandibular joint. Cranio. 1984;3(1):46–57.
Sindelar BJ, Alonzo TA. The effects of intraoral splints on the masticatory system of pigs. J Oral Rehabil. 2003;30(8):823–31.
Stapelmann H, Turp J. The NTI-ss device for the therapy of bruxism, temporomandibular disorders, and headache – where do we stand? A qualitative systematic review of the literature. BMC Oral Health. 2008;8(22):1–23.
Stoustrup P, Kristensen KD, Verna C, Kuseler A, Pedersen TK, Herlin T. Intra-articular steroid injection for temporomandibular joint arthritis in juvenile idiopathic arthritis: a systematic review on efficacy and safety. Semin Arthritis Rheum. 2013;43:63–70.
Swift JQ, Roszkowski MT. The use of opioid drugs in Management of Chronic Orofacial Pain. J Oral Maxillofac Surg. 1998;56:1081–5.
Ta LE, Dionne RA. Treatment of painful temporomandibular joints with cyclooxygenase-2 inhibitor: a randomized placebo controlled comparison of celecoxib to naproxen. Pain. 2004;111:13–21.
Tabrizi R, Karagah T, Arabion H, Soleimanpour MR, Soleimanpour M. Outcomes of arthrocentesis for the treatment of internal derangement pain: with or without corticosteroids? J Craniofac Surg. 2014;25(6):571–5.
Tolvanen M, Oikarinenvj WJ. A 30 year follow-up study of temporo-mandibular joint menisectomies: a report on five patients. Br J Oral Maxillofac. 1988;26(4):311–6.
Tomaz-Morales JF, Lucena LB, Mota IA, Pereira AK, Lucena BT, Castro RD, Alves GA. Temporomandibular disorder is more prevalent among patients with pri-

mary headaches in a tertiary outpatient clinic. Arg Neuropsiquiatr. 2015;73(11):913–7.

Truelove E, Huggins KH, Manci L, Dworkin SF. The efficacy of traditional, low-cost and nonsplint therapies for temporomandibular disorder. J Am Dent Assoc. 2006;137(8):1099–107.

Tsukiyama Y, Kazuyoshi B, Clark GT. An evidenced-base assessment of occlusal adjustment as a treatment for temporomandibular disorders. J Prostho Dent. 2001;86(1):10–6.

Tuchman M, Barrett JA, Donevan S, Hedberg TG, Taylor CP. Central sensitization and Cavα2δ ligands in chronic pain syndromes: pathologic processes and pharmacologic effect. J Pain. 2010;11(12):1241–9.

Tuncer AB, Ergun N, Tuncer AH, Karahan S. Effectiveness of manual therapy and home physical therapy in patients with temporomandibular disorders: a randomized controlled trial. J Bodywork Move. 2013;17:302–8.

Turner JA, Dworkin SF, Manci L, Huggins KH, Truelove EL. The roles of beliefs, catastrophizing, and coping in the functioning of patients with temporomandibular disorders. Pain. 2001;92:41–51.

Velly AM, Look JO, Carlson C, et al. The effect of catastrophizing and depression on chronic pain – a prospective cohort study of temporomandibular muscle and joint pain disorders. Pain. 2011;152:2377–83.

Wassell RW, Verhees L, Lawrence K, Davies S, Lobbezzoo F. Over-the-counter (OTC) bruxism splints available on the internet. Br Dent J. 2014;216(11):1–10.

Wilkes CH. Surgical treatment of internal derangement of the temporomandibular joint. A long term study. Arch Otolaryngol Head Neck Surg. 1991; 117(1):64–72.

Wolford LM, Pitta MC, Reiche-Fischel O, Franco PF. TMJ Concepts/techmedica custom-made TMJ total joint prosthesis: 5 year follow-up study. Int J Oral Maxillofac Surg. 2003;32(3):268–74.

Wolford LM, Mercuri LG, Schneiderman ED, Movahed R, Allen W. Twenty-year follow-up study on a patient-fitted temporomandibular joint prosthesis: the techmedica/TMJ Concepts device. J Oral Maxillofac Surg. 2015;73(5):952–60.

Yang S, Eaton CB, McAlindon TE, Lapane KL. Effects of glucosamine and chondroitin on treating knee osteoarthritis: an analysis with marginal structural models. Arthritis Rheumatol. 2015;67(3):714–23.

Yi P, Pryzbylkowski P. Opioid induced hyperalgesia. Pain Med. 2015;16:S32–6.

Yoshida H, Sakata T, Hayashi T, Shirao K, Oshiro N, Morita S. Evaluation of mandibular condylar movement exercise for patients with internal derangement of the temporomandibular joint on initial presentation. Br J Oral Maxillofac Surg. 2010;49:310–3.

Zeidler H, Kaltwasser JP, Leanard JP, Kohlmann T, Sigmund R, Degner F, Hettich M. Prescription and tolerability of meloxicam in day to day practice postmarketing observational cohort study of 13,307 patient in Germany. J Clin Rheumat. 2002;8(6):305–15.

Psychosocial Considerations in TMD

10

Emily J. Bartley, John E. Schmidt Jr,
Charles R. Carlson, and Roger B. Fillingim

Abstract

Temporomandibular disorders represent a group of complex painful conditions, whose etiology and persistence are driven by a complex mosaic of influences, including psychological factors. This chapter addresses the importance of psychological contributions to TMD. Evidence is reviewed demonstrating not only that increased psychological symptoms are observed in people with TMD, but also the premorbid psychological functioning predicts future development of TMD. In addition, psychiatric diagnoses that can influence TMD symptoms and responses to treatment are discussed. Finally, the nature and effectiveness of psychological interventions for TMD are reviewed, and issues that impact interpretation of these findings are considered.

10.1 Introduction

Temporomandibular disorders (TMDs) represent a complex set of painful conditions characterized by orofacial pain and altered masticatory functioning. Similar to other chronic pain conditions, considerable information indicates that TMDs are associated with a variety of psychosocial factors, including psychological stress, increased affective distress, behavioral changes, and maladaptive pain coping (Fillingim et al. 2011c; Suvinen et al. 2005). While adverse psychological consequences of chronic pain have long been appreciated, increasing evidence suggests that premorbid psychosocial factors predict the onset and persistence of TMD, such that the associations between TMD and psychosocial function

E.J. Bartley, PhD • R.B. Fillingim, PhD (✉)
College of Dentistry and Pain Research & Intervention Center of Excellence, University of Florida, Gainesville, FL, USA
e-mail: ebartley@dental.ufl.edu; rfilling@ufl.edu

J.E. Schmidt Jr, PhD
Department of Psychology, Naval Post-Graduate Dental School, Navy Medicine Professional Development Center Walter Reed National Military Medical Center, Bethesda, MD, USA
e-mail: john.e.schmidt.civ@mail.mil

C.R. Carlson, PhD
Department of Psychology, University of Kentucky, Lexington, KY, USA
e-mail: ccarl@email.uky.edu

© Springer International Publishing AG 2018
H.A. Gremillion, G.D. Klasser (eds.), *Temporomandibular Disorders*,
https://doi.org/10.1007/978-3-319-57247-5_10

appear to be bidirectional (Aggarwal et al. 2010a; Fillingim et al. 2013; Garofalo et al. 1998). Given their importance in the development and expression of TMD, psychosocial factors reflect potentially important treatment targets.

This chapter addresses psychosocial considerations in TMD. After briefly highlighting some important conceptual issues related to the influence of psychosocial processes in TMD, we will discuss findings regarding psychosocial factors that are associated with TMD, including findings from case-control studies, as well as data from prospective studies that examine psychosocial factors as predictors of TMD onset and persistence. Next, we summarize the findings regarding psychological interventions for TMD and discuss several methodological and conceptual issues that impact the interpretation of this literature. We conclude the chapter with a brief summary and several recommendations for future research.

Conceptual Issues It is important to consider the relevance of psychosocial factors to TMD in the context of the broader biopsychosocial model (Fig. 10.1). The biopsychosocial model (discussed in more detail below) posits that the experience of pain and its manifestations across time are sculpted by complex and dynamic interactions among biological, psychological, and social factors. One corollary of this model is that the factors that influence chronic pain, including TMD, are almost never purely "biological" or "psychosocial." Rather, biological processes (e.g., cerebral activation, inflammation) directly impact psychological function (e.g., mood/affect, pain coping) and vice versa. The categorization of variables as biological versus psychological represents a distinction of convenience and is typically more related to the methods used to assess these processes than to the actual mechanisms themselves. This also has important implications from a treatment perspective, as it is important to recognize that psychological interventions can directly and robustly affect biological mechanisms that contribute to pain. Explaining this to patients can greatly increase their motivation to engage in psychological interventions, thereby enhancing compliance and expectations for positive outcomes. These issues will be revisited with specific examples in the sections below.

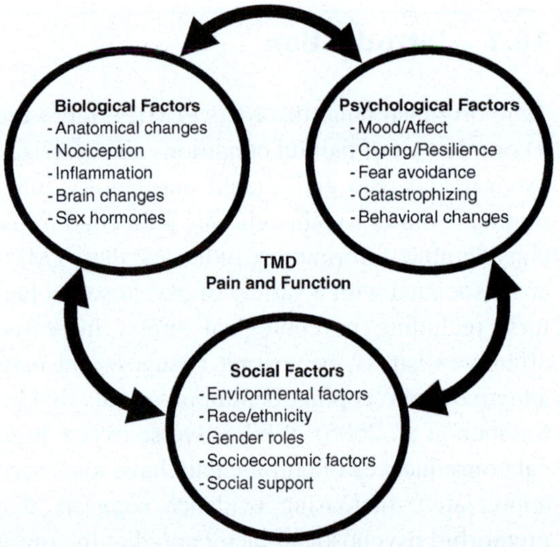

Fig. 10.1 Biopsychosocial model of pain applied to TMD. This model posits that TMD-related pain and function are sculpted by complex and dynamic interactions among biological, psychological, and social factors

The biopsychosocial model also conveys that a mosaic of biological, psychological, and social factors contributes to pain, although the relative importance of each set of factors and their interactions vary considerably across patients and over time. This renders invalid the historical clinical exercise of determining whether a given patient's pain is "biological" or "psychological" in nature—it is always both. Hence, the clinician's task is to try and understand the multitude of biopsychosocial factors that are contributing to a patient's symptoms and to develop a treatment plan that adequately addresses these factors.

It is also important to note that most previous research examining psychosocial contributions to TMD has focused on psychosocial risk factors and adverse psychological outcomes in TMD. However, there is increasing recognition that protective psychological processes, or resilience factors, may provide a buffer from the adverse effects of chronic pain. In addition, building resilience has become the focus of psychological interventions for pain in recent years. Thus, the increasing emphasis on positive psychology not only has important conceptual and mechanistic implications but also could greatly influence the development of psychological interventions for TMD, as we will discuss in more detail below.

10.2 Psychosocial Factors Related to TMD

Associations between TMD and psychological factors have been explored for over 40 years (Molin et al. 1973). Early research with patients reporting a TMD condition found a strong association between TMDs and psychological factors such as depression, anxiety, and perceived stress (Keefe and Dolan 1986; Carlson et al. 1993; Vassend et al. 1995; Beaton et al. 1991; Rudy et al. 1995). These studies were typically retrospective studies even though several had pain-free healthy control groups for comparisons. The relationships among psychological factors and TMD conditions have been explored in many subsequent studies with small and large samples of patients (Mckinney et al. 1990; Carlson et al. 1998; Fillingim et al. 1996; Schmidt and Carlson 2009; Manfredini et al. 2010; Pankhurst 1997). Several areas of dysfunction in patients with TMD conditions were identified in these early studies. Among the most prevalent concerns in the psychological domain were high levels of anxiety and depression. Difficulties with physical functioning were also associated with the presence of a TMD condition with patients consistently reporting significant sleep dysfunction and fatigue (Carlson et al. 1998; Yatani et al. 2002). Patients with TMD conditions also presented with higher autonomic reactivity and arousal compared to controls (Schmidt and Carlson 2009; Eisenlohr-Moul et al. 2015; Chen et al. 2013). In addition, the presence of a TMD condition was associated with reduced social support (Schmidt and Carlson 2009). All of these factors highlight the complexity and broad impact of a chronic TMD condition on daily functioning and quality of life. Management of many TMD conditions is typically a complex problem and not a straightforward dental care issue. Therefore, treating these conditions through the clinical application of the biopsychosocial model has proven to be a most effective methodology.

The biopsychosocial model as posited by Engel (1977) brought a much needed reevaluation of the biomedical model of disease management (Engel 1977). Prior to Engel's seminal thesis, many health-care providers focused specifically on treating the biological insult or injury and managing physical symptoms. Engel challenged clinicians and scientists to think more broadly by considering all aspects of the patient's life. In Engel's view, to discount the importance and impact of a person's psychological and social characteristics on disease was to fall well short of appropriate and effective care. In the study and treatment of orofacial pains, the biopsychosocial model has been used to improve diagnosis and treatment planning as presented by Okeson (2014). In Okeson's framework, education and management of TMD conditions are accomplished by considering the somatosensory and psychosocial domains of functioning. The pain classification developed by Dworkin and LeResche (Dworkin and Leresche 1992), advanced by Okeson (2014), and further refined by the Diagnostic Criteria for TMD (DC/TMD) (Schiffman et al. 2014) is presented on two axes with physical conditions on Axis I (e.g., musculoskeletal pains, neuropathic pains) and psychosocial conditions on Axis II (e.g., mood symptoms, somatic symptoms). The use of this classification approach for symptom management and treatment highlights the importance of assessing and understanding psychosocial factors in developing effective treatment plans.

Psychological factors have consistently been shown to be associated with TMD clinical symptoms, especially pain, disability, and symptom chronicity, in both retrospective and cross-sectional studies. However, the temporality of these associations remained difficult to elucidate until recently with the application of larger population-based and well-controlled longitudinal studies. A primary aim of these studies was to determine if the presence of significant psychological distress was predictive of the onset and chronicity of a TMD condition. In a 3-year prospective cohort study of 171 healthy females, Slade et al. (2007) identified painful new-onset TMD conditions in 8.8% of the sample. Predictors from baseline assessment of these new cases included depression, perceived stress, and mood state. A much larger study based on data from the population-based Study of Health in Pomerania followed a sample of over 3000 participants for about 9 years (Kindler et al. 2012). New-onset TMD conditions were found in 4.1% of the sample, and baseline depression and anxiety were both predictive of subsequent development of a TMD condition. These and other studies (Leresche 1997; Aggarwal et al. 2010b) have looked carefully at possible predictors of TMD with the goal of improving the identification of potential TMD cases early rather than late when the problem becomes chronic, significantly worse, and more challenging to manage.

More recently, increased knowledge of TMD conditions was acquired with the initiation of the OPPERA (Orofacial Pain: Prospective Evaluation and Risk Assessment) study. The primary goal of the OPPERA study was to identify psychological and physiological risk factors, clinical characteristics, and associated genetic mechanisms that influence the development of TMDs (Dworkin 2011). Two issues of *The Journal of Pain* were dedicated to the presentation of findings from the OPPERA study (2011, volume 12, number 11, supplement 3; and 2013, volume 14, number 12, supplement 2).

The initial analyses of baseline psychosocial data from the OPPERA study (Fillingim et al. 2011a) included TMD cases and TMD-free controls. The analyses of baseline data corroborated previous findings and further emphasized the importance of assessing psychosocial characteristics in TMD patients. The TMD cases in this study presented with higher depression, higher anxiety, higher somatization, and higher-negative affect and reported higher perceived stress. In a follow-up study using TMD-free study, participants (2737 participants provided follow-up data) assessed an average of 2.8 years after baseline; Fillingim et al. (2013) found new-onset TMD conditions in 9% of the sample. The development of a TMD condition was predicted by negative mood, psychological distress, perceived stress, and somatization. The strongest predisposing psychosocial risk factors for the development of TMD were global psychological symptoms, particularly somatic symptoms. The results of the studies demonstrate the importance of assessing and treating psychological distress in patients with new-onset and chronic TMD conditions. TMDs are typically accompanied by significant psychological distress, which may both predict and contribute to the chronicity of the TMD condition. The specific psychological factors are discussed in detail below, including psychiatric disorders as well as subclinical variations of psychological symptoms that occur in the general population. It is important to recognize that much of the literature described above, including the OPPERA studies, has demonstrated associations between elevated psychological symptomatology (e.g., depressed or anxious mood) and TMD, even in the absence of actual psychiatric conditions. Below, we discuss both these subclinical variations in psychological functioning as well as psychiatric conditions, as both issues are highly relevant to the clinical management of TMD.

Depression Symptoms of depression are the most prevalent psychological concern in patients with TMD conditions (Liao et al. 2011; Giannakopoulos et al. 2010). Therefore, it is important for the clinician to have a sound understanding of symptoms, diagnostic criteria, assessment, and potential impact that clinically significant depression may have on treatment of TMD. The diagnostic criteria for a major depressive disorder (MDD) as found in the Diagnostic and Statistical Manual of Mental Disorders V (American Psychiatric Association 2013) are provided in Table 10.1.

Symptoms of depression are strongly associated with pain severity and pain sensitivity in chronic pain populations (Gerrits et al. 2015). The relationship between depression and perception or sensation of pain is difficult to elucidate and has been a major focus of research (Klauenberg et al. 2008). To explore the possible associations among experimentally stimulated pain perception and depression, Boettger and colleagues compared patients diagnosed with MDD

Table 10.1 DSM-V diagnostic criteria for major depressive disorder (MDD)

(A) For a diagnosis of major depressive episode, five (or more) of the following symptoms have been present during the same 2 week period and represent a change from previous functioning. One of the symptoms must be either (a) depressed mood or (b) loss of interest or pleasure
(1) Depressed mood most of the day, nearly every day, as indicated by either subjective report (e.g., feels sad, empty, hopeless) or observation made by others (e.g., appears tearful). In children and adolescents, this may be irritable mood
(2) Markedly diminished interest or pleasure in all, or almost all, activities most of the day, nearly every day
(3) Significant weight loss when not dieting or weight gain (e.g., a change of more than 5% of body weight in a month) or decrease or increase in appetite nearly every day. For children, they may not gain an expected amount of weight
(4) Insomnia or hypersomnia nearly every day
(5) Psychomotor agitation or retardation nearly every day (observable by others, not merely subjective feelings of restlessness or being slowed down)
(6) Fatigue or loss of energy nearly every day
(7) Feelings of worthlessness or excessive or inappropriate guilt (which may be delusional) nearly every day (not merely self-reproach or guilt about being sick)
(8) Diminished ability to think or concentrate, or indecisiveness, nearly every day (either by subjective account or observable by others)
(9) Recurrent thoughts of death (not just fear of dying), recurrent suicidal ideation without a specific plan, or a suicide attempt or a specific plan for committing suicide
(B) The symptoms cause clinically significant distress or impairment in social, occupational, or other important areas of functioning
(C) The episode is not attributable to the physiological effects of a substance or to another medical condition
(D) The occurrence of the major depressive episode is not better explained by schizoaffective disorder, schizophrenia, schizophreniform disorder, delusional disorder, or other specified and unspecified schizophrenia spectrum and other psychotic disorders
(E) There has never been a manic episode or a hypomanic episode

to matched controls (matched on age, gender, and handedness) using the Thermal Grill Illusion (TGI) (Boettger et al. 2013). The TGI describes a painful and unusual sensation evoked by alternating warm and cold stimuli (Craig and Bushnell 1994). Participants with MDD presented with higher heat and cold pain thresholds and reported lower overall pain VAS ratings to the TGI stimuli compared to controls (Boettger et al. 2013). In contrast, Strigo and colleagues reported that people with MDD had lower heat pain thresholds and showed greater affective bias compared to controls, in that their ratings of heat pain unpleasantness substantially exceeded those of controls (Strigo et al. 2008). These results further demonstrate the complexity of the relationship between depression and pain perception and highlight the need for further research in this area.

Patients struggling with chronic pain conditions, such as TMD, are generally more socially isolated, experience sleep dysfunction and increased daytime fatigue, and report difficulty with attention and mental focus. All of these characteristics are also among the diagnostic criteria for a depressive disorder (see Table 10.1). Further, pain perception in chronic pain patients may exacerbate negative affect via an increase in catastrophizing (Roth et al. 2005) and cognitive distortions (Richardson et al. 2009). The associations among negative affect and maladaptive cognitive attributes have also been identified in patients with TMD conditions (Turner et al. 2005a). For example, in a large prospective cohort study, Velly and colleagues (Velly et al. 2011) followed 480 participants with TMD over an 18-month period. Baseline catastrophizing was strongly associated with increased pain intensity and with disability at the 18-month follow-up assessment. Both depression and catastrophizing are factors that may potentially complicate treatment adherence and effectiveness; thus these psychologically based concerns should be assessed for and treated concurrently with the TMD condition.

Table 10.2 DSM-V diagnostic criteria for generalized anxiety disorder (GAD)

(A) Excessive anxiety and worry (apprehensive expectation), occurring more days than not for at least 6 months, about a number of events or activities (such as work or school performance)
(B) The individual finds it difficult to control the worry
(C) The anxiety and worry are associated with three (or more) of the following six symptoms (with at least some symptoms present for more days than not for the past 6 months)
(1) Restlessness or feeling keyed up or on edge
(2) Being easily fatigued
(3) Difficulty concentrating or mind going blank
(4) Irritability
(5) Muscle tension
(6) Sleep disturbance (difficulty falling or staying asleep, or restless unsatisfying sleep)
(D) The anxiety, worry, or physical symptoms cause clinically significant distress or impairment in social, occupational, or other important areas of functioning
(E) The disturbance is not attributable to the physiological effects of a substance (e.g., a drug of abuse, medication) or another medical condition (hyperthyroidism)
(F) The disturbance is not better explained by another mental disorder

Anxiety The prevalence of anxiety symptoms and diagnosable anxiety disorders in TMD conditions is significantly higher than the general population. While anxiety is often concurrent with symptoms of depression, the presentation of anxiety symptoms, the impact on TMD, and the challenge to treatment can be much different. In fact, in the most recent iteration of the Diagnostic and Statistical Manual of Mental Disorders, an anxiety qualifier was added to the diagnostic criteria for major depression to capture patients with a depressive disorder concurrent with anxiety symptoms that may exacerbate negative affect (American Psychiatric Association 2013). Clinicians working with TMD will likely encounter patients experiencing generalized anxiety disorder and post-traumatic stress disorder (Okeson 2014). Generalized anxiety disorder (GAD) is characterized by persistent, excessive, and often unrealistic worry about events or activities. For these patients, the worry is out of control and the worst expectations are feared in any given situation. The worry can be focused on daily events and activities, can be unrelenting, and can significantly interfere with daily living, social activities, and management of health-care concerns. The prevalence of GAD in the US population is approximately 3%, with a lifetime prevalence rate of 5%. The sex ratio is approximately two-thirds female. Specific symptoms of GAD as found in the Diagnostic and Statistical Manual of mental disorders V (American Psychiatric Association 2013) are summarized in Table 10.2.

In the OPPERA (Fillingim et al. 2013) and other studies (Kindler et al. 2012), anxiety, as defined by the State-Trait Anxiety Scale (Spielberger et al. 1983), was identified as a predictor of TMD development. Retrospective studies with patients consistently identify anxiety as an important target for comprehensive treatment, however, less so than significant symptoms of depression (Reiter et al. 2015; Giannakopoulos et al. 2010). Yet, this may not be the case when the problem in coping is due to a trauma resulting in symptoms of post-traumatic stress disorder (PTSD).

Traumatic Stress and Post-Traumatic Stress Disorder The experience of a traumatic stressor and symptoms of post-traumatic stress disorder (PTSD) are frequently reported by patients with TMD conditions, and recent studies have explored the prevalence of traumatic events and PTSD symptom severity in this population (Bertoli et al. 2007; Sherman et al. 2005; De Leeuw et al. 2005a, b). Stressful life events and PTSD symptoms were also found to be predictors of the development of TMD conditions in the OPPERA study (Fillingim et al. 2013). In the DSM-V, PTSD is included under the category of trauma- and stress-related disorders, with the main criteria being the exposure to actual or threatened death, injury, or sexual violence, intrusion symptoms (e.g., flashbacks, distressing dreams and memories) associated with the event, persistent avoidance of reminders of the trauma, negative cognitions and mood alterations, and elevations in arousal and reactivity associated with the trauma.

In a retrospective study of 600 TMD patients, de Leeuw and colleagues found that over half the sample reported at least one traumatic stressor. Most often reported stressors included the serious injury or death of a family member or close friend, followed by severe auto accident and sudden injury/serious accident (De Leeuw et al. 2005a). Traumatic stressors in patients with TMD conditions are often associated with pain severity, affective distress, and disability. These associations are even stronger for those patients meeting criteria for PTSD (Sherman et al. 2005; De Leeuw et al. 2005a). In another study by de Leeuw and colleagues, 14.7% of the sample (total sample $n = 1478$) met diagnostic criteria for PTSD (De Leeuw et al. 2005a). Pain severity, affective distress, and sleep dysfunction were significantly higher in patients meeting PTSD criteria, compared to patients reporting a traumatic stressor but not meeting criteria, as well as to those patients reporting no traumatic stressor. In a similar project examining the symptoms of PTSD among consecutively seen patients with TMD conditions, Sherman and colleagues (2005) found that among 183 patients, 23% of the sample received a current or full lifetime diagnosis of PTSD using a structured clinical interview and the PTSD Symptom Checklist (PCL). In this study, symptoms of PTSD were associated with pain severity and affective distress.

Given the prevalence of traumatic life events and PTSD among patients with TMDs, clinicians should have a clear understanding of the diagnostic criteria for PTSD (American Psychiatric Association 2013). Screening for PTSD symptomatology should be included as part of baseline assessment procedures, and clinicians should make appropriate referrals for psychological treatment as needed. Further, health-care providers should be cognizant of the strong associations among PTSD symptoms, pain severity, and affective distress and be mindful of how PTSD symptoms may interfere with treatment effectiveness and adherence in patients with TMDs.

Somatic Symptoms and Related Disorders Somatic symptoms and related disorders are a cluster of disorders characterized by somatic symptoms that are either highly distressing or result in significant disruption in daily functioning. Examples of somatic symptoms can include pain, fatigue, or neurological symptoms (e.g., seizures, dizziness, or paralysis). Primary disorders include somatic symptom disorder, illness anxiety disorder, conversion disorder, and factitious disorder. The most commonly observed diagnosis using the new DSM-V criteria will most likely be somatic symptom disorder with predominant pain (previously pain disorder in the DSM-IV). To meet diagnostic criteria, the individual must experience excessive thoughts, feelings, and behaviors related to the somatic symptoms with a typical course of at least 6 months of persistent symptoms. The somatic symptoms may or may not be associated with another medical condition and often can represent a diagnostic label for clinicians to use when they do not have an explanation for the physical symptoms that the patient is reporting. Diagnostic criteria emphasize the psychosocial aspect of somatic symptoms and related disorders by incorporating affective, cognitive, and behavioral components into the criteria in addition to the biological complaint, regardless of the medical explanation. This definition allows for a more comprehensive clinical picture of the patient's complaint.

In contrast to diagnoses of somatic symptom disorders, most studies of TMD have examined somatic symptom reports using questionnaires that provide continuous information regarding the breadth and severity of somatic symptoms. The most often used assessment tool has been the somatization subscale of the Symptom Check List-90-Revised (SCL-90-R). The SCL-90-R was originally developed by Derogatis in 1977 and revised in 1994 (Derogatis 1994) and assesses multiple aspects of psychopathology and overall psychological functioning. However, care should be exercised when using this instrument in chronic pain patients. Research has identified problems with the validity of the individual subscales in studies of patients with chronic pain (Hardt et al. 2000). In studies where the entire SCL-90-R has been used, patients with TMD conditions consistently present with significantly higher levels of somatic symptoms, depression, and anxiety when compared to matched pain-free controls (Carlson et al. 2001; Schmidt and Carlson 2009; Mcgregor et al. 1996). Somatic symptoms assessed by the SCL-90-R include cardiovascular, gastrointestinal, respiratory, pain, and other symptoms with strong autonomic mediation. The presence of high levels of somatic symptoms in TMD patients suggests the involvement of central mechanisms influencing autonomic tone and should provide clues to the treating clinician that peripherally based treatments alone are less likely to be effective. Rather, a multidisciplinary treatment approach integrating physical treatment modalities with psychological intervention is strongly encouraged.

Personality Disorders From a broad perspective, personality disorders are enduring patterns of pervasive and inflexible behavior based on how an individual relates to others and the nature of those interactions. Onset typically occurs in adolescence and early adulthood, and behaviors deviate markedly from the expectations of the individual's culture and societal norms. Personality disorders are stable over time and commonly lead to distress or impairment in daily functioning. Given the challenging nature of working with patients with a diagnosable personality disorder, additional information will be provided on each disorder as presented in the DSM-V.

Personality disorders are grouped into three clusters based on descriptive similarities (Table 10.3). Cluster A includes paranoid, schizoid, and schizotypal personality disorders. The paranoid individual will present as suspicious and distrustful of others, which can include relationships with health-care providers. Schizoid individuals are isolated, have limited range of emotional expression, and lack a desire for intimacy. Several of these characteristics are also shared with the schizotypal individual such as limited emotional expression, but these individuals also present with distorted thought patterns which may include very unusual behavior. The Cluster A disorders are relatively uncommon with prevalence ranging from 0.3% up to 4.9% in one national epidemiological study (Kessler et al. 2005).

Table 10.3 DSM-V diagnostic features across personality disorder clusters

Cluster A	
Paranoid personality disorder	Distrust and suspiciousness such that other's motives are interpreted as malevolent
Schizoid personality disorder	Detachment from social relationships and a restricted range of emotional expression
Schizotypal personality disorder	Discomfort in close relationships, cognitive or perceptual distortions, and behavior eccentricities
Cluster B	
Antisocial personality disorder	Disregard for, and violation of, the rights of others.
Borderline personality disorder	Instability in interpersonal relationships, self-image, and affects and marked impulsivity
Histrionic personality disorder	Excessive emotionality and attention seeking
Narcissistic personality disorder	Grandiosity, need for admiration, and lack of empathy
Cluster C	
Avoidant personality disorder	Social inhibition, feelings of inadequacy, and hypersensitivity to negative evaluation
Dependent personality disorder	Submissive and clinging behavior related to an excessive need to be taken care of
Obsessive-compulsive personality disorder	Preoccupation with orderliness, perfectionism, and control

The Cluster B disorders include antisocial, borderline, histrionic, and narcissistic personality disorders. Individuals with antisocial personality disorder are characterized as having little or no regard for others, are often deceitful, and fail to conform to lawful behavior. Conversely, borderline personality disorder is distinguished by instability in interpersonal relationships, emotion, and self-image. An individual with borderline personality disorder can be extremely difficult to manage from a clinical perspective, and referral for appropriate mental health care is strongly encouraged. Prevalence of borderline personality disorder has been found to be 6% in primary care settings and up to 10% in outpatient mental health facilities. Cluster B also includes histrionic and narcissistic personality disorders. Patients with histrionic personality disorder present with excessive emotional expression and attention-seeking behavior, and maintaining professional boundaries with the clinician can be a challenge for them. Conversely, narcissistic personality disorder is a condition whereby patients present with a grandiose sense of self-importance believing he or she is special and deserves special treatment with a superior sense of entitlement.

Avoidant, dependent, and obsessive-compulsive personality disorders comprise Cluster C. The common characteristic among these disorders is pervasive fear and anxiety in daily functioning. In general, the individual with avoidant personality disorder will be socially inhibited, feel socially inadequate, and be overly sensitive to any criticism or disapproval. On the other hand, individuals with dependent personality disorder will present with a pervasive need to be taken care of, leading to submissive and clinging behavior including fears of abandonment. Generally, these individuals will continue to pursue treatment regardless of the outcome or clinical improvement. Patients with obsessive-compulsive personality disorder (OCPD) are preoccupied with order, perfection, and mental and interpersonal control that overshadows daily functioning. Individuals with OCPD are typically not open to new ideas and concepts regarding treatment, focusing instead on details, lists, and perfectionism.

Research focusing on personality disorders and TMD conditions is minimal in the published literature. A primary reason for the lack of research may be due to personality disorder assessment, which can be time-consuming and require resources not found at a typical orofacial pain center. However, research focusing on personality disorders and chronic pain has demonstrated comorbidity (Vendrig 2000; Tragesser et al. 2010; Conrad et al. 2007). Individuals with personality disorders present with marginal and nonadaptive coping styles that decompensate when challenged with injury, pain, or other life issues. The diathesis-stress model fits this conceptual idea well and has been tested in different chronic pain populations (Conrad et al. 2007; Weisberg and Keefe 1997). Overall, individuals with personality disorders can be very challenging to work with in any healthcare setting and perhaps even more so when managing a chronic TMD condition. Pervasive and stable personality abnormalities may interfere with proper assessment and diagnosis, treatment planning, and patient adherence to treatment recommendations.

10.3 Mechanisms Underlying TMD

Oral Parafunction Oral parafunction is a generalized term capturing any oral behavior or habit that occurs outside the range of normal, healthy functioning of muscles and structure in the orofacial region. Oral parafunctions can include bruxism, teeth clenching or grinding, tongue thrusting, fingernail biting, chewing nonfood items such as pens/pencils, or any other habitual use of the orofacial muscles, muscles of mastication, and structural regions not related to normal eating, drinking, speaking, movement, and posture.

Oral parafunction has long been considered as a potential source of pain, dysfunction, and the development and maintenance of TMD conditions. Patients with TMD conditions have consistently demonstrated an association between TMD symptoms and oral parafunction (Gavish et al. 2000; Van Der Meulen et al. 2006) including parafunctional clenching for up to hours at a time (Glaros 1996). To improve the understanding of the relationship between parafunction and a TMD condition in a TMD patient sample, ecological momentary assessment has been used to collect perceived clenching/grinding behavior randomly throughout the day during study participation. In these studies (Glaros et al. 2005a, b; Chen et al. 2007), patients with myofascial pain and arthralgia reported significantly more nonfunctional tooth contact compared to non-TMD control participants. These results strongly suggest that patients with TMD conditions engage in higher levels of parafunction, which may in turn contribute to the severity and chronicity of the condition.

The potential association between parafunctional activity and developing TMD pain has also been explored in pain-free participants (Glaros and Burton 2004; Glaros et al. 1998; Svensson and Arendt-Nielsen 1996). In these studies, participants were randomized to either an "increase" or "decrease" muscle activity group. Those assigned to the "increase" group were instructed to maintain masseter and right/left temporalis EMG muscle activity above a threshold of 10 microvolts for 17–20 min by light clenching. The "decrease" group was instructed to maintain the same muscle groups below 2 microvolts. The muscle training took place over five consecutive days with muscle activity assessed using surface EMG. Participants in the "increase" group were more likely to be diagnosed with TMD pain after training. Pain VAS scores were significantly higher in the "increase" group participants compared to the "decrease" group participants, and masseter EMG activity was significantly correlated with reported pain severity (Glaros and Burton 2004). These findings are supportive of the view that long-term, low-level parafunction activity may lead to pain and a TMD condition meeting RDC criteria.

More recently, Ohrbach and colleagues explored the role of oral parafunction in the development of TMD conditions as part of the OPPERA study (Ohrbach et al. 2013). The large sample of 2737 participants was followed for nearly 3 years, and 260 people were identified as having developed first-onset TMD. Parafunctional behaviors were assessed using the Oral Behaviors Checklist (Markiewicz et al. 2006) which provides a total score based on the frequency of 21 different parafunctional behaviors including clenching/grinding teeth; pressing, holding, or tightening facial muscles; holding jaw forward or to the side; biting or chewing tongue or cheeks/lips; and biting objects such as hair, pencils, fingernails. Patients responded to each item on a five-point Likert scale from "none of the time" to "all of the time." Oral parafunction was found to be a strong predictor of developing a TMD problem, with those at highest risk engaging in numerous parafunctional behaviors extensively either by engaging in a large number of parafunctional behaviors or frequently engaging in a small number of parafunctional behaviors. Ohrbach and colleagues speculated that the presence of an underlying central dysregulation (e.g., persistent psychophysiological reactivity, overactive motor system) may be contributing to the association between oral parafunction and the development and chronicity of a TMD condition (Ohrbach et al. 2013). These behavior patterns and habits are often a target for change in multidisciplinary treatment for TMD conditions. In fact, by learning to be aware of clenching patterns and to allow these muscle groups to relax, patients may report significant reductions in TMD.

Coping/Catastrophizing Pain coping refers to cognitive and behavioral strategies that individuals employ to manage pain and reduce its negative impact on functioning and quality of life. People with pain use multiple coping strategies. Active coping strategies are generally considered adaptive (e.g., distraction, calming self-statements, seeking emotional support), while more passive approaches tend to be maladaptive, such as pain catastrophizing (pain catastrophizing is a negative cognitive and attentional approach to pain, characterized by magnification, rumination, and helplessness (Sullivan et al. 2001)). Abundant evidence demonstrates that pain coping influences pain-related outcomes, including outcomes among people with TMD. For example, individuals with TMD have been shown to report decreased use of adaptive coping and increased use of maladaptive coping compared to people without TMD (Ferrando et al. 2004; Fillingim et al. 2011b). Moreover, in TMD sufferers measures of catastrophizing predict increased pain severity and pain-related interference (Aaron et al. 2006; Litt et al. 2004, 2009). Thus, increasing active coping and decreasing catastrophizing are primary goals of cognitive behavioral interventions for TMD pain, as described further below.

Resilience Factors Recent years have witnessed a proliferation of studies examining psychosocial factors that promote successful adaptation (i.e., resilience) to pain. In a broad sense, resilience is a dynamic construct involved in health promotion and serves as a model to understand how people achieve physical and psychosocial well-being despite ongoing adversity. In general, people with greater resilience have a greater capacity for adaptive physiological and emotional recovery, persist in valued and meaningful activities in spite of stressful circumstances, and experience enhanced personal growth as a consequence of adverse events (Sturgeon and Zautra 2010). A number of studies have identified several psychosocial factors that promote pain-related resilience including positive affect, optimism, hope, sense of purpose/meaning in life, self-efficacy, benefit finding, and positive social interactions, among others (Sturgeon and Zautra 2010, 2013).

While most research in TMD has focused on the identification of maladaptive factors that confer risk to negative functioning and symptom burden, there is also evidence supporting the influence of resilience in this population. For instance, higher optimism had a buffering effect on ischemic pain sensitivity and unpleasantness ratings (Costello et al. 2002). Further, Brister and colleagues (Brister et al. 2006) found that TMD patients with greater self-efficacy reported higher physical and psychological functioning (i.e., lower pain, disability, emotional distress), as well as greater use of adaptive pain coping strategies. Similarly, increased self-efficacy for pain was significantly associated with overall improvements in pain, depression, and jaw opening from baseline to 3-month follow-up after usual dental care with or without cognitive behavioral treatment (Turner et al. 1995). Taken together, these findings suggest that greater levels of psychological resilience may mitigate the negative effects of persistent pain. In contrast to the prevailing risk model, considering protective factors associated with pain adaptation may provide new opportunities for improving treatment outcomes in TMD.

10.4 Psychological Interventions for TMD

Standard of care for TMD typically involves pharmacotherapy and/or intraoral splint therapy, as well as self-management strategies including heat/ice packs, soft diet, and patient education. However, evidence for the long-term effectiveness of these treatments is unimpressive (List and Axelsson 2010). Over the past four decades, psychosocial factors (e.g., anxiety, depression, stress) have been recognized as robust contributors to TMD onset and persistence. Moreover, it is generally accepted that both physical and psychosocial factors interact in TMD pathophysiology (i.e., biopsychosocial model, see Fig. 10.1 above). Based on this biopsychosocial conceptualization of TMD pain, several behavioral and psychological treatments have been applied in TMD management. In the next section, we outline some of the more common therapeutic modalities (i.e., electromyography, hypnosis, cognitive behavioral therapy) that have been implemented over recent years.

Electromyographic Biofeedback While a number of factors are postulated in the pathogenesis of TMD, it is generally acknowledged that psychological stress is a significant contributor to symptomatology. The assumption underlying this association is that heightened stress increases parafunctional oral habits (i.e., clenching, bruxism) and muscle hypertrophy, thus facilitating joint damage and maintaining the symptoms commonly observed in TMD (Gameiro et al. 2006). Given the notion that stress-induced muscle hyperactivity is implicated in the development and maintenance of TMD, electromyography (EMG) combined with relaxation and biofeedback therapy has been used as a treatment tool to normalize muscle activity and reduce pain. The primary objective of EMG biofeedback (BF) is to reduce muscle hyperactivity through increased proprioceptive awareness of muscle tension. Surface electrodes are typically attached to the masseter muscle, although placement can also target the temporalis and/or frontalis muscles, and muscle electrical activity is converted into signals on a computer screen for visual feedback. Over a series of contractions and relaxation of the muscles, patients learn to regulate periods of muscle tension. When used in conjunction with relaxation, the reduction in physiological arousal from indices of sympathetic nervous system activation becomes a key target in treatment (i.e., biofeedback-assisted relaxation training [BART]). Progressive muscle relaxation (PMR) is a commonly paired technique, which often involves systematically tensing and relaxing large muscle groups of the body with the intent to increase discernibility between muscular tension and relaxation (Jacobson 1938). While PMR is frequently combined with biofeedback, treatment can also involve diaphragmatic breathing (breathing through contraction of the diaphragm), autogenic relaxation (suggestive technique to promote feelings of warmth and heaviness associated with decreased sympathetic activity), and guided imagery (generation of positive mental images) to promote a relaxed state and reduce physiological responses that enhance autonomic arousal (e.g., skin conductance, heart rate).

To this end, a handful of studies have reported on the efficacy of BF in TMD—either assessing post-intervention effects within the same group or comparing outcomes with a no-treatment control. For instance, Carlsson and Gale (Carlsson and Gale 1977) conducted six to 18 sessions of masseter BF in 11 patients, ceasing treatment only when patients had no additional improvement in their ability to relax or reduce pain. Of the 11 patients, nine reported reductions in TMD pain, while the other two reported null effects. Using a manipulation to induce stress, Dahlstrom and colleagues (Dahlstrom et al. 1982) found that EMG activity, self-reported discomfort, and mandibular dysfunction were lower in TMD patients after six weekly BF sessions; however, there was no significant change in anxiety. In an examination of bruxism, defined as episodes of tonic daytime and nighttime muscle activity recorded by EMG, Sato and colleagues (Sato et al. 2015) randomized 12 men to either a BF group or a no-treatment control condition. After 3 weeks with BF training, participants in the BF group exhibited decreased daytime and nighttime EMG activity compared to baseline and the no-treatment condition. A few studies have compared BF with oral splint therapy with mixed results. Dahlstrom and colleagues compared 6 weeks of oral splint therapy with BF and found that both groups equally reduced pain and muscle tension at the 1- and 12-month follow-up periods (Dahlstrom et al. 1985). In contrast, Hijzen and colleagues observed that BF led to greater improvements in clinical dysfunction, pain, and range of motion relative to either an oral splint or no-treatment control groups (Hijzen et al. 1986). When adding BF to other TMD treatments including jaw posture instruction and a prosthetic guide (similar to an oral splint), Erlandson and Poppen found that BF added to the prosthesis and instructional groups produced greater improvements in range of motion, palpation, and self-reported pain, as well as EMG activity, when compared to BF alone (Erlandson and Poppen 1989). In a subsequent study by Turk and colleagues, the comparative efficacy of oral splint therapy versus BF/stress management (SM) was evaluated in two separate investigations. In the first study, patients underwent oral splint therapy and BF/SM for 6 weeks, with more robust improvements in pain observed in the oral splint group immediately after treatment. However, at the 6-month follow-up, the BF/SM group sustained improvements in pain and depression, whereas the oral splint group relapsed. In the second study, three groups consisting of oral splint therapy, BF/SM, and the combined treatment of oral splint with BF/SM were compared with one another. Overall, the authors found that the combined group was more effective in reducing pain and depression at the 6-month follow-up than the two independent treatments (Turk et al. 1993).

Hypnosis and Relaxation Hypnosis has been utilized as a treatment for pain over the past century, with several randomized-controlled clinical trials (RCTs) noting its efficacy in acute pain, medical procedures, and even chronic pain reduction over placebo (Elkins et al. 2007). The procedure involves sustaining highly focused attention, whereby suggestions for deep relaxation and comfort are induced (i.e., hypnotic induction). Commonly, imagery and visualization are incorporated in the process, and posthypnotic suggestions for analgesia are traditionally given to promote pain relief beyond the session. It is suggested that hypnosis reduces pain through mechanisms underlying attention control and dissociation (Hilgard 1973). Although hypnosis and relaxation (e.g., progressive muscle relaxation, diaphragmatic breathing) are similar in many respects, hypnosis is considered to be a heightened state of concentration in which openness to suggestion and responsiveness is essential to the success of the technique.

Despite the large body of literature reporting on the effects of hypnosis and relaxation in pain, limited evidence addresses these methods in TMD. In an early investigation, Gessel and Alderman found that 6 of 11 patients exhibited improvement in their TMD symptoms after relaxation training (Gessel and Alderman 1971). In contrast, splint therapy was more effective in improving pain and maximal oral opening in a study by Okeson and colleagues, when compared to relaxation. However, it is important to note that participants in this study listened to a 20 min relaxation tape once daily, rather than training being instituted by a professional (Okeson et al. 1983). Simon and Lewis examined the effectiveness of six hypnosis sessions on TMD pain and found that patients exhibited decreases in pain frequency and duration, pain intensity, as well as medical outcome use, effects which were maintained at the 6-month follow-up (Simon and Lewis 2000). A 5-session hypnorelaxation group was compared with occlusal splint therapy and a condition receiving TMD education/advice in a subsequent study by Winocur and colleagues (Winocur et al. 2002). The hypnorelaxation group received progressive muscle relaxation as well as self-hypnosis, while the education condition was provided information and support on their condition. The authors found that both hypnorelaxation and oral splint therapy were effective in reducing sensitivity to palpation, when compared to support/advice; however, hypnorelaxation participants reported significantly greater decreases in pain intensity (Winocur et al. 2002). Taken together, these studies provide some support for the use of hypnosis and relaxation in the treatment of TMD; however, small samples sizes, lack of standardization procedures, and methodological limitations hinder conclusions that can be drawn in terms of their efficacy.

Cognitive Behavioral Therapy Over the past few decades, cognitive behavioral therapy (CBT) has become a widely accepted psychotherapy approach for the treatment of pain (Ehde et al. 2014). Guided by the tenets of the biopsychosocial model, the primary goals of CBT are to target maladaptive cognitive and behavioral processes that maintain chronic pain, with the belief that a person's thoughts influence their behaviors and emotions. Specifically, negative thoughts about pain can induce avoidance of pleasant activities and facilitate overall deconditioning and emotional distress, such as anxiety and depression. Thus, with the assistance of a therapist, patients engage in exercises that downregulate negative cognitions and emotions and increase behavioral activation toward regularly enjoyed activities that are typically avoided due to pain. Structured relaxation, activity pacing, goal setting, assertive communication, pleasant activity scheduling, and cognitive restructuring are primary techniques used to increase adaptive pain coping, decrease stress, and attenuate exacerbation of pain flares. Educating the patient on their pain condition also plays a significant role in the treatment process (Thorne 2004).

In general, research supports the efficacy of CBT in the treatment of pain, with small-to-medium effect sizes reported in a number of outcomes (Hofmann et al. 2012), and improvements in functioning are often maintained over long-term follow-up beyond the effects of standard medical care (Turner et al. 2006). In the context of TMD, multiple studies have demonstrated positive effects of CBT on pain-related outcomes. Dworkin and colleagues tested whether a two-session CBT intervention added to usual care was more effective in reducing TMD symptoms than usual care alone (occlusal splint, pharmacotherapy, nutrition and parafunctional behavior modification, cold/heat packs). While groups were equivalent in their improvements in pain, pain interference, jaw opening, and affective functioning at the 3-month follow-up, patients in the CBT group reported greater declines in pain intensity and interference at 12 months (Dworkin et al. 1994). In a subsequent study by the same authors (Dworkin et al. 2002a), usual care was compared with a three-session self-care treatment (implementing cognitive behavioral techniques) tailored to the patient's level of psychosocial functioning. At the 12-month follow-up, the self-care group exhibited significant declines in pain, pain interference, and pain associated with muscle palpation, but there were no changes in range of motion. Although depression and somatization decreased more for the self-care group, these effects were only marginally significant. Dworkin and colleagues also compared the efficacy of a six-session CBT protocol with usual care. The CBT group exhibited significant decreases in pain intensity, pain interference, and ability to control pain at posttreatment, while there were no group differences in range of motion or palpation pain. In contrast to their earlier studies, groups were comparable in outcomes at the 12-month follow-up (Dworkin et al. 2002b).

In a series of RCTs by Turner and colleagues, this group used a daily diary approach to evaluate the efficacy of a brief (4-biweekly sessions) CBT treatment compared with standard self-management care. Overall, greater improvements in pain-related beliefs (perceived control, harm beliefs), catastrophizing, and coping (cognitive coping, relaxation use) were observed in the CBT group at posttreatment; however, there were no differences across CBT and self-management in pain, jaw use limitations, or daily activity interference (Turner et al. 2005b). In a subsequent analysis at 1 year, the CBT group exhibited greater improvement in pain-related beliefs, pain intensity, depression, jaw functioning, and activity interference (Turner et al. 2006). The authors found that baseline to 6-month changes in perceived pain control beliefs and self-efficacy mediated the effects of CBT on 1-year outcomes (Turner et al. 2007). Litt and colleagues found that compared to standard care alone, 6 weeks of standard care plus CBT produced significantly greater reductions in pain and catastrophizing at posttreatment, as well as greater increases in adaptive coping strategies, self-efficacy, and perceived control (Litt et al. 2009). The results for pain were largely maintained after 1 year; however, there were no group differences in depression or pain interference. The authors found that readiness to engage in therapy, somatization, and high self-efficacy moderated decreased pain over time, while somatization was a significant moderator of treatment on pain interference (Litt et al. 2010). While the overall findings of these studies are mixed, the results seem to suggest that CBT is most effective for pain and emotional functioning, relative to parafunctional habits. Further, long-term effects appear to be more robust than immediate posttreatment findings.

Habit Reversal Habit control has garnered some attention in the treatment of TMD, with the premise being to reduce muscle hyperactivity associated with maladaptive oral habits (e.g., clenching, bruxism, lip/fingernail biting) that facilitate pain. The technique was pioneered in the 1970s to treat a variety of disorders including tics, nervous habits, stuttering, and parafunctional behaviors believed to be associated with muscular tension (Woods and Miltenberger 1995; Azrin and Nunn 1973; Miltenberger et al. 1998). The main tenets of habit control are first to make the patient more aware of their involuntary oral habits and then provide them with an adaptive competing response that will extinguish the unwanted behavior. An example of this would be to induce deep breathing exercises or relaxation upon the commencement of the maladaptive behavior. Occasionally, positive self-statements, contingent rewards, and cognitive restructuring are implemented to reinforce training (Gramling et al. 1996; Townsen et al. 2001). When compared to no-treatment or a control group, some studies have found habit reversal to be effective for pain (Gramling et al. 1996; Townsen et al. 2001; Peterson et al. 1993; Glaros et al. 2007) and range of motion (Peterson et al. 1993); however, results have been mixed for oral habit frequency (Townsen et al. 2001; Gramling et al. 1996). There is also efficacy supporting habit reversal in the reduction of depression but not for other psychological outcomes such as anxiety, somatization, and psychological adjustment (Gramling et al. 1996). While some of these findings are encouraging, it has also been suggested that habit reversal reduces pain to the same magnitude as intraoral splint therapy (Glaros et al. 2007).

Combined Therapies Versus Usual Care or No Treatment Some studies have combined therapeutic modalities to enhance treatment outcomes and provide a more comprehensive approach to treating TMD. For instance, Brooke and colleagues offered eight sessions of BF/relaxation plus stress coping skills therapy (i.e., assertive training, rational emotive therapy, and stress inoculation) to 13 patients recalcitrant to conservative therapy (physiotherapy, medication, oral splint). After 8 weeks, all but one participant exhibited improvements in pain, jaw functioning (joint sounds, parafunctional movements), and pterygoid muscle tenderness assessed via intraoral palpation with the "index finger pushed upward behind the maxillary tuberosity" (Brooke et al. 1977). In a six-session combined BF/CBT format, Gatchel and colleagues found that when compared to non-intervention, the treatment group exhibited greater decrements in pain intensity and psychological distress, as well as improved adaptive coping skills after 1 year (Gatchel et al. 2006). Similarly, Ferrando and colleagues observed that hypnosis/CBT was superior to usual care in reducing pain frequency, medication use, pain intensity, somatization, and anxiety; these outcomes remained stable at the 9-month follow-up (Ferrando et al. 2012). In contrast to these findings, a later study found equivalent improvement in pain, parafunctional limitations, and psychological outcomes at the 8-week posttreatment period when comparing BF/CBT with occlusal splint therapy. However, pain coping skills were significantly improved for the combined group at the 6-month follow-up, and effect sizes for treatment-related changes tended to be larger in the combined group for all outcome variables (Shedden Mora et al. 2013). In a pilot study, the efficacy of a group-based relaxation program was evaluated in 24 patients with TMD (Vranceanu et al. 2013). After undergoing 4 weeks of medical treatment (i.e., pain education, pharmacotherapy, occlusal splint, jaw stretching), participants were enrolled in an 8-week relaxation group consisting of imagery, mindfulness, contemplation, yoga, single-pointed focus meditation, and CBT. Posttreatment gains were found in mental and physical health functioning, self-reported pain measures, range of motion, pressure pain thresholds, and palpation pain. However, no-treatment changes were observed in psychological symptoms or perceived stress.

Treatment Versus an Active Comparator Two studies investigated the benefit of combining psychological treatments. For instance, Stenn and colleagues examined whether BF added to a CBT/relaxation group was more effective in reducing TMD symptoms than a program only including relaxation and CBT. While the participants receiving BF reported lower pain after treatment, there were no discernible group differences in masseter muscle tension (Stenn et al. 1979). Subsequently, Olson and Malow reported that participants receiving combined psychotherapy and frontalis BF exhibited greater reductions in muscle tenderness when compared to frontalis or masseter BF alone; however, there were no group differences in pain (Olson and Malow 1987).

Other studies have evaluated the effectiveness of different psychological interventions compared to each other. For example, Moss and colleagues found that relaxation was generally superior to BF in improving jaw pain and muscle tension (Moss et al. 1983). Conversely, Funch and Gale observed no significant group effects for TMD pain across 12 weeks of BF and relaxation therapy at posttreatment or at the

2-year follow-up (Funch and Gale 1984). Stam and colleagues examined the efficacy of a hypnosis/coping skills group with PMR/coping skills and a no-treatment control group. When compared to the control group, patients in both intervention groups had lower pain and improvement in parafunctional behaviors; however, there were no group differences across the active treatments (Stam et al. 1984). In a series of RCTs, BF, CBT, and combined BF/CBT were compared with one another and with a no-treatment control at 12-week (Mishra et al. 2000) and 1-year follow-up (Gardea et al. 2001). Overall, pain decreased across all treatment groups; however, the BF group showed the greatest improvement at posttreatment. Interestingly, there were no short-term effects across the active treatment groups for mood disturbance (Mishra et al. 2000). At the 1-year evaluation, all treatment groups exhibited improvements in pain, disability, and mandibular functioning, yet the largest treatment gains were found in the combined group. In light of these findings, the authors postulated that biofeedback may provide immediate benefits due to its focus on physical pain, while the targeting of psychosocial-based outcomes in CBT takes longer to produce positive effects (Gardea et al. 2001). In a more recent study by Abrahamsen and colleagues, hypnosis was found to be superior to PMR in reducing pain and improving coping strategies, whereas masseter palpation pain was lower in the relaxation group. Both groups improved equally in oral functioning (i.e., jaw opening, chewing limitations), pain-related sleep disturbance, and psychological outcomes (i.e., somatization, OCD, anxiety) (Abrahamsen et al. 2009).

Other Therapeutic Approaches Among the multiple factors underlying TMD, it has been suggested that autonomic dysregulation is a significant contributor to pain and concomitant symptoms in chronic TMD. In an attempt to address this potential causative factor, Carlson and Bertrand developed and applied a biobehavioral intervention (i.e., physical self-regulation) to directly target and enhance self-regulatory processes associated with psychophysiological functioning (Carlson and Bertrand 1995). Treatment consists of multiple components, including pain education, monitoring of muscle functioning, training in proprioceptive awareness of head/neck posture, postural relaxation, diaphragmatic breathing, sleep hygiene, and lifestyle management of symptoms (i.e., physical activity, diet, fluid intake). In an RCT evaluating physical self-regulation (PSR) compared to occlusal splint therapy/self-care strategies, Carlson and colleagues administered PSR for two sessions over a period of 3 weeks, with assessments at 6 and 26 weeks posttreatment (Carlson et al. 2001). While improvements in pain severity, range of motion, and affective distress were comparable in both groups at posttreatment, the authors found that the PSR group showed greater pain reduction and mandibular opening at the follow-up period. The large effect size comparing PSR to dental treatment at the long-term follow-up ($d = .96$) was considered to be clinically meaningful (Sauer et al. 2010).

Although not yet addressed in TMD, encouraging evidence supports the efficacy of other psychosocial and behaviorally based interventions in the treatment of chronic pain. Examples of these treatments include in vivo graded exposure, mindfulness meditation, and resilience-based therapy. In the context of graded exposure, fear avoidance beliefs are suggested to be a perpetuating factor of pain chronicity and disability, as well as maintaining harm expectancies associated with pain and physical activity (Fritz et al. 2001; Leeuw et al. 2007). Thus, treatments targeting pain-related fear and avoidance are gaining momentum in their clinical utility. This approach generally involves the patient developing a hierarchy of least to most avoided physical activities, and through a series of graded exposure exercises, the patient gradually confronts each activity until reductions in fear occur (Vlaeyen et al. 2012). In the context of TMD, this might involve exposure to jaw movements or consumption of foods that evoke fear. Likewise, mindfulness meditation has emerged as a viable therapy in a number of health-related conditions including depression, anxiety, stress, cardiovascular disease, eating disorders, and pain (Song et al. 2014; Baer 2003; Parswani et al. 2013; Grossman et al. 2004). Derived from Buddhist principles, mindfulness involves increasing nonjudgmental awareness and sustained self-regulated attention on the immediate experience. Cultivating an openness to experience and focus on the here and now are fundamental principles in mindfulness, with techniques such as body scan, mindful breathing, and sitting meditation being common practices. With respect to pain, patients are encouraged to explore sensations of pain and distress while suspending a judgmental frame of mind on the experience. Through this process, mindfulness uncouples the sensory and affective dimensions of pain, thereby reducing pain-related suffering through cognitive reappraisal (Kabat-Zinn 1982). Essentially, the patient becomes a passive observer in the pain experience rather than succumbing to active resistance. Meta-analytic studies of mindfulness meditation in chronic pain have shown small-to-moderate effects on depression, anxiety, and perceived pain control; however, these effects may not be as robust for pain intensity (Song et al. 2014; Bawa et al. 2015).

In contrast to treatments taking on a pathology-approach to pain and targeting the reduction of deficits or negative symptoms, resilience-based treatments emphasize augmenting personal strengths and resilience factors to promote positive coping. As mentioned previously, resilience is the process of successful adaptation after adversity or severe stress (Norris 2010), and evidence supports this facet in the promotion of mental well-being, pain acceptance, and physical health (Sturgeon and Zautra 2010). While scant, there is a growing body of literature investigating the effects of brief, therapeutic approaches that foster resilience in pain and affective functioning (Berg et al. 2008; Hanssen et al. 2013; Howell et al. 2014). Therefore, the ability to sustain resilience through enhancement of positive affect may offer a new approach to tackling the complexities of TMD and its associated burden.

10.5 Summary of Findings from Studies of Psychological Interventions for TMD

There is general agreement in the scientific community that psychosocial and behavioral modalities are effective in the treatment of chronic pain; however, their use in TMD management is often not considered by medical/dental providers. Recent reviews and meta-analytic studies (Crider et al. 2005; Zhang et al. 2015; Roldan-Barraza et al. 2014; Aggarwal et al. 2011; Medlicott and Harris 2006; Randhawa et al. 2016) suggest that relaxation and BF may be more effective than placebo and intraoral splint therapy in reducing pain (Medlicott and Harris 2006). When comparing across CBT, habit control, and BF in comparison to usual care, a Cochrane review (Aggarwal et al. 2011) revealed that there is overall weak evidence for the support of psychosocial interventions for TMD treatment, namely, due to high bias and a relative dearth of studies that could be pooled. However, subgroup analysis of individual interventions revealed the greatest support for CBT in terms of long-term positive effects on depression, pain, and activity interference. In general, the consensus from these studies is that there needs to be more sophisticated research that includes a lower risk of bias, larger samples sizes, better control or comparison groups, and standardized methodology. As such, the overall low quality of some of the existing research limits the conclusions that can be drawn regarding efficacy and prompts the need for more well-designed randomized clinical trials that draw on the results of promising behaviorally based interventions.

10.6 Interpreting Findings Regarding Psychological Interventions for TMD

The above summary of the literature regarding psychological contributions to TMD clearly indicates that psychological factors are associated with risk of TMD development and persistence. Moreover, among individuals with chronic TMD, increased psychological symptomatology is associated with greater clinical pain and pain-related interference. These findings have provided the rationale for testing the effectiveness of psychological interventions in persons with TMD. As reviewed above, compared to no treatment or to an active control condition (e.g., education), most forms of psychological intervention produce greater reductions in pain and psychological symptoms among TMD patients. However, on average, the effects of these psychological interventions appear somewhat underwhelming, as these treatments produce modest effects on clinical pain and, not surprisingly, somewhat greater effects on psychological outcomes. Given the robust associations between psychological functioning and TMD symptoms, one might expect psychological therapies to produce more impressive effects. Indeed, many providers would report much greater effects of psychological interventions based on their clinical experience. In order to address this paradox, below we discuss several methodological and conceptual issues that are important to consider when interpreting the existing findings regarding the effectiveness of psychological interventions in individuals with TMD.

Clinical Trial Design Several aspects of clinical trial design could significantly influence findings regarding the effectiveness of psychological treatments (see Table 10.4). As is true in all clinical trials, issues such as sample size, inclusion/exclusion criteria, treatment fidelity, blinding, control conditions, and data analytic approach could affect the magnitude of the observed effects. Indeed, Fricton and colleagues (Fricton et al. 2010) recently examined the quality of clinical trials for six types of treatments for TMD, including psychological therapies, and concluded "much of the evidence base for TMJD treatments may be susceptible to systematic bias and most past studies should be interpreted with caution" (p. 139). In particular, RCTs of TMD frequently fell short on issues related to sample size determination, statistical methods, and randomization methods. Thus, overall low design quality could reduce the ability of RCTs for TMD to validly identify treatment effects. Notably, the authors did observe that over time the quality of RCTs for TMD is improving. However, there are several issues more specific to TMD that could also contribute to reduced effect sizes in clinical trials.

TMD Natural History In contrast to conditions like cancer or autoimmune disorders, TMD is typically not a progressive condition destined to increase in severity without successful treatment. In fact, TMD in many cases is self-limiting. In a previous longitudinal study, Ohrbach and Dworkin (Ohrbach and Dworkin 1998) observed that nearly three quarters of people with chronic TMD showed at least some improvement over a

Table 10.4 Important considerations in interpreting clinical trials of psychological treatments for TMD

Design issue	Comments
General clinical trial design issues (e.g., sample size, control condition, randomization, statistical analyses)	Many TMD trials show high risk of bias, particularly regarding sample size determination, statistical methods, and randomization methods (Fricton ref)
Natural history of TMD	TMD is not a progressive condition. Rather, symptoms fluctuate considerably, and many patients show considerable improvement over time regardless of treatment (Ohrbach ref)
Inclusion/exclusion criteria	Classification of TMD varies considerably across studies. Also, patients with comorbid pain conditions and significant psychological symptoms are often excluded
Different interventions target different TMD symptoms	Interventions such as hypnosis, biofeedback, and relaxation target pain more directly, while other treatments, such as CBT and mindfulness, primarily target psychological processes
Standardized versus tailored treatments	Treatments in clinical trials tend to be standardized across patients, while clinical practice typically modifies treatments based on patients' needs and responses to therapy

5-year period, with nearly half showing complete resolution of pain. In addition, TMD pain is often episodic and characterized by epochs of more severe pain interspersed with periods of low or no pain (Van Grootel et al. 2005). Because of this episodic and sometimes remitting nature of TMD, patients enrolled in both the control and active treatment conditions may show significant reduction in symptoms over the treatment period, obfuscating any potential treatment effect. Indeed, patients are more likely to seek treatment during times of increased symptoms, increasing the probability of reduced pain at future time points due to regression to the mean (Whitney and Von Korff 1992). Similarly, enrollment in a clinical trial may be more likely during times of increased symptom severity, in which case regression to the mean would predict that many patients could show reduction in symptoms over the course of the trial independent of any treatment effect.

Inclusion/Exclusion Criteria There is considerable variability in the TMD case classification that is used for inclusion into clinical trials. Many TMD clinical trials include patients who meet well-validated diagnostic criteria based on the Research Diagnostic Criteria (RDC) for TMD or its more recent evolution, the Diagnostic Criteria for TMD (DC/TMD) (Schiffman et al. 2014). However, other trials fail to apply specific diagnostic criteria, which lead to differences in the patient populations across studies. In addition, many (but not all) trials apply a pain severity (e.g., average pain >40/100 over the past week) criterion to avoid floor effects, potentially increasing the likelihood of regression to the mean, as noted above. Regarding exclusion criteria, trials often exclude patients with certain comorbidities, including other pain conditions (e.g., fibromyalgia) and psychiatric disorders. In addition, individuals taking certain classes of medications such as opioids and antidepressants are often excluded. While helpful for reducing heterogeneity, these exclusions can have the unintended consequence of excluding patients who stand to benefit most from psychological interventions, those with comorbid pain conditions and significant psychological symptomatology. Indeed, these are the very patients who are most likely to receive psychological treatments in standard clinical practice. Thus, the inclusion/exclusion criteria applied in many clinical trials can render the findings less generalizable to typical clinical practice.

Targets of Psychological Treatments As reviewed above, there are multiple psychological interventions for TMD, and different treatments target different domains of TMD-related symptomatology, thus, these treatments may impact TMD symptoms in substantially different ways. Some therapies are designed to directly target TMD pain, such as hypnosis and its analgesic suggestions. In contrast, relaxation and biofeedback therapies indirectly target pain based on the assumption that excessive masticatory muscle activity contributes to TMD pain; therefore, reductions in muscle activity will reduce pain. Relaxation-based therapies may also confer more general benefits that enhance physical and psychological well-being, which could also favorably impact pain. This may help explain why previous systematic reviews have found some evidence supporting the pain-relieving effects of hypnosis and relaxation. However, other psychological therapies primarily target psychological function, which may produce trickle down effects that improve pain. For example, cognitive behavioral interventions focus on altering maladaptive thoughts and behaviors, which may lead to enhanced emotional functioning and positive behavioral changes that subsequently reduce pain severity. This more indirect path to pain reduction helps explain why CBT often produces greater effects on psychological functioning than on pain severity. Similarly, mindfulness-based interventions emphasize nonjudgmental awareness of the pain experience, which is intended to reduce the counterproductive urgency to achieve relief that often accompanies pain and leads to increased stress and frustration. Unfortunately, RCTs of mindfulness for TMD are generally lacking. Understanding the differing targets of psychological interventions is important in interpreting their effects. Indeed, treatments are likely to show greater effects on the aspects of TMD symptomatology that they directly target, which may help explain why the pain-reducing effects of some treatments are less impressive than their effects on psychological outcomes.

Need to Test Tailored Treatments RCTs of psychological interventions for TMD typically deliver highly standardized therapies and strive to ensure that all patients in a given condition are treated similarly. Moreover, the dosing and duration of treatments in clinical trials are likewise predefined and standardized across patients. In contrast, psychological treatments delivered in the course of clinical practice tend to change over time and are ideally tailored to the needs of the patient. That is, if a patient is not responding well to a given therapy, a provider is likely to alter the treatment by increasing the dose, adding another treatment or switching to an altogether new therapy. Historically, this has not been typical in RCTs of psychological interventions. However, interest in tailoring psychological treatments to patient characteristics is increasing, and a recent systematic review provides some support for this approach (Kotiranta et al. 2014). Moreover, there is increasing use of adaptive clinical trial designs, which allow modifications to the trial to increase its efficiency and flexibility (Chow 2014). While these approaches do not generally involve tailoring interventions on a per patient basis, some adaptive designs do allow patient selection and treatment switching, which can approximate personalized treatment approaches. Thus, in the future, more clinical trials could be designed to test the effectiveness of psychological therapies that are targeted to patients based on their specific characteristics and needs.

Taken together, these conceptual and methodological issues illustrate the challenges associated with developing an evidence base that accurately reflects the effectiveness of psychological interventions for TMD pain. Future research should use more sophisticated methodologies to determine the effectiveness of both existing and developing psychological treatments for TMD and to inform optimal tailoring of these treatments based on patient characteristics. Furthermore, efforts should be made to extend through large-scale replication trials the promising and clinically significant outcomes for psychological- and behavioral-based interventions already present in the literature.

10.7 Summary

The findings discussed throughout this chapter clearly demonstrate the robust influence that psychological processes have in TMD. Psychological factors not only influence the severity of TMD symptoms, but they also represent premorbid risk factors for future development of TMD. Importantly, psychological resilience factors can improve psychological and physical functioning in people with TMD and may protect against development of chronic TMD symptoms. Thus, TMD is best conceptualized within the framework of the biopsychosocial model, which should also guide treatment selection. Indeed, numerous psychological and behavioral interventions have demonstrated at least some benefit for patients with TMD; therefore, a multimodal approach to treatment that is tailored to the patient's specific biopsychosocial profile is optimal. Future research is needed to better identify the psychological interventions that are most effective for TMD and to elucidate the mechanisms whereby these interventions produce their benefits.

References

Aaron LA, Turner JA, Mancl LA, Sawchuk CN, Huggins KH, Truelove EL. Daily pain coping among patients with chronic temporomandibular disorder pain: an electronic diary study. J Orofac Pain. 2006;20:125–37.

Abrahamsen R, Zachariae R, Svensson P. Effect of hypnosis on oral function and psychological factors in temporomandibular disorders patients. J Oral Rehabil. 2009;36:556–70.

Aggarwal VR, Lovell K, Peters S, Javidi H, Joughin A, Goldthorpe J. Psychosocial interventions for the management of chronic orofacial pain. Cochrane Database Syst Rev. 2011;11:Cd008456.

Aggarwal VR, Macfarlane GJ, Farragher TM, Mcbeth J. Risk factors for onset of chronic oro-facial pain--results of the North Cheshire oro-facial pain prospective population study. Pain. 2010a;149:354–9.

Aggarwal VR, Macfarlane GJ, Farragher TM, Mcbeth J. Risk factors for onset of chronic oro-facial pain--results of the North Cheshire oro-facial pain prospective population study. Pain. 2010b;149:354–9.

American Psychiatric Association. Diagnostic and statistical manual of mental disorders. American Psychiatric Association: Washington, DC; 2013.

Azrin NH, Nunn RG. Habit-reversal: a method of eliminating nervous habits and tics. Behav res Ther. 1973;11:619–28.

Baer RA. Mindfulness training as a clinical intervention: a conceptual and empirical review. Clin Psychol Sci Pract. 2003;10:125–43.

Bawa FL, Mercer SW, Atherton RJ, Clague F, Keen A, Scott NW, Bond CM. Does mindfulness improve outcomes in patients with chronic pain? Systematic review and meta-analysis. Br J Gen Pract. 2015;65:E387–400.

Beaton RD, Egan KJ, Nakagawa-Kogan H, Morrison KN. Self-reported symptoms of stress with temporomandibular disorders: comparisons to healthy men and women. J Prosthet Dent. 1991;65:289–93.

Berg CJ, Snyder CR, Hamilton N. The effectiveness of a hope intervention in coping with cold pressor pain. J Health Psychol. 2008;13:804–9.

Bertoli E, De Leeuw R, Schmidt JE, Okeson JP, Carlson CR. Prevalence and impact of post-traumatic stress disorder symptoms in patients with masticatory muscle or temporomandibular joint pain: differences and similarities. J Orofac Pain. 2007;21:107–19.

Boettger MK, Grossmann D, Bar KJ. Thresholds and perception of cold pain, heat pain, and the thermal grill illusion in patients with major depressive disorder. Psychosom Med. 2013;75:281–7.

Brister H, Turner JA, Aaron LA, Mancl L. Self-efficacy is associated with pain, functioning, and coping in patients with chronic temporomandibular disorder pain. J Orofac Pain. 2006;20:115–24.

Brooke RI, Stenn PG, Mothersill KJ. The diagnosis and conservative treatment of myofascial pain dysfunction syndrome. Oral Surg Oral med Oral Pathol. 1977;44:844–52.

Carlson CR, Bertrand P. Self-regulation training manual. University Press: Lexington, KY; 1995.

Carlson CR, Bertrand PM, Ehrlich AD, Maxwell AW, Burton RG. Physical self-regulation training for the management of temporomandibular disorders. J Orofac Pain. 2001;15:47–55.

Carlson CR, Okeson JP, Falace DA, Nitz AJ, Curran SL, Anderson D. Comparison of Psychologic and physiologic functioning between patients with masticatory muscle pain and matched controls. J Orofac Pain. 1993;7:15–22.

Carlson CR, Reid KI, Curran SL, Studts J, Okeson JP, Falace D, Nitz A, Bertrand PM. Psychological and physiological parameters of masticatory muscle pain. Pain. 1998;76:297–307.

Carlsson SG, Gale EN. Biofeedback in the treatment of long-term temporomandibular joint pain an outcome study. Biofeedback Self Regul. 1977;2:161–71.

Chen CY, Palla S, Erni S, Sieber M, Gallo LM. Nonfunctional tooth contact in healthy controls and patients with myogenous facial pain. J Orofac Pain. 2007;21:185–93.

Chen H, Nackley A, Miller V, Diatchenko L, Maixner W. Multisystem dysregulation in painful temporomandibular disorders. J Pain. 2013;14:983–96.

Chow SC. Adaptive clinical trial design. Annu Rev Med. 2014;65:405–15.

Conrad R, Schilling G, Bausch C, Nadstawek J, Wartenberg HC, Wegener I, Geiser F, Imbierowicz K, Liedtke R. Temperament and character personality profiles and personality disorders in chronic pain patients. Pain. 2007;133:197–209.

Costello NL, Bragdon EE, Light KC, Sigurdsson A, Bunting S, Grewen K, Maixner W. Temporomandibular disorder and optimism: relationships to ischemic pain sensitivity and interleukin-6. Pain. 2002;100:99–110.

Craig AD, Bushnell MC. The thermal grill illusion: unmasking the burn of cold pain. Science. 1994;265:252–5.

Crider A, Glaros AG, Gevirtz RN. Efficacy of biofeedback-based treatments for temporomandibular disorders. Appl Psychophysiol Biofeedback. 2005;30:333–45.

Dahlstrom L, Carlsson GE, Carlsson SG. Comparison of effects of electromyographic biofeedback and occlusal splint therapy on mandibular dysfunction. Scand J Dent Res. 1982;90:151–6.

Dahlstrom L, Carlsson SG, Gale EN, Jansson TG. Stress-induced muscular activity in mandibular dysfunction: effects of biofeedback training. J Behav Med. 1985;8:191–200.

De Leeuw R, Bertoli E, Schmidt JE, Carlson CR. Prevalence of post-traumatic stress disorder symptoms in orofacial pain patients. Oral Surg Oral Med Oral Pathol Oral Radiol Endod. 2005a;99:558–68.

De Leeuw R, Schmidt JE, Carlson CR. Traumatic stressors and post-traumatic stress disorder symptoms in headache patients. Headache. 2005b;45:1365–74.

Derogatis LR. Symptom Checklist-90-R. Minneapolis, MN: National Computer Symptoms; 1994.

Dworkin SF. The Oppera study: act one. J Pain. 2011; 12:T1–3.

Dworkin SF, Huggins KH, Wilson L, Mancl L, Turner J, Massoth D, Leresche L, Truelove E. A randomized clinical trial using research diagnostic criteria for temporomandibular disorders-axis II to target clinic cases for a tailored self-care TMD treatment program. J Orofac Pain. 2002a;16:48–63.

Dworkin SF, Leresche L. Research diagnostic criteria for temporomandibular disorders: review, criteria, examinations and specifications, critique. J Craniomandib Disord. 1992;6:301–55.

Dworkin SF, Turner JA, Mancl L, Wilson L, Massoth D, Huggins KH, Leresche L, Truelove E. A randomized clinical trial of a tailored comprehensive care treatment program for temporomandibular disorders. J Orofac Pain. 2002b;16:259–76.

Dworkin SF, Turner JA, Wilson L, Massoth D, Whitney C, Huggins KH, Burgess J, Sommers E, Truelove

E. Brief group cognitive-behavioral intervention for temporomandibular disorders. Pain. 1994;59:175–87.

Ehde DM, Dillworth TM, Turner JA. Cognitive-behavioral therapy for individuals with chronic pain: efficacy, innovations, and directions for research. Am Psychol. 2014;69:153–66.

Eisenlohr-Moul TA, Crofford LJ, Howard TW, Yepes JF, Carlson CR, De Leeuw R. Parasympathetic reactivity in fibromyalgia and temporomandibular disorder: associations with sleep problems, symptom severity, and functional impairment. J Pain. 2015;16:247–57.

Elkins G, Jensen MP, Patterson DR. Hypnotherapy for the management of chronic pain. Int J Clin Exp Hypn. 2007;55:275–87.

Engel GL. The need for a new medical model: a challenge for biomedicine. Science. 1977;196:129–36.

Erlandson, P. M., Jr. & Poppen, R. 1989. Electromyographic biofeedback and rest position training of masticatory muscles in myofascial pain-dysfunction patients. J Prosthet Dent, 62, 335–338.

Ferrando M, Andreu Y, Galdon MJ, Dura E, Poveda R, Bagan JV. Psychological variables and temporomandibular disorders: distress, coping, and personality. Oral SurgOral MedOral PatholOral RadiolEndod. 2004;98:153–60.

Ferrando M, Galdon MJ, Dura E, Andreu Y, Jimenez Y, Poveda R. Enhancing the efficacy of treatment for temporomandibular patients with muscular diagnosis through cognitive-behavioral intervention, including hypnosis: a randomized study. Oral Surg Oral med Oral Pathol Oral Radiol. 2012;113:81–9.

Fillingim RB, Maixner W, Kincaid S, Sigurdsson A, Harris MB. Pain sensitivity in patients with temporomandibular disorders: relationship to clinical and psychosocial factors. Clin J Pain. 1996;12:260–9.

Fillingim RB, Ohrbach R, Greenspan JD, Knott C, Diatchenko L, Dubner R, Bair E, Baraian C, Mack N, Slade GD, Maixner W. Psychological factors associated with development of TMD: the Oppera prospective cohort study. J Pain. 2013;14:T75–90.

Fillingim RB, Ohrbach R, Greenspan JD, Knott C, Dubner R, Bair E, Baraian C, Slade GD, Maixner W. Potential psychosocial risk factors for chronic TMD: descriptive data and empirically identified domains from the Oppera case-control study. J Pain. 2011a;12:T46–60.

Fillingim RB, Ohrbach R, Greenspan JD, Knott C, Dubner R, Bair E, Baraian C, Slade GD, Maixner W. Potential psychosocial risk factors for chronic TMD: descriptive data and empirically identified domains from the Oppera case-control study. J Pain. 2011b;12:T46–60.

Fillingim RB, Slade GD, Diatchenko L, Dubner R, Greenspan JD, Knott C, Ohrbach R, Maixner W. Summary of findings from the Oppera baseline case-control study: implications and future directions. J Pain. 2011c;12:T102–7.

Fricton JR, Ouyang W, Nixdorf DR, Schiffman EL, Velly AM, Look JO. Critical appraisal of methods used in randomized controlled trials of treatments for temporomandibular disorders. J Orofac Pain. 2010;24:139–51.

Fritz JM, George SZ, Delitto A. The role of fear-avoidance beliefs in acute low back pain: relationships with current and future disability and work status. Pain. 2001;94:7–15.

Funch DP, Gale EN. Biofeedback and relaxation therapy for chronic temporomandibular joint pain: predicting successful outcomes. J Consult Clin Psychol. 1984;52:928–35.

Gameiro GH, Da Silva Andrade A, Nouer DF, Ferraz De Arruda Veiga MC. How may stressful experiences contribute to the development of temporomandibular disorders? Clin Oral Investig. 2006;10:261–8.

Gardea MA, Gatchel RJ, Mishra KD. Long-term efficacy of biobehavioral treatment of temporomandibular disorders. J Behav med. 2001;24:341–59.

Garofalo JP, Gatchel RJ, Wesley AL, Ellis E. Predicting chronicity in acute temporomandibular joint disorders using the research diagnostic criteria. J Am Dent Assoc. 1998;129:438–47.

Gatchel, R. J., Stowell, A. W., Wildenstein, L., Riggs, R. & Ellis, E., 3rd 2006. Efficacy of an early intervention for patients with acute temporomandibular disorder-related pain: a one-year outcome study. J Am Dent Assoc, 137, 339–347.

Gavish A, Halachmi M, Winocur E, Gazit E. Oral habits and their association with signs and symptoms of temporomandibular disorders in adolescent girls. J Oral Rehabil. 2000;27:22–32.

Gerrits MM, Van Marwijk HW, Van Oppen P, Van Der Horst H, Penninx BW. Longitudinal association between pain, and depression and anxiety over four years. J Psychosom res. 2015;78:64–70.

Gessel AH, Alderman MM. Management of myofascial pain dysfunction syndrome of the temporomandibular joint by tension control training. Psychosomatics. 1971;12:302–9.

Giannakopoulos NN, Keller L, Rammelsberg P, Kronmuller KT, Schmitter M. Anxiety and depression in patients with chronic temporomandibular pain and in controls. J Dent. 2010;38:369–76.

Glaros AG. Awareness of physiological responding under stress and nonstress conditions in temporomandibular disorders. Biofeedback Self Regul. 1996;21:261–72.

Glaros AG, Baharloo L, Glass EG. Effect of parafunctional clenching and estrogen on temporomandibular disorder pain. Cranio. 1998;16:78–83.

Glaros AG, Burton E. Parafunctional clenching, pain, and effort in temporomandibular disorders. J Behav med. 2004;27:91–100.

Glaros AG, Kim-Weroha N, Lausten L, Franklin KL. Comparison of habit reversal and a behaviorally-modified dental treatment for temporomandibular disorders: a pilot investigation. Appl Psychophysiol Biofeedback. 2007;32:149–54.

Glaros AG, Williams K, Lausten L. The role of parafunctions, emotions and stress in predicting facial pain. J Am Dent Assoc. 2005a;136:451–8.

Glaros AG, Williams K, Lausten L, Friesen LR. Tooth contact in patients with temporomandibular disorders. Cranio. 2005b;23:188–93.

Gramling SE, Neblett J, Grayson R, Townsend D. temporomandibular disorder: efficacy of an oral habit reversal treatment program. J Behav Ther Exp Psychiatry. 1996;27:245–55.

Grossman P, Niemann L, Schmidt S, Walach H. Mindfulness-based stress reduction and health benefits: a meta-analysis. J Psychosom res. 2004;57:35–43.

Hanssen MM, Peters ML, Vlaeyen JW, Meevissen YM, Vancleef LM. Optimism lowers pain: evidence of the causal status and underlying mechanisms. Pain. 2013;154:53–8.

Hardt J, Gerbershagen HU, Franke P. The symptom check-list, SCL-90-R: its use and characteristics in chronic pain patients. Eur J Pain. 2000;4:137–48.

Hijzen TH, Slangen JL, Van Houweligen HC. Subjective, clinical and EMG effects of biofeedback and splint treatment. J Oral Rehabil. 1986;13:529–39.

Hilgard ER. A neodissociation interpretation of pain reduction in hypnosis. Psychol Rev. 1973;80:396–411.

Hofmann SG, Asnaani A, Vonk IJ, Sawyer AT, Fang A. The efficacy of cognitive behavioral therapy: a review of meta-analyses. Cognit Ther Res. 2012;36:427–40.

Howell AJ, Jacobson RM, Larsen DJ. 2014. Enhanced psychological health among chronic pain clients engaged in hope-focused group counseling. Couns Psychol

Jacobson E. Progressive relaxation. Chicago, IL: University Of Chicago Press; 1938.

Kabat-Zinn J. An outpatient program in behavioral medicine for chronic pain patients based on the practice of mindfulness meditation: theoretical considerations and preliminary results. Gen Hosp Psychiatry. 1982;4:33–47.

Keefe FJ, Dolan E. Pain behavior and pain coping strategies in low back pain and myofascial pain dysfunction syndrome patients. Pain. 1986;24:49–56.

Kessler RC, Birnbaum H, Demler O, Falloon IRH, Gagnon E, Guyer M, Howes MJ, Kendler KS, Shi L, Walters E, Wu EQ. The prevalence and correlates of non-affective psychosis in the National Comorbidity Survey Replication (NCS-R). Biol Psychiatry. 2005;58:668–76.

Kindler S, Samietz S, Houshmand M, Grabe HJ, Bernhardt O, Biffar R, Kocher T, Meyer G, Volzke H, Metelmann HR, Schwahn C. Depressive and anxiety symptoms as risk factors for temporomandibular joint pain: a prospective cohort study in the general population. J Pain. 2012;13:1188–97.

Klauenberg S, Maier C, Assion HJ, Hoffmann A, Krumova EK, Magerl W, Scherens A, Treede RD, Juckel G. Depression and changed pain perception: hints for a central disinhibition mechanism. Pain. 2008;140:332–43.

Kotiranta U, Suvinen T, Forssell H. Tailored treatments in temporomandibular disorders: where are we now? A systematic qualitative literature review. J Oral Facial Pain Headache. 2014;28:28–37.

Leeuw M, Goossens ME, Linton SJ, Crombez G, Boersma K, Vlaeyen JW. The fear-avoidance model of musculoskeletal pain: current state of scientific evidence. J Behav Med. 2007;30:77–94.

Leresche L. Epidemiology of temporomandibular disorders: implications for the investigation of etiologic factors. Crit Rev Oral Biol Med. 1997;8:291–305.

Liao CH, Chang CS, Chang SN, Lane HY, Lyu SY, Morisky DE, Sung FC. The risk of temporomandibular disorder in patients with depression: a population-based cohort study. Community Dent Oral Epidemiol. 2011;39:525–31.

List T, Axelsson S. Management of TMD: evidence from systematic reviews and meta-analyses. J Oral Rehabil. 2010;37:430–51.

Litt MD, Shafer D, Napolitano C. Momentary mood and coping processes in TMD pain. Health Psychol. 2004;23:354–62.

Litt MD, Shafer DM, Ibanez CR, Kreutzer DL, Tawfik-Yonkers Z. Momentary pain and coping in temporomandibular disorder pain: exploring mechanisms of cognitive behavioral treatment for chronic pain. Pain. 2009;145:160–8.

Litt MD, Shafer DM, Kreutzer DL. Brief cognitive-behavioral treatment for TMD pain: long-term outcomes and moderators of treatment. Pain. 2010;151:110–6.

Manfredini D, Winocur E, Ahlberg J, Guarda-Nardini L, Lobbezoo F. Psychosocial impairment in temporomandibular disorders patients. RDC/ TMD Axis II findings from a multicentre study. J Dent. 2010;38:765–72.

Markiewicz MR, Ohrbach R, Mccall WD. Oral behaviors checklist: reliability of performance in targeted waking-state behaviors. J Orofac Pain. 2006;20:306–16.

Mcgregor NR, Butt HL, Zerbes M, Klineberg IJ, Dunstan RH, Roberts TK. Assessment of pain (distribution and onset), symptoms, SCL-90-R inventory responses, and the association with infectious events in patients with chronic orofacial pain. J Orofac Pain. 1996;10:339–50.

Mckinney MW, Londeen TF, Turner SP, Levitt SR. Chronic TM disorder and non-TM disorder pain: a comparison of behavioral and psychological characteristics. Cranio. 1990;8:40–6.

Medlicott MS, Harris SR. A systematic review of the effectiveness of exercise, manual therapy, electrotherapy, relaxation training, and biofeedback in the management of temporomandibular disorder. Phys Ther. 2006;86:955–73.

Miltenberger RG, Fuqua RW, Woods DW. Applying behavior analysis to clinical problems: review and analysis of habit reversal. J Appl Behav Anal. 1998;31:447–69.

Mishra KD, Gatchel RJ, Gardea MA. The relative efficacy of three cognitive-behavioral treatment approaches to temporomandibular disorders. J Behav Med. 2000;23:293–309.

Molin C, Schalling D, Edman G. Psychological studies of patients with mandibular pain dysfunction syndrome. 1. Personality traits in patients and controls. Sven Tandlak Tidskr. 1973;66:1–13.

Moss RA, Wedding D, Sanders SH. The comparative efficacy of relaxation training and masseter EMG feedback in the treatment of TMJ dysfunction. J Oral Rehabil. 1983;10:9–17.

Norris FH. Behavioral science perspective on resilience. The Community and Regional Resilience Institute (CARRI). Oak Ridge Natl Lab. 2010;10:3–10.

Ohrbach R, Bair E, Fillingim RB, Gonzalez Y, Gordon SM, Lim PF, Ribeiro-Dasilva M, Diatchenko L, Dubner R, Greenspan JD, Knott C, Maixner W, Smith SB, Slade GD. Clinical orofacial characteristics associated with risk of first-onset TMD: the OPPERA prospective cohort study. J Pain. 2013;14:T33–50.

Ohrbach R, Dworkin SF. Five-year outcomes in TMD: relationship of changes in pain to changes in physical and psychological variables. Pain. 1998;74:315–26.

Okeson JP. Psychologic factors and oral and facial pain. Bell's oral and facial pain 7th ed. Quintessence Publishing, Hanover Park, IL. 2014; pp. 503–523.

Okeson JP, Moody PM, Kemper JT, Haley JV. Evaluation of Occlusal splint therapy and relaxation procedures in patients with temporomandibular disorders. J Am Dent Assoc. 1983;107:420–4.

Olson RE, Malow RM. Effects of biofeedback and psychotherapy on patients with myofascial pain dysfunction who are nonresponsive to conventional treatments. Rehabil Psychol. 1987;32:195–204.

Pankhurst CL. Controversies in the aetiology of temporomandibular disorders. Part 1. Temporomandibular disorders: all in the mind? Prim Dent Care. 1997;4:25–30.

Parswani MJ, Sharma MP, Iyengar SS. Mindfulness-based stress reduction program in coronary heart disease: A randomized control trial. Int J Yoga. 2013;6:111–7.

Peterson AL, Dixon DC, Talcott GW, Kelleher WJ. Habit reversal treatment of temporomandibular disorders: a pilot investigation. J Behav Ther Exp Psychiatry. 1993;24:49–55.

Randhawa K, Bohay R, Cote P, Van Der Velde G, Sutton D, Wong JJ, Yu H, Southerst D, Varatharajan S, Mior S, Stupar M, Shearer HM, Jacobs C, Taylor-Vaisey A. The effectiveness of noninvasive interventions for temporomandibular disorders: a systematic review by the ontario protocol for traffic injury management (OPTIMa) collaboration. Clin J Pain. 2016;32:260–78.

Reiter S, Emodi-Perlman A, Goldsmith C, Friedman-Rubin P, Winocur E. Comorbidity between depression and anxiety in patients with temporomandibular disorders according to the research diagnostic criteria for temporomandibular disorders. J Oral Facial Pain Headache. 2015;29:135–43.

Richardson EJ, Ness TJ, Doleys DM, Banos JH, Cianfrini L, Richards JS. Depressive symptoms and pain evaluations among persons with chronic pain: catastrophizing, but not pain acceptance, shows significant effects. Pain. 2009;147:147–52.

Roldan-Barraza C, Janko S, Villanueva J, Araya I, Lauer HC. A systematic review and meta-analysis of usual treatment versus psychosocial interventions in the treatment of myofascial temporomandibular disorder pain. J Oral Facial Pain Headache. 2014;28:205–22.

Roth RS, Geisser ME, Theisen-Goodvich M, Dixon PJ. Cognitive complaints are associated with depression, fatigue, female sex, and pain catastrophizing in patients with chronic pain. Arch Phys med Rehabil. 2005;86:1147–54.

Rudy TE, Turk DC, Kubinski JA, Zaki HS. Differential treatment responses of TMD patients as a function of psychological characteristics. Pain. 1995;61:103–12.

Sato M, Iizuka T, Watanabe A, Iwase N, Otsuka H, Terada N, Fujisawa M. Electromyogram biofeedback training for daytime clenching and its effect on sleep bruxism. J Oral Rehabil. 2015;42:83–9.

Sauer SE, Burris JL, Carlson CR. New directions in the management of chronic pain: self-regulation theory as a model for integrative clinical psychology practice. Clin Psychol rev. 2010;30:805–14.

Schiffman E, Ohrbach R, Truelove E, Look J, Anderson G, Goulet JP, List T, Svensson P, Gonzalez Y, Lobbezoo F, Michelotti A, Brooks SL, Ceusters W, Drangsholt M, Ettlin D, Gaul C, Goldberg LJ, Haythornthwaite JA, Hollender L, Jensen R, John MT, De Laat A, De Leeuw R, Maixner W, Van Der Meulen M, Murray GM, Nixdorf DR, Palla S, Petersson A, Pionchon P, Smith B, Visscher CM, Zakrzewska J, Dworkin SF. Diagnostic criteria for temporomandibular disorders (DC/TMD) for clinical and research applications: recommendations of the international RDC/TMD consortium network* and orofacial pain special interest groupdagger. J Oral Facial Pain Headache. 2014;28:6–27.

Schmidt JE, Carlson CR. A controlled comparison of emotional reactivity and physiological response in masticatory muscle pain patients. J Orofac Pain. 2009;23:230–42.

Shedden Mora MC, Weber D, Neff A, Rief W. Biofeedback-based cognitive-behavioral treatment compared with occlusal splint for temporomandibular disorder: a randomized controlled trial. Clin J Pain. 2013;29:1057–65.

Sherman JJ, Carlson CR, Wilson JF, Okeson JP, Mccubbin JA. Post-traumatic stress disorder among patients with orofacial pain. J Orofac Pain. 2005;19:309–17.

Simon EP, Lewis DM. Medical hypnosis for temporomandibular disorders: treatment efficacy and medical utilization outcome. Oral Surg Oral Med Oral Pathol Oral Radiol Endod. 2000;90:54–63.

Slade GD, Diatchenko L, Bhalang K, Sigurdsson A, Fillingim RB, Belfer I, Max MB, Goldman D, Maixner W. Influence of psychological factors on risk of temporomandibular disorders. J Dent res. 2007;86:1120–5.

Song Y, Lu H, Chen H, Geng G, Wang J. Mindfulness intervention in the management of chronic pain and psychological comorbidity: a meta-analysis. Int J Nurs Sci. 2014;1:215–23.

Spielberger CD, Gorusch RL, Lushene R, Vagg PR, Jacobs GA. Manual for the state-trait anxiety inventory (Form Y1). Palo Alto, CA: Consulting Psychologists Press; 1983.

Stam HJ, Mcgrath PA, Brooke RI. The effects of a cognitive-behavioral treatment program on temporo-mandibular pain and dysfunction syndrome. Psychosom med. 1984;46:534–45.

Stenn PG, Mothersill KJ, Brooke RI. Biofeedback and a cognitive behavioral approach to treatment of myofascial pain dysfunction syndrome. Behav Ther. 1979;10:29–36.

Strigo IA, Simmons AN, Matthews SC, Craig AD, Paulus MP. Increased affective bias revealed using experimental graded heat stimuli in young depressed adults: evidence of "emotional allodynia". Psychosom Med. 2008;70:338–44.

Sturgeon JA, Zautra AJ. Resilience: a new paradigm for adaptation to chronic pain. Curr Pain Headache Rep. 2010;14:105–12.

Sturgeon JA, Zautra AJ. Psychological resilience, pain catastrophizing, and positive emotions: perspectives on comprehensive modeling of individual pain adaptation. Curr Pain Headache Rep. 2013;17:317.

Sullivan MJ, Thorn B, Haythornthwaite JA, Keefe F, Martin M, Bradley LA, Lefebvre JC. Theoretical perspectives on the relation between catastrophizing and pain. Clin J Pain. 2001;17:52–64.

Suvinen TI, Reade PC, Kemppainen P, Kononen M, Dworkin SF. Review of aetiological concepts of temporomandibular pain disorders: towards a biopsychosocial model for integration of physical disorder factors with psychological and psychosocial illness impact factors. Eur JPain. 2005;9:613–33.

Svensson P, Arendt-Nielsen L. Effects of 5 days of repeated submaximal clenching on masticatory muscle pain and tenderness: an experimental study. J Orofac Pain. 1996;10:330–8.

Thorne BE. Cognitive therapy for chronic pain: a step-by-step guide. New York, NY: Guilford Press; 2004.

Townsen D, Nicholson RA, Buenaver L, Bush F, Gramling S. Use of a habit reversal treatment for temporomandibular pain in a minimal therapist contact format. J Behav Ther Exp Psychiatry. 2001;32:221–39.

Tragesser SL, Bruns D, Disorbio JM. Borderline personality disorder features and pain: the mediating role of negative affect in a pain patient sample. Clin J Pain. 2010;26:348–53.

Turk DC, Zaki HS, Rudy TE. Effects of intraoral appliance and biofeedback/stress management alone and in combination in treating pain and depression in patients with temporomandibular disorders. J Prosthet Dent. 1993;70:158–64.

Turner JA, Brister H, Huggins K, Mancl L, Aaron LA, Truelove EL. Catastrophizing is associated with clinical examination findings, activity interference, and health care use among patients with temporomandibular disorders. J Orofac Pain. 2005a;19:291–300.

Turner JA, Holtzman S, Mancl L. Mediators, moderators, and predictors of therapeutic change in cognitive-behavioral therapy for chronic pain. Pain. 2007;127:276–86.

Turner JA, Mancl L, Aaron LA. Brief cognitive-behavioral therapy for temporomandibular disorder pain: effects on daily electronic outcome and process measures. Pain. 2005b;117:377–87.

Turner JA, Mancl L, Aaron LA. Short-and long-term efficacy of brief cognitive-behavioral therapy for patients with chronic temporomandibular disorder pain: a randomized, controlled trial. Pain. 2006;121:181–94.

Turner JA, Whitney C, Dworkin SF, Massoth D, Wilson L. Do changes in patient beliefs and coping strategies predict temporomandibular disorder treatment outcomes? Clin J Pain. 1995;11:177–88.

Van Der Meulen MJ, Lobbezoo F, Aartman IH, Naeije M. Self-reported oral parafunctions and pain intensity in temporomandibular disorder patients. J Orofac Pain. 2006;20:31–5.

Van Grootel RJ, Van Der Glas HW, Buchner R, De Leeuw JR, Passchier J. Patterns of pain variation related to myogenous temporomandibular disorders. Clin J Pain. 2005;21:154–65.

Vassend O, Krogstad BS, Dahl BL. Negative affectivity, somatic complaints, and symptoms of temporomandibular disorders. J Psychosom Res. 1995;39:889–99.

Velly AM, Look JO, Carlson C, Lenton PA, Kang W, Holcroft CA, Fricton JR. The effect of catastrophizing and depression on chronic pain--a prospective cohort study of temporomandibular muscle and joint pain disorders. Pain. 2011;152:2377–83.

Vendrig AA. The Minnesota multiphasic personality inventory and chronic pain: a conceptual analysis of a long-standing but complicated relationship. Clin Psychol Rev. 2000;20:533–59.

Vlaeyen J, Morley S, Linton SJ, Boersma K, De Jong J. Pain-related fear: exposure based treatment for chronic pain. IASP Press, Washington, DC 2012.

Vranceanu AM, Shaefer JR, Saadi AF, Slawsby E, Sarin J, Scult M, Benson H, Denninger JW. The relaxation response resiliency enhancement program in the management of chronic refractory temporomandibular joint disorder: results from a pilot study. J Musculoskelet Pain. 2013;21:224–30.

Weisberg JN, Keefe FJ. Personality disorders in the chronic pain population - basic concepts, empirical findings, and clinical implications. Pain Forum. 1997;6:1–9.

Whitney CW, Von Korff M. Regression to the mean in treated versus untreated chronic pain. Pain. 1992;50:281–5.

Winocur E, Gavish A, Emodi-Perlman A, Halachmi M, Eli I. Hypnorelaxation as treatment for myofascial pain disorder: a comparative study. Oral Surg Oral Med Oral Pathol Oral Radiol Endod. 2002;93:429–34.

Woods DW, Miltenberger RG. Habit reversal: a review of applications and variations. J Behav Ther Exp Psychiatry. 1995;26:123–31.

Yatani H, Studts J, Cordova M, Carlson CR, Okeson JP. Comparison of sleep quality and clinical and Psychologic characteristics in patients with temporomandibular disorders. J Orofac Pain. 2002;16:221–8.

Zhang Y, Montoya L, Ebrahim S, Busse JW, Couban R, Mccabe RE, Bieling P, Carrasco-Labra A, Guyatt GH. Hypnosis/relaxation therapy for temporomandibular disorders: a systematic review and meta-analysis of randomized controlled trials. J Oral Facial Pain Headache. 2015;29:115–25.

The manufacturer's authorised representative in the EU is Springer
Nature Customer Service Centre GmbH, Europaplatz 3, 69115 Heidelberg,
Germany. If you have any concerns regarding our products, please
contact ProductSafety@springernature.com

Printed and bound by CPI Group (UK) Ltd, Croydon, CR0 4YY
01/10/2026
02225905-0005